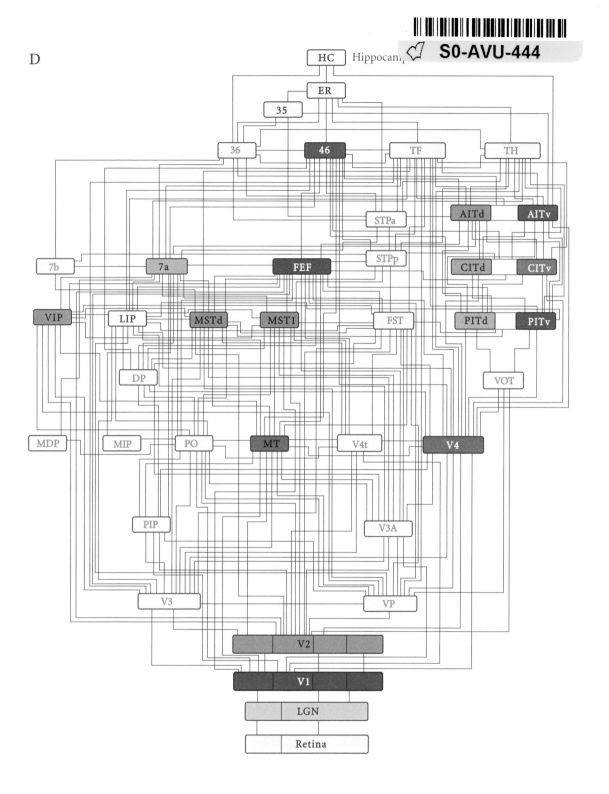

D

S0-AVU-444

(A) Lateral (left) and medial (right) view of the human brain. (B) Two similar views and (C) an unfolded and flattened map of the macaque's monkey brain. All non-white areas are involved with visual processing. The human and monkey brains are drawn at different scales. (D) Organizational chart of the monkey's visual system. Optical information flows from the retina in a quasi-hierarchical manner through a large number of cortical areas. Most of the links are reciprocal. Only the retina, LGN, V1, and V2 are drawn with some of their substructures. (B)-(D) are modified from Van Essen and Gallant (1994) and Felleman and Van Essen (1991). For more anatomical information, see http://brainmap.wustl.edu.

The Quest for Consciousness

A Neurobiological Approach

The Quest for Consciousness

A Neurobiological Approach

CHRISTOF KOCH

ROBERTS AND COMPANY PUBLISHERS
Englewood, Colorado

Roberts & Company Publishers
4660 South Yosemite Street
P. O. Box 9154
Englewood, Colorado 80111
Internet: www.roberts-publishers.com
Telephone: (303) 221-3325

Ordering information: (800) 351-1161
Fax: (516) 422-4097
Internet: www.roberts-publishers.com

Publisher: *Ben Roberts*
Production Manager: *Leslie Galen, Integre Technical Publishing Co., Inc.*
Manuscript Editor: *John Murdzek*
Designer: *Mark Ong, Side by Side Studios*
Compositor: *Integre Technical Publishing Co., Inc.*
Illustrator: *Emiko-Rose Paul, Echo Medical Media*
Printer and Binder: *Malloy Incorporated*

Copyright © 2004 by Roberts & Company Publishers

About the type: Minion is a 1990 Adobe Originals typeface by Robert Slimbach. Minion is inspired by classical, old-style typefaces of the late Renaissance, a period of elegant, beautiful, and highly readable type designs. Created primarily for text setting, Minion combines the aesthetic and functional qualities that make text type highly readable with the versatility of digital technology.

About the paper: Finch Opaque is a smooth, bright stock with high opacity, making it readable and well suited for half-tones and illustrations.

Reproduction or translation of any part of this work beyond that permitted by Section 107 or 108 of the 1976 United States Copyright Act without the permission of the copyright owner is unlawful. Requests for permission or further information should be addressed to the Permissions Department, Roberts & Company Publishers.

Library of Congress Cataloging-in-Publication Data

Koch, Christof.
    The quest for consciousness : a neurobiological approach / Christof Koch.
       p. cm.
Includes bibliographical references and index.
    ISBN 0-9747077-0-8 (hardcover)
    1. Consciousness–Physiological aspects. 2. Neurobiology–Research. I. Title.
QP411.K63 2004
153–dc22
                              2003023807

Printed in the United States of America
10 9 8 7 6 5 4 3 2

I dedicate this book to

FRANCIS CRICK

Friend, Mentor, and Scientist

Contents

Foreword by Francis Crick

We do not know in advance what are the right questions to ask, and we often do not find out until we are close to the answer.

From Steven Weinberg

It is a pleasure to write an informal introduction to this unusual and excellent book. Most of the ideas in it have been developed by Christof and myself in continual collaboration, as our joint papers show, and Christof has involved me in much of the writing of it, though the hard work, and the breezy, informal yet well-reasoned style are all his own. So mine is not an unbiased assessment.

I strongly recommend it to the main audience for which it is intended, which is, in round terms, not merely neuroscientists, but scientists of all sorts with an interest in consciousness.

Consciousness is the major unsolved problem in biology. That there is no present consensus on the general nature of the solution is made clear by Christof in Chapter 1. How do what philosophers call "qualia," the redness of red and the painfulness of pain, arise from the concerted actions of nerve cells, glial cells and their associated molecules? Can qualia be explained by what we now know of modern science, or is some quite different kind of explanation needed? And how to approach this seemingly intractable problem?

In the past dozen years there has been an enormous flood of books and papers about consciousness. Before that the behaviorist approach, and, surprisingly, much of the initial phase of cognitive science which replaced it, effectively stifled almost all serious discussion of the subject.

What is different about this book? Rather than another closely argued and largely sterile discussion of the root of the mind-body problem, our strategy has been to try first to find the neuronal correlates of consciousness (often called the NCC). Because of our emphasis on the behavior of neurons we have concentrated mainly on topics that can be studied in the macaque monkey, while including parallel work on humans. Thus, both language and dreams receive little or no emphasis. How would you study a monkey's dreams?

We have also avoided some of the more difficult aspects of consciousness, such as self-consciousness and emotion, and concentrated instead on perception, especially visual perception. And we have tried to approach visual perception at a number of levels, from visual psychology, brain scans, neurophysiology and neuroanatomy, down to neurons, synapses, and molecules.

This involves digesting an enormous number of experimental observations, some of which inevitably will turn out to be wrong or misleading, while at the same time trying out various theoretical hypotheses. These ideas are seldom totally novel, though the combination of them may be new.

Thus, parts of the book are necessarily heavy on "facts." This is especially true of the chapters on the details of the macaque visual system, but Christof has a recapitulation at the end of each chapter (except for Chapter 19, which is a recapitulation of most of the book), so that the reader can, the first time round, skip some of the details.

Another unusual feature is that, for a book with so many facts, it is a delight to read. Christof's informal style, which would be strictly banned by the editors of scientific journals, carries the reader along. It also conveys quite a bit about Christof's background and tastes, from his love of dogs to his very catholic love of music, with quotations ranging from Aristotle to Woody Allen, and from Lewis Carroll to Richard Feynman and Bertie Wooster.

While easy to read, Christof has provided, in the convenient footnotes and references, a guide to both broad surveys and key papers, so that the interested reader can easily begin to explore the very extensive literature on almost all the relevant topics.

Solving the problem of consciousness will need the labors of many scientists, of many kinds, though it is always possible that there will be a few crucial insights and observations. The book is designed as an introduction for scientists, especially younger ones, with the hope that it will lead them to contribute to the field. A few years ago one could not use the word "consciousness" in a paper for, say, *Nature* or *Science*, nor in a grant application. But thankfully, times are changing, and the subject is now ripe for intensive exploration. Read on!

Preface

We must know. We will know.

Epitaph on the gravestone of David Hilbert, German mathematician

I had already taken an aspirin, but the toothache persisted. Lying in bed, I couldn't sleep because of the pounding in my lower molar. Trying to distract myself from this painful sensation, I pondered why it hurt. I knew that an inflammation of the tooth pulp sent electrical activity up one of the branches of the trigeminal nerve that ends in the brainstem. After passing through further switching stages, pain was ultimately generated by activity of nerve cells deep inside the forebrain. But none of this explained why it felt like anything! How was it that sodium, potassium, calcium, and other ions sloshing around my brain caused this awful feeling? This mundane manifestation of the venerable mind-body problem, back in the summer of 1988, has occupied me to the present day.

The mind-body dilemma can be expressed succinctly by the question, "How can a physical system, such as the brain, experience anything?" If, for example, a temperature sensor coupled to a computer becomes really hot, the processor may turn on a red alarm light. Nobody would claim, however, that the flow of electrons onto the gate of the transistor that closes the light switch causes the machine to have a bad day. How is it, then, that neural activity can give rise to the sensation of a burning pain? Is there something magical about the brain? Does it have to do with its architecture, with the type of neurons involved, or with its associated electro-chemical activity patterns?

The matter becomes even more mysterious with the realization that much, if not most, of what happens inside my skull isn't accessible to introspection. Indeed, most of my daily actions—tying my shoes, driving, running, climbing, simple conversation—work on autopilot, while my mind is busy dealing with more important things. How do these behaviors differ neurologically from those that give rise to conscious sensations?

In this book, I seek answers to these questions within a neuroscientific framework. I argue for a research program whose supreme aim is to discover the neuronal correlates of consciousness, the NCC. These are the smallest set

xv

of brain mechanisms and events sufficient for some specific conscious feeling, as elemental as the color red or as complex as the sensual, mysterious, and primeval sensation evoked when looking at the jungle scene on the book jacket. Characterizing the NCC is one of the ultimate scientific challenges of our times.

To get to the heart of the matter, I need to be as close as I can to where the rubber meets the road, in the interstitial spaces between phenomenal experience and corporeal brain matter. These regions have been best explored in visual perception, which is why this book focuses on seeing, though not exclusively. I survey the relevant anatomical, neurophysiological, psychological, and clinical data and weave these into a larger tapestry that constitutes a novel framework for thinking about the neuronal basis of consciousness.

This book is intended for anybody curious about an ancient debate that has recaptured the imagination of today's philosophers, scientists, engineers, doctors, and thinking people in general. What is consciousness? How does it fit into the natural order of things? What is it good for? Is it unique to humans? Why do so many of our actions bypass consciousness? Answers to these questions will determine a new image of what it is to be human. This image, which is slowly emerging even now, contradicts many of the traditional images of which we have grown fond. Who knows where this quest will take us? As Lord Dunsany wrote, "Man is a small thing and the night is large and full of wonder."

The ideas expressed in these pages are the fruits of an intensive collaboration with Francis Crick at the Salk Institute in La Jolla, California, just north of San Diego. We first met in 1981 in Tübingen, Germany, while debating with Tomaso Poggio over the function of dendritic spines. When I subsequently moved to the Massachusetts Institute of Technology in Cambridge and devised, with Shimon Ullman, ways to explain visual attention on the basis of artificial neural networks, Shimon and I visited Francis for a stimulating and vigorous week-long exchange of ideas. The pace of our interaction intensified when I became a professor at the California Institute of Technology in Pasadena, a two-hour drive from La Jolla.

Francis's interest in the biological basis of consciousness, which he traces back to the days after the Second World War, converged with my unbridled enthusiasm for thinking about visual attention and awareness within a computational framework and mapping that onto neurobiological circuits. Our joint speculations took on concrete form with the rediscovery of oscillatory and synchronized spiking activity in the cat visual cortex in the late 1980s. Francis and I published our first paper, "Towards a neurobiological theory of consciousness," in 1990. As new data became available and our point of view evolved to encompass multiple aspects of consciousness, we kept up a steady pace of publications. Over the last five years, I spent two to three days each month in

Francis's home. For reasons of his own, Francis chose not to be a co-author of this book. Nevertheless, to emphasize the joint ownership of the main ideas expressed herein, I frequently write "we" or "us" to mean "Francis and I." I know this is somewhat unusual, but ours is an unusual collaboration.

Although I have retained my enthusiasm, acquired in youth, for certain Greek and Germanic philosophers—Plato, Schopenhauer, Nietzsche, and the young Wittgenstein—my writing style strives to follow the Anglo-Saxon tradition of clarity. *The Economist*'s guide to writing summarizes it as, "say it as simply as possible." I try to be unambiguous in distinguishing what is known from what is mere speculation. I provide references to the literature in ample footnotes. These also allude to complexities that may not be of interest to the general reader. The first time a technical term is mentioned, it is italicized, and further explained in the glossary.

If you are new to these questions, I suggest you begin by reading the introductory chapter and the interview at the very end, which summarizes in an informal manner my thinking on a range of topics. The novel technical material is contained in Chapters 2, 9, 11, 13, and 15, while Chapters 14 and 18 are in a more speculative vein.

I use this book for an introductory class on the neurobiology of consciousness. Teaching material, including homework and streaming media versions of all of my lectures, can be found at www.klab.caltech.edu/cns120.

I would here like to acknowledge everybody who made this book possible.

Foremost, of course, is Francis Crick. Without his constant guidance, insight, and creativity, this book simply would not have happened. All the basic ideas found here have been published over the years with Francis. He read and commented upon numerous versions of the manuscript. I dedicate the book to Francis and his searing, uncompromising search for the truth, no matter where it takes him, and to his wisdom and his ability to gracefully accept the unavoidable. I do not know anybody else like him.

Over the years, I have benefited, again and again, from the gracious hospitality and wonderful cooking of Odile Crick, Francis's wife, and have had too few occasions to reciprocate. It was she who suggested the title of the book during one of our frequent lunches on their sun-drenched patio in La Jolla.

The research program carried out in my laboratory is intense, time-consuming, and deeply satisfying. It is also quite expensive. Over the years, I have enjoyed the unstinting support of a number of institutions. First and foremost is the California Institute of Technology, under the leadership of David Baltimore. What an oasis—an ivory tower—perfectly suited to the search for the truth with a capital 'T.' External funding has been provided by the National Science Foundation, the National Institute of Health, the National Institute of

Mental Health, the Office of Naval Research, the Defense Advanced Research Project Agency, the W.M. Keck Foundation, the McDonnell-Pew Foundation, the Alfred Sloan Foundation, the Swartz Foundation, and the Gordon and Betty Moore Foundation.

Thanks to my students, post-doctoral fellows, and colleagues, who along with my son Alexander and my daughter Gabriele, read portions of the book and provided insightful feedback: Larry Abbott, Alex Bäcker, Randolph Blake, Edward Callaway, Michael Herzog, Karen Heyman, Anya Hurlbert, Gabriel Kreiman, Gilles Laurent, David Leopold, Nikos Logothetis, Wei Ji Ma, John Maunsell, Earl Miller, David Milner, Anthony Movshon, William Newsome, Bruno Olshausen, Leslie Orgel, Carl Pabo, Javier Perez-Orive, Tomaso Poggio, John Reynolds, Robert Rodieck, David Sheinberg, Wolf Singer, Larry Squire, Nao Tsuchiya, Endel Tulving, Elizabeth Vlahos, Brian Wandell, Patrick Wilken, and Semir Zeki.

I have much profited by discussions regarding the conceptual basis of my research program with philosophers Tim Bayne, Ned Block, David Chalmers, Pat Churchland, Dan Dennett, Ilya Farber, and Alva Noë.

I have been blessed by nine enthusiastic readers of the entire manuscript: John Murdzek, a professional developmental editor, and eight consciousness aficionados—Tim Bayne, Joseph Bogen, Constanze Hofstötter, Oliver Landolt, Ernst Niebur, Parashkev Nachev, Javier Perez-Orive, and Rufin Van Rullen. Three colleagues, Bruce Bridgeman, McKell Carter, and Ilya Farber, took the time and the immense effort to carefully proofread the entire manuscript. The perseverance and never-ending stream of suggestions of all these readers eliminated many infelicities, both small and large, and immensely improved the readability of the book. Thank you very much. My editor, Ben Roberts, masterfully steered the entire process from raw manuscript to the final tome you hold in your hands. A true bibliophile, he insisted at all times on the highest standards for both form and content. The art, from the gorgeous cover to the endpages, the figures in the text, and the font and overall layout of the book were designed by Emiko-Rose Paul and her team at Echo Medical Media and by Mark Stuart Ong. Leslie Galen from Integre Technical Publishing proofread every single character between the two bookends and oversaw the entire production process. I could not have asked for a better team of professionals.

When all is said and done, there remains my immediate family, without whom I am lost: Edith, Alexander, Gabriele, and our canine companions, Trixie, Nosy, and Bella. I have no idea why I am so lucky as to be with all of you.

And now, esteemed reader, I invite you to enjoy the book.

Pasadena, August 2003

CHAPTER ONE

Introduction to the Study of Consciousness

Consciousness is what makes the mind-body problem really intractable...
Without consciousness the mind-body problem would be much less
interesting. With consciousness it seems hopeless.

From *What Is It Like to Be a Bat?* by Thomas Nagel

In Thomas Mann's unfinished novel, *Confessions of Felix Krull, Confidence Man,* Professor Kuckuck comments to the Marquis de Venosta on the three fundamental and mysterious stages of creation. Foremost is the creation of something—namely, the universe—out of nothing. The second act of genesis is the one that begat life from inorganic, dead matter. The third mysterious act is the birth of consciousness[1] and conscious beings, beings that can reflect upon themselves, out of organic matter. Humans and at least some animals not only detect light, move their eyes, and perform other actions, but also have "feelings" associated with these events. This remarkable feature of the world cries out for an explanation. Consciousness remains one of the key puzzles confronting the scientific worldview.

1.1 | WHAT NEEDS TO BE EXPLAINED?

Throughout recorded history, men and women have wondered how we can see, smell, reflect upon ourselves, and remember. How do these sensations arise? The fundamental question at the heart of the mind-body problem is, what is the relation between the conscious mind and the electro-chemical interactions

---

[1] The word consciousness derives from the Latin *conscientia,* composed of *cum* (with or together) and *scire* (to know). Until the early 17th century, consciousness was used in the sense of moral knowledge of right or wrong, what is today referred to as *conscience.*

in the body that give rise to it?[2] How do the salty taste and crunchy texture of potato chips, the unmistakable smell of dogs after they have been in the rain, or the feeling of hanging on tiny fingerholds on a cliff a couple of meters above the last secure foothold, emerge from networks of neurons? These sensory qualities, the building blocks of conscious experience, have traditionally been called *qualia*. The puzzle is, how can a physical system have qualia?

Furthermore, why is a particular quale the way it is and not different? Why does red look the way it does, quite distinct from the sensation of seeing blue? These are not abstract, arbitrary symbols; they represent something *meaningful* to the organism. Philosophers talk about the mind's capacity to represent or to be *about* things. How meaning arises from electrical activity in the vast neural networks making up the brain remains a deep mystery. The structure of these networks, their connectivity, surely plays a role, but how so?[3]

How is it that humans and animals can have experiences? Why can't people live, and beget, and raise children without consciousness? From a subjective vantage point, this would resemble not being alive at all, like sleepwalking through life. Why, then, from the point of view of evolution, does consciousness exist? What survival value is attached to subjective, mental life?

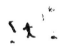

In Haitian lore, a zombie is a dead person who, by the magical power of a sorcerer, must act out the wishes of the person controlling him. In philosophy, a *zombie* is an imaginary being who behaves and acts just like a normal person but has absolutely no conscious life, no sensations, and no feelings. A particularly insidious zombie will even lie, claiming that she is experiencing something when she is not.

The fact that it is so difficult to imagine such a scenario is living proof of the fundamental importance of consciousness to daily life. Following René Descartes's famous remark—made in the context of establishing his existence—I can ascertain with certainty that "I am conscious." Not always,

---

[2]No consensual usage of objective and subjective terms has emerged across disciplines. I adopt the following convention throughout the book: *detection* and *behavior* are objective terms that can be operationalized (see, Dennett, 1991), as in "the retina detects the red flash, and the observer presses her finger in response." Detection and behavior can occur in the absence of consciousness. I use *sensation, perception, seeing, experience, mind,* and *feeling* in their subjective senses, as in "conscious sensation" and so on. While I'm on the topic of convention, here is another one. Throughout the book, I use *awareness* and *consciousness* (or *aware* and *conscious*) as synonyms. Some scholars distinguish between these two on ontological (Chalmers, 1996), conceptual (Block, 1995), or psychological (Tulving, 1995) grounds. At this point, little empirical evidence justifies such a distinction (see, however, Lamme, 2003). I might have to revise this standpoint in the future. Curiously, the contemporary scientific literature discourages the usage of the word consciousness, while awareness is acceptable. This is more a reflection of sociological trends than deep insight.

[3]The exact relationship between qualia and meaning is unclear (see the anthology by Chalmers, 2002).

not in a dreamless sleep or while under anesthesia, but often: when I read, talk, climb, think, discuss, or just sit and admire the beauty of the world.[4]

The mystery deepens with the realization that much of what goes on in the brain bypasses consciousness. Electrophysiological experiments prove that furious activity in legions of neurons can fail to generate a conscious percept or memory. In a reflex action, you will instantly and vigorously shake your foot if you detect an insect crawling over it, even though the realization of what is happening only comes later on. Or your body reacts to a fearful sight, a spider or gun, before it's been consciously registered: Your palms become sweaty, your heartbeat and blood pressure increase, and adrenaline is released. All this happens before you know that you are afraid, or why. Many relatively complex sensory-motor behaviors are similarly rapid and nonconscious. Indeed, the point of training is to teach your body to quickly execute a complex series of movements—returning a serve, evading a punch, or tying shoelaces—without thinking about it. Nonconscious processing extends to the highest echelons of the mind. Sigmund Freud argued that childhood experiences—especially those of a traumatic nature—can profoundly determine adult behavior in a way that is not accessible to consciousness. Much high-level decision making and creativity occurs without conscious thought, a topic treated in more depth in Chapter 18.

So much of what constitutes the ebb and flow of daily life takes place outside of consciousness. Some of the best evidence for this comes from the clinic. Consider the strange case of the neurological patient D.F. She is unable to see shapes or recognize pictures of everyday objects, yet she can catch a ball. Even though she can't tell the orientation of a thin mail box-like slit (is it horizontal?) she can deftly post a letter into the slit (Figure 13.2). By studying such patients, neuropsychologists have inferred the existence of *zombie agents in the brain that bypass awareness; that is, they don't involve consciousness* (recall that in the second footnote to this chapter, I equate awareness with consciousness). These agents are dedicated to stereotypical tasks, such as shifting the eyes or positioning the hand. They usually operate fairly rapidly and don't have access to explicit memory. I'll return to these themes in Chapters 12 and 13.

Why, then, isn't the brain just a large collection of specialized zombie agents? Life might be boring if it were, but since such agents work effortlessly and

---

[4]Strictly speaking, I don't know whether you are conscious or not. You might even be a zombie! However, because you act and speak just as I do, because your brain is similar to mine, and because you and I share the same evolutionary heritage, I sensibly assume that you are also conscious. At present, our scientific understanding of consciousness is insufficient to prove this, but everything about the natural world is compatible with this assumption. *Mental solipsism* denies this and argues that only the subject himself is truly conscious while everybody else is a zombie. This seems implausible and also rather arbitrary. After all, why should I, out of all the people in the world, be singled out for consciousness?

rapidly, why is consciousness needed at all? What is its function? In Chapter 14, I argue that consciousness gives access to a general-purpose and deliberate processing mode for planning and contemplating a future course of action. Without consciousness, you would be worse off.

Consciousness is an intensely private matter. A sensation cannot be directly conveyed to somebody else but is usually circumscribed in terms of other experiences. Try to explain your experience of seeing red. You'll end up relating it to other percepts, such as "red as a sunset" or "red as a Chinese flag" (this task becomes next to impossible when communicating to a person blind from birth). You can talk meaningfully about the relationships among different experiences but not about any single one. This too needs to be explained.

Here, then, is the charter for our quest: To understand how and why the neural basis of a specific conscious sensation is associated with that sensation rather than with another, or with a completely nonconscious state; why sensations are structured the way they are, how they acquire meaning, and why they are private; and, finally, how and why so many behaviors occur without consciousness.

1.2 | A SPECTRUM OF ANSWERS

Philosophers and scientists have pondered the mind-body problem in its present form since the publication of René Descartes's *Traité de l'homme* in the mid-17th century. Until the 1980s, however, the vast majority of work in the brain sciences made no references to consciousness. In the last two decades, philosophers, psychologists, cognitive scientists, clinicians, neuroscientists, and even engineers have published dozens of monographs and books aimed at "discovering," "explaining," or "reconsidering" consciousness. Much of this literature is either purely speculative or lacks any detailed scientific program for systematically discovering the neuronal basis of consciousness and, therefore, does not contribute to the ideas discussed in this book.

Before introducing the approach my long-time collaborator Francis Crick and I have taken to address these problems, I will survey the philosophical landscape to familiarize readers with some of the possible categories of answers that people have considered. Keep in mind that only cartoon-like pocket sketches of these positions are provided here.[5]

---

[5]I can't possibly do justice to the sophisticated nature of these arguments. Anyone interested in all the subtle twists and turns is urged to consult the philosophical anthologies by Block, Flanagan, and Güzeldere (1997) and by Metzinger (1995). The textbook by the philosopher Patricia Churchland (2002) surveys different aspects of the mind-body problem with an emphasis on the relevant neuroscience. I also recommend the compact and readable monograph by Searle (1997). For the reverberations of these discussions among theologians, see Brown, Murphy, and Malony (1998) and the thoughtful McMullin (2000).

Consciousness Depends on an Immaterial Soul

Plato, the patriarch of Western philosophy, is widely credited with the concept of a person as an immortal soul imprisoned in a mortal body. He also proposed that ideas have a real existence and are eternal. These Platonic views were subsequently absorbed into the New Testament and form the basis of the classical Roman Catholic doctrine of a *soul*. The belief that at the heart of consciousness lies a transcendent and immortal soul is widely shared by many religions and faiths throughout the world.[6]

In modern times, Descartes distinguished between *res extensa*—physical substance with spatial extent that includes the animal spirits running through nerves and filling the muscles—and *res cogitans*, thinking substance. He argued that *res cogitans* is unique to humans and gives rise to consciousness. Descartes's ontological division constitutes the very definition of *dualism*: two forms of substances, matter and soul stuff. Weaker forms of dualism had been proposed earlier by Aristotle and by Thomas Aquinas. The most famous modern defenders of dualism are the philosopher Karl Popper and the neurophysiologist and Nobel laureate John Eccles.

While logically consistent, strong dualist positions are dissatisfying from a scientific viewpoint. Particularly troublesome is the mode of interaction between the soul and the brain. How and where is this supposed to take place? Presumably, this interaction would have to be compatible with the laws of physics. This, however, would require an exchange of energy that needs to be accounted for. And what happens to this spooky substance, the soul, once its carrier, the brain, dies? Does it float around in some hyperspace, like a ghost?[7]

The concept of an immaterial essence can be saved by postulating that the soul is immortal and completely independent of the brain. This leaves it as something ineffable, undetectable, a "ghost in the machine," to use a phrase coined by Gilbert Ryle, outside of science.

---

[6]Being raised in a devout Roman Catholic family, I have much sympathy for this point of view. Flanagan's book (2002) explores the clash between the notion of soul (and free will) and the modern scientific view that tends to deny both (see also Murphy, 1998).

[7]Popper and Eccles (1977) argued that brain-soul interactions are camouflaged by Heisenberg's uncertainty principle, according to which it is impossible to know precisely both the position and the momentum of a microscopic system, such as an electron, at the same time. In 1986, Eccles postulated that the conscious mind interferes with the release probability of vesicles at synapses in a way that does not violate conservation of energy yet is sufficient to influence the brain's behavior. These ideas have not been received with enthusiasm by the scientific community. Yet what is refreshing about the Popper and Eccles (1977) monograph is that they take consciousness seriously. They assume that sensations are a product of evolution that cries out for some function (see, in particular, Eccles, 1991). This was a remarkable sentiment after so many decades of behaviorism that disregarded consciousness entirely.

Consciousness Cannot Be Understood by Scientific Means

Quite a different philosophical tradition is the *mysterian*[8] position, which claims that human beings are unable to comprehend consciousness because it is just too complex. This limitation is either a principled, formal one (how can any system completely understand itself?) or a practical one, expressed as a pessimism about the human mind's inability to perform the necessary massive conceptual revisions (what chance does an ape have of understanding general relativity?).

Other philosophers assert that they don't see how the physical brain can generate consciousness and that, therefore, any scientific program to explore the physical basis of consciousness is doomed to failure. This is an argument from ignorance: The current absence of a compelling argument for a link between the brain and the conscious mind cannot be taken as evidence that such a link does not exist. Of course, to answer these critics, science will have to come up with the relevant concepts and evidence to support this link.

Although scientists may never fully comprehend—even in principle, let alone in practice—the workings of brains and the genesis of consciousness, it is premature to conclude so now. Neuroscience is a young discipline, accumulating new knowledge with ever-more-refined methods at a breathtaking pace. Before much of this development has run its course, there is no reason to come to this defeatist conclusion. Just because one particular scholar is unable to understand how consciousness might arise does not mean that it must be beyond all human comprehension!

Consciousness Is Illusory

Another type of philosophical reaction to the mind-body dilemma is to deny that there is any real problem at all. The most lively contemporary exponent of this rather counterintuitive notion—originating in the behaviorist tradition—is the philosopher Daniel Dennett from Tufts University. In *Consciousness Explained*, he argues that consciousness as most people conceive of it is an elaborate illusion, mediated by the senses in collusion with motor output, and supported by social constructions and learning. While acknowledging that people claim that they are conscious and that this persistent, but erroneous, belief needs to be explained, he denies the inner reality of the ungraspable aspects of qualia. He thinks that the usual way of thinking about consciousness is wildly wrong. Dennett seeks to explain the *third-person account* of con-

---

[8]The term *mysterian* originates with Flanagan (1992), who used it to characterize the approaches of Lucas (1961), Nagel (1974), and McGinn (1991).

sciousness while rejecting those aspects of the *first-person account* that render it resistant to reduction.[9]

Having dental pain is about expressing, or wanting to express, certain behaviors: To stop chewing on that side of the mouth, to run away and hide until the pain has subsided, to grimace, and so on. These "reactive dispositions," as he calls them, are real. But not the badness of the pain, according to Dennett. That elusive feeling doesn't exist.[10]

Given the centrality of subjective feelings to everyday life, it would require extraordinary factual evidence before concluding that qualia and feelings are illusory. Philosophical arguments, based on logical analysis, even when fortified by results from cognitive psychology, are not powerful enough to deal with the real brain with all of its subtleties in a decisive manner. The philosophical method is at its best when formulating questions, but does not have much of a track record at answering them. The provisional approach I take in this book is to consider first-person experiences as brute facts of life and seek to explain them.[11]

Consciousness Requires Fundamentally New Laws

Some have called for new scientific laws to explain the puzzle of consciousness, rather than just more facts and principles about the brain. Roger Penrose, at Oxford University, argues in the wonderful *The Emperor's New Mind* that present-day physics is incapable of explaining the intuitive powers of mathematicians—and, by extension, of people at large. Penrose believes that a yet-to-be-formulated theory of quantum gravity will explain how human con-

---

[9] A third-person account recognizes only objective events, such as light of a certain wavelength impinging upon the retina, causing the person to exclaim "I see red," while the first-person account is concerned with subjective events, such as the sensation of red. The late Francisco Varela labeled the program of mapping first-person experiences onto the brain *neurophenomenology* (Varela, 1996).

[10] I refer the reader to Dennett's book (1991), and to Dennett and Kinsbourne (1992). See Ryle (1949) for an antecedent in the behavioral tradition. For an update on his views, consult Dennett (2001). In his 1991 book, Dennett rightly takes aim at the notion of a *Cartesian theater*, a single place in the brain where conscious perception must occur (note that this does not exclude the possibility of a distributed set of neuronal processes that express consciousness at any one point in time). He proposes a *multiple drafts* model to account for various puzzling aspects of consciousness, such as the nonintuitive role of time in the organization of experience. Dennett's writing is characterized by his skillful use of colorful metaphors and analogies, of which he is overly fond. It is difficult to relate these to specific neuronal mechanisms.

[11] These are deep waters. Dennett retorts that innocently accepting feelings as facts to be explained is giving a hostage to fortune; that to talk about real qualia is a highly ideological move akin to presupposing the existence of "real magic," full of epistemological implications (Dennett, 2004).

sciousness can carry out processes that no possible digital (Turing) computer could implement. In conjunction with the anesthesiologist Stuart Hameroff, at the University of Arizona at Tucson, Penrose has proposed that microtubules, self-assembling cytoskeletal proteins found throughout all cells in the body, are critically involved in mediating coherent quantum states across large populations of neurons.[12]

While Penrose has generated a vigorous debate regarding the extent to which mathematicians can be said to have access to certain noncomputable truths and whether these can be instantiated by computers, it remains utterly mysterious how quantum gravity could explain how consciousness occurs in certain classes of highly organized matter. Both consciousness and quantum gravity have enigmatic features, but to conclude that one is therefore the cause of the other seems rather arbitrary. Given the lack of any evidence for macroscopic quantum-mechanical effects occurring in the brain, I will not pursue this idea further.

The philosopher David Chalmers, at the University of Arizona at Tucson, has sketched an alternative proposal in which information has two aspects: a physically realizable aspect that is used in computers, and a phenomenal or experiential aspect that is inaccessible from the outside. In his view, any information-processing system, from a thermostat to a human brain, can be conscious in at least some rudimentary sense (although Chalmers admits that it probably doesn't feel like much "to be a thermostat"). While the audacity of endowing all systems that represent information with experience has a certain appeal and elegance, it is not clear to me how Chalmers's hypothesis could be tested scientifically. For now, this modern-day *panpsychism* can only be accepted as a provocative hypothesis. Over time, though, a theory couched in the language of probabilities and information theory might well prove necessary to understand consciousness. Even if Chalmers's framework is accepted, a more quantitative structure must be worked out. Do certain types of processing architectures, such as massive parallel versus serial, facilitate the development of consciousness? Does the richness of experience relate to the amount or

---

[12] Penrose's books (Penrose, 1989, 1994) are among the most lucid and best-written accounts of Turing machines, Gödel's theorems, computing, and modern physics I have read. However, given that both monographs nominally deal with the human mind and brain, they are equally remarkable for the almost complete absence of any serious discussion of psychology and neuroscience. Hameroff and Penrose (1996) outline their proposal that microtubules, a major component of cellular scaffolding, are critical to the processes underlying consciousness. The Achilles' heel of this idea is the lack of any biophysical mechanism that would permit neurons, and not just any cells in the body, to rapidly form highly specific coalitions across large regions of the brain on the basis of quantum-coherency effects. All of this is supposed to take place, of course, at body temperature, a rather hostile environment for sustaining quantum coherency over macroscopic scales. See Grush and Churchland (1995) for a telling criticism.

organization of memory (shared or not, hierarchical or not, static or dynamic memory, and so on)?[13]

While I cannot rule out that explaining consciousness may require fundamentally new laws, I currently see no pressing need for such a step.

Consciousness Requires Behavior

The *inactive* or *sensorimotor* account of consciousness stresses the fact that a nervous system can't be considered in isolation. It is part of a body living in a habitat that has acquired, through myriad sensorimotor interactions over its lifetime, knowledge about the way that the world (including its own body) acts. This knowledge is put to skillful use in the body's ongoing encounters with the world. Proponents of this view acknowledge that the brain supports perception but claim that neural activity is not sufficient for consciousness, and that it is futile to look for physical causes or correlates of consciousness. The behaving organism embedded in a particular environment is what generates feelings.[14]

While proponents of the enactive point of view rightly emphasize that perception usually takes place within the context of action, I have little patience for their neglect of the neural basis of perception. If there is one thing that scientists are reasonably sure of, it is that brain activity is both necessary and sufficient for biological sentience. Empirical support for this fact derives from many sources. For instance, in dreaming, a highly conscious state, almost all voluntary muscles are inhibited. That is, each night, most of us have episodes of phenomenal feelings yet fail to move.[15] Another example is that direct brain stimulation with electrical or magnetic pulses triggers simple percepts, such as flashes of colored light, the basis for ongoing research in neuroprosthetic devices for the blind. Also, many patients are unfortunate enough to lose the use of their motor system, either during short-lived episodes[16] or permanently,[17] yet continue to experience the world.

---

[13]I definitely recommend at least browsing through Chalmers's (1996) book, in particular his Chapter 8. For a theoretical approach toward consciousness based on measures of complexity and information theory, see Tononi and Edelman (1998) and Edelman and Tononi (2000). Nagel (1988) examines panpsychism.

[14]The manifesto of this movement is O'Regan and Noë, (2001). See also Noë (2004) and Järvilehto (2000). Historical antecedents of the enactive movement in philosophy and psychology are (Merleau-Ponty, 1962) and (Gibson, 1966) respectively.

[15]The eyes move, of course, during periods of heightened dream activity. Revonsuo (2000) and Flanagan (2000) overview the form and putative functions of dream content.

[16]A transient form of paralysis is one of the characteristic features of *narcolepsy*, a neurological disorder. Triggered by a strong emotion—laughter, embarrassment, anger, excitement—the afflicted subject suddenly loses skeletal muscle tone without becoming unconscious. Such *cataplectic* attacks can last for minutes and leave the patient collapsed on the floor, utterly unable to move or to signal, but fully aware of her surroundings (Guilleminault, 1976; Siegel, 2000).

[17]The most dramatic of these have *locked-in syndrome* (Feldman, 1971; see also Celesia, 1997).

I conclude that action is not necessary for consciousness. Of course, this is not to argue that motion of the body, eyes, limbs, and so on, isn't important in shaping awareness. It is! Yet behavior is not strictly necessary for qualia to occur.

Consciousness Is an Emergent Property of Certain Biological Systems

The working hypothesis of this book is that consciousness emerges from neuronal features of the brain.[18] Understanding the material basis of consciousness is unlikely to require any exotic new physics, but rather a much deeper appreciation of how highly interconnected networks of a large number of heterogeneous neurons work. The abilities of coalitions of neurons to learn from interactions with the environment and from their own internal activities are routinely underestimated. Individual neurons themselves are complex entities with unique morphologies and thousands of inputs and outputs. Their interconnections, the *synapses*, are molecular machines that come equipped with learning algorithms that modify their strength and dynamics across many timescales. Humans have little experience with such a vast organization. Hence, even biologists struggle to appreciate the properties and power of the nervous system.

A reasonable analogy can be made with the debate raging at the turn of the 20th century concerning vitalism and the mechanisms underlying heredity. How can mere chemistry store all the information needed to specify a unique individual? How can chemistry explain how splitting a single frog embryo at the two-cell stage gives rise to two tadpoles? Doesn't this require some *vitalistic* force, or new law of physics, as Erwin Schrödinger postulated?

The central difficulty faced by researchers at the time was that they could not imagine the great specificity inherent in individual molecules. This is perhaps best expressed by William Bateson, one of England's leading geneticists

---

Take the case of Jean-Dominique Bauby, editor of the French fashion magazine *Elle*, who retained nothing but the ability to move his eyes up and down following a massive stroke. He composed an entire book on his inner experiences using eye movements as a form of Morse code. Bauby's 1997 *Le Scaphandre et le Papillon* (translated as *The Diving-Bell and the Butterfly*) is a strangely uplifting and inspirational volume written under appalling circumstances. If his last link with the world, his vertical eye movements, had been severed, Bauby would have been condemned to living a fully conscious life while appearing all but dead! He and other such patients perceive the world consciously, although this has never been systematically studied. *Frozen addicts*, referred to in footnote 24 in Chapter 7, are yet another living proof that complete lack of mobility and consciousness can coexist.

[18] A system has emergent properties if these are not possessed by its parts. There are no mystical, new-age overtones to this. In that sense, the laws of heredity emerge from the molecular properties of DNA and other macromolecules, or the initiation and propagation of the action potential in axonal fibers, emerge from the attributes of voltage-dependent ionic channels inserted into the neuronal membrane. For a general introduction to the problem of emergence, see Beckermann, Flohr, and Kim (1992).

in the early part of the 20th century. His 1916 review of *The Mechanism of Mendelian Heredity*, a book by the Nobel laureate Thomas Hunt Morgan and his collaborators, states:

> The properties of living things are in some way attached to a material basis, perhaps in some special degree to nuclear chromatin; and yet it is inconceivable that particles of chromatin or of any other substance, however complex, can possess those powers which must be assigned to our factors or gens. The supposition that particles of chromatin, indistinguishable from each other and indeed almost homogeneous under any known test, can by their material nature confer all the properties of life surpasses the range of even the most convinced materialism.

What Bateson and others did not know at the time, given the technology available, was that chromatin (that is, the chromosomes) is only homogeneous statistically, being composed of roughly equal amounts of the four nucleic bases, and that the exact linear sequence of the nucleotides encodes the secrets of heredity. Geneticists underestimated the ability of these nucleotides to store prodigious amounts of information. They also underestimated the amazing specificity of protein molecules, which has resulted from the action of natural selection over a few billion years of evolution. These mistakes must not be repeated in the quest to understand the basis of consciousness.

Once again, I assume that the physical basis of consciousness is an emergent property of specific interactions among neurons and their elements. Although consciousness is fully compatible with the laws of physics, it is not feasible to predict or understand consciousness from these.

1.3 | MY APPROACH IS A PRAGMATIC, EMPIRICAL ONE

In order to make progress on these difficult questions without getting bogged down in diversionary skirmishes, I will have to make some assumptions without justifying them in too much detail. These provisional working hypotheses might well need to be revised or even rejected later on. The physicist turned molecular biologist Max Delbrück advocated "The Principle of Limited Sloppiness" when it comes to experiments. He recommended trying things in a rough and ready manner to see whether they might work out. I apply this principle to the realm of ideas about the brain.

A Working Definition

Most everyone has a general idea of what it means to be conscious. According to the philosopher John Searle, "Consciousness consists of those states of sentience, or feeling, or awareness, which begin in the morning when we awake from a dreamless sleep and continue throughout the day until we fall into a coma or die or fall asleep again or otherwise become unconscious."[19] If I ask you to describe what you see and you respond in an appropriate manner, I will assume for now that you are conscious. Some form of attention is required, but is not sufficient. Operationally, consciousness is needed for nonroutine tasks that require retention of information over seconds.

Although fairly vague, this provisional definition is good enough to get started. As the science of consciousness advances, it will need to be refined and expressed in more fundamental neuronal terms. Until the problem is better understood, a more formal definition of consciousness is likely to be either misleading or overly restrictive, or both. If this seems evasive, try defining a *gene*. Is it a stable unit of hereditary transmission? Does a gene have to code for a single enzyme? What about structural and regulatory genes? Does a gene correspond to one continuous segment of nucleic acid? What about introns? And wouldn't it make more sense to define a gene as the mature mRNA transcript after all the editing and splicing have taken place? So much is now known about genes that any simple definition is likely to be inadequate. Why should it be any easier to define something as elusive as consciousness?[20]

Historically, significant scientific progress has commonly been achieved in the absence of formal definitions. For instance, the phenomenological laws of electrical current flow were formulated by Ohm, Ampère, and Volta well before the discovery of the electron in 1892 by Thompson. For the time being, therefore, I adopt the above working definition of consciousness and will see how far I can get with it.

Consciousness Is Not Unique to Humans

It is plausible that some species of animals—mammals, in particular—possess some, but not necessarily all, of the features of consciousness; that they see, hear, smell, and otherwise experience the world. Of course, each species has its own unique sensorium, matched to its ecological niche. But I assume that

---

[19] The definition, taken from Searle (1997), leaves out an entire domain of conscious experiences that are usually not remembered: vivid dreams that can't be distinguished from real life. More elaborate definitions of consciousness are no more helpful. For instance, Schiff and Plum (2000), two neurologists who treat severely neurologically impaired patients, state: "At its least, normal human consciousness consists of a serially time-ordered, organized, restricted, and reflective awareness of self and the environment. Moreover, it is an experience of graded complexity and quantity." While useful clinically, this definition presupposes notions of awareness, the self, and so on. The *Oxford English Dictionary* is no better, having eight entries under 'consciousness' and twelve under 'conscious.'

[20] See Keller (2000) and Ridley (2003) for the checkered history of the term "genes" and Churchland (1986, 2002) and, in particular, the essay by Farber and Churchland (1995), for the role of definitions in science.

these animals have feelings, have subjective states. To believe otherwise is presumptuous and flies in the face of all experimental evidence for the continuity of behaviors between animals and humans. We are all Nature's children.

This is particularly true for monkeys and apes, whose behavior, development, and brain structure are remarkably similar to those of humans (it takes an expert to distinguish a cubic millimeter of monkey brain tissue from the corresponding chunk of human brain tissue). In fact, the best way to study stimulus awareness today relies on correlating neuronal responses of trained monkeys to their behavior. Given this likeness, appropriate experiments on nonhuman primates—carried out in a humane and ethical manner—are a powerful resource for discovering the mechanisms underlying consciousness.[21]

Of course, humans do differ fundamentally from all other organisms in their ability to talk. True language enables *homo sapiens* to represent and disseminate arbitrarily complex concepts. Language leads to writing, representative democracy, general relativity, and the Macintosh computer, activities and inventions that are beyond the capabilities of our animal friends. The primacy of language for most aspects of civilized life has given rise to a belief among philosophers, linguists, and others that consciousness is impossible without language and that, therefore, only humans can feel and introspect. While this might be true, to a limited extent, about self-consciousness (as in, "I know that I am seeing red"), all of the evidence from split-brain patients, autistic children, evolutionary studies, and animal behavior is fully compatible with the position that at least mammals experience the sights and sounds of life.[22]

At present, it is unknown to what extent conscious perception is common to *all* animals. It is probable that consciousness correlates to some extent with the complexity of the organism's nervous system. Squids, bees, fruit flies, and even roundworms are all capable of fairly sophisticated behaviors. Perhaps they too possess some level of awareness; perhaps they too can feel pain, experience pleasure, and see.

---

[21] A few words on some of the approximately 200 primate species, of which humans are but one member. The order of *primates* is divided into two suborders, *prosimians* (literally, "before monkeys") and *anthropods*, encompassing monkeys, apes and humans. There are two superfamilies of monkeys, which have distinct geographical distributions, *New World* and *Old World monkeys*. Old World monkeys, which include *baboons* and *macaques*, have larger and more convoluted brains than New World monkeys, are easily bred in captivity, and are not endangered. They are popular as a model system for human brain organization. *Gorillas, orangutans* and the two species of *chimpanzees* constitute the *great apes.* Given their highly developed cognitive abilities and kinship to humans, little invasive research is carried out on apes. Most of what is known about their brains derives from postmortem studies.

[22] The belief that only humans are conscious and that animals are mere automatons, advocated most famously by Descartes, used to be widespread. After Darwin and the rise of evolutionary explanations, it became less so. However, even today some argue that language is a sine qua non for consciousness (Macphail, 1998). Griffin (2001) is the classical reference surveying consciousness throughout the animal kingdom.

How Can Consciousness Be Approached in a Scientific Manner?

Consciousness takes many forms, but it seems best to begin with the form that is easiest to investigate. Studying vision has several advantages over studying other senses, at least when it comes to understanding consciousness.

First, humans are visual creatures. This is reflected in the large amount of brain tissue dedicated to the analysis of images, and in the importance of seeing in daily life. If you have a cold, for instance, your nose becomes stuffy and you may lose your sense of smell, but this impairs you only mildly. A transient loss of vision, as occurs during snow blindness on the other hand, devastates you.

Second, visual percepts are vivid and rich in information. Pictures and movies are highly structured, yet easy to manipulate using computer-generated graphics.

Third, as noted already by the young philosopher Arthur Schopenhauer in 1813, vision is more easily deceived than any of the other senses. This manifests itself in a sheer endless number of illusions. Take *motion-induced blindness:* a bunch of randomly moving blue lights are superimposed onto three highly salient but stationary yellow spots. Fixate anywhere on the display, and after a while one, two, or even all three disks simply disappear.[23] Gone! It is an amazing sight: The swirling blue cloud wipes the yellow spots from sight, even though the spots continue to stimulate the retina. Following a brief eye movement the spots reappear. While such sensory phenomena are far removed from "intentionality," the "aboutness of consciousness," "free will," and other concepts dear to philosophers, understanding the neuronal basis of visual illusions can teach much about the physical basis of consciousness in the brain. In the early days of molecular biology, Delbrück focused on the genetics of phages, simple viruses that prey on bacteria. You might have thought that the way phages pass information on to their descendants is irrelevant to human heredity. Yet this is not the case. Likewise, Eric Kandel's belief that the lowly marine snail *Aplysia* has much to teach us about the molecular and cellular strategies underlying memory has proven to be prophetic.[24]

Last, and most important, the neuronal basis of many visual phenomena and illusions has been investigated throughout the animal kingdom. Perceptual neuroscience has advanced to such a point that reasonably sophisticated computational models have been constructed and have proven their worth in guiding experimental agendas and summarizing the data.

I therefore concentrate on visual sensation or awareness. Antonio Damasio, the eminent neurologist at the University of Iowa, refers to such sensory forms

---

[23] Motion-induced blindness was discovered by Bonneh, Cooperman, and Sagi (2001).
[24] Kandel (2001).

of awareness as *core consciousness*, and differentiates these from *extended consciousness*.[25] Core consciousness is all about the here and now, while extended consciousness requires a sense of self—the self-referential aspect that for many people epitomizes consciousness—and of the past and the anticipated future.

My research program neglects, for now, these and other aspects such as language and emotions. This is not to say that they are not critically important to humans. They are. Aphasics, children with severe autism, or patients who have lost their sense of self are severely impaired, confined to hospitals or nursing homes. For the most part, however, they can still see and feel pain. Extended consciousness shares with sensory consciousness the same mysterious stance, but it is much less amenable to experimental investigations since these capabilities can't easily be studied in laboratory animals, making access to the underlying neurons difficult.

Underlining my choice is the tentative assumption that all the different aspects of consciousness (smell, pain, vision, self-consciousness, the feeling of willing an action, of being angry and so on) employ one or perhaps a few common mechanisms. Figuring out the neuronal basis for one modality, therefore, will simplify understanding them all. From an introspective point of view, this hypothesis is quite radical. What is the commonality between a sound, a sight, and a smell? Their content feels quite different, yet all three have that magical buzz about them. Given the way natural selection works, it is likely that the subjective sensations associated with each are caused by similar neuronal events and circuits.

I allude to nonvisual lines of work, too, such as olfaction and Pavlovian conditioning, particularly if they have features that make them easy to study in the laboratory. Given the desirability of relating consciousness to the firing activity of individual neurons and their arrangements, it will be imperative to carry out relevant experiments in behaving mice. The amazing development of ever-more-powerful molecular biology tools permits scientists to manipulate rodent brains in a deliberate, delicate, and reversible manner, something currently not possible in primates.

Altered states of consciousness—hypnosis, out-of-body experiences, lucid dreaming, hallucination, meditation, and so on—are not covered in this book. While all are fascinating case studies of the human condition, it is difficult

---

[25] See Damasio's book (1999). A pithy formulation of his ideas can be found in Damasio (2000). The cognitive psychologist Endel Tulving at the University of Toronto refers to percepts as involving *noetic* (knowing) consciousness, in contrast to *autonoetic* (self-knowing) consciousness that is characteristic of episodic memory (Tulving, 1985). Edelman and Tononi (2000) refer to *primary* and *higher-order* consciousness, and Block refers to phenomenal consciousness on the one hand and reflective and self-consciousness on the other (Block, 1995).

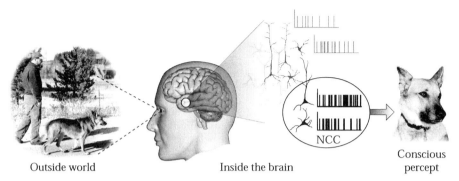

Outside world   Inside the brain   Conscious percept

FIGURE 1.1 *The Neuronal Correlates of Consciousness* The NCC are the minimal set of neural events—here synchronized action potentials in neocortical pyramidal neurons—sufficient for a specific conscious percept.

to access their underlying neuronal representations (can a monkey be hypnotized?). A comprehensive theory of consciousness will ultimately have to account for these unusual phenomena.[26]

1.4 | THE NEURONAL CORRELATES OF CONSCIOUSNESS

Francis and I are bent on discovering the *neuronal correlates of consciousness* (NCC). Whenever information is represented in the NCC you are conscious of it. The goal is to discover *the minimal set of neuronal events and mechanisms jointly sufficient for a specific conscious percept* (Figure 1.1). The NCC involve the firing activity of neurons in the forebrain.[27] As detailed in the next chapter, by firing activity I mean the sequences of pulses, about a tenth of a volt in amplitude and 0.5–1 msec in duration, that neurons emit when they are excited. These binary *spikes* or *action potentials* can be treated as the principal output of forebrain neurons. Stimulating the relevant cells with some yet-to-

---

[26]Blackmore (1982), Grüsser and Landis (1991), and Blanke et al. (2002) describe the psychology and neurology of out-of-body experiences, a fascinating phenomenon that has, until recently, been almost entirely co-opted by new age mystics. Hallucinations, internally generated percepts in the awake state that can't be distinguished from externally generated percepts, are a hallmark of schizophrenia and other mental disorders. Their neuronal basis is being explored using brain imaging (Frith, 1996; Flytche et al., 1998; Manford and Andermann, 1998; Vogeley, 1999).

[27]I follow a tripartite division of the vertebrate brain into the *forebrain*, the *midbrain*, and the *hindbrain*. The forebrain consists, by and large, of the neocortex, the basal ganglia, hippocampus, amygdala, olfactory bulb, and the thalamus and its associated structures. The hindbrain includes the pons, medulla, and the cerebellum.

be-invented technology that replicates their exact spiking pattern should trigger the same percept as using natural images, sounds, or smells. As I emphasized a few pages earlier, I assume that consciousness depends on what is inside the head, not necessarily on the behavior of the organism.

The notion of the NCC is significantly more subtle than illustrated by the figure, and must also specify over what range of circumstances and data the correlation between neuronal events and conscious percept holds. Is the relationship true only when the subject is awake? What about dreams or various pathologies? Is the relationship the same for all animals? These complications are taken up in Chapter 5.

Using the NCC in this way implies that if I am aware of an event, the NCC in my head must directly express this. *There must be an explicit correspondence between any mental event and its neuronal correlates.* Another way of stating this is that any change in a subjective state must be associated with a change in a neuronal state.[28] Note that the converse need not necessarily be true; two different neuronal states of the brain may be mentally indistinguishable.

It is possible that the NCC are not expressed in the spiking activity of some neurons but, perhaps, in the concentration of free, intracellular calcium ions in the postsynaptic dendrites of their target cells.[29] Or the invisible partners of neurons, *glia* cells that support, nurture and maintain nerve cells and their environment in the brain, might be directly involved (although this is unlikely[30]). But whatever the correlates are, they must map directly, rather than indirectly, onto conscious perception because the NCC are all that are needed for that particular experience.

---

[28] This stance implies that in the absence of a physical carrier, consciousness can't exist. Put succinctly: No matter, never mind.

[29] The proposition that the NCC are closely related to subcellular processes is not as outlandish as it may sound. Cellular biophysicists have realized over the past years that the distribution of calcium ions within neurons represents a crucial variable for processing and storing information (Koch, 1999). Calcium ions enter spines and dendrites through voltage-gated channels. This, along with their diffusion, buffering, and release from intracellular stores, leads to rapid local modulations of the calcium concentration. The concentration of calcium can, in turn, influence the membrane potential (via calcium-dependent membrane conductances) and—by binding to buffers and enzymes—turn on or off intracellular signaling pathways that initiate plasticity and form the basis of learning. The dynamics of calcium in thick dendrites and cell bodies spans the right time scale (on the order of hundreds of milliseconds) for perception. Indeed, it has been established experimentally in the cricket that the concentration of free, intracellular calcium in the omega interneuron correlates well with the degree of auditory masking, a time-dependent modulation of auditory sensitivity in these animals (Sobel and Tank, 1994).

[30] *Glia* cells are as numerous as neurons but lack their glamor. Their behavior is sluggish and they show little of the elaborate sensitivity associated with neurons (Laming et al., 1998). This is why they are unlikely to play a direct role in perception. Some glia cells exhibit all-or-none propagating calcium events, akin to action potentials, except that they occur over seconds (Cornell-Bell et al., 1990; Sanderson, 1996).

The NCC may be associated with some special type of activity in one or more sets of neurons with some special pharmacological, anatomical, and biophysical properties that must exceed some threshold and last for some minimal amount of time.

As I shall argue in Chapter 14, it is quite unlikely that consciousness is a mere epiphenomenon. Rather consciousness enhances the survival of its carrier. This means that the NCC activity must affect other neurons in some manner. This post-NCC activity influences other neurons that ultimately cause some behavior. This activity can also feed back to the NCC neurons and to previous stages in the hierarchy, significantly complicating matters.

Discovering the NCC would constitute a major step forward on the road to a final understanding of consciousness. Identification of the NCC would enable neuroscientists to manipulate its cellular substrate on the basis of pharmacological intervention and genetic manipulation. It may be possible to fashion transgenic mice whose NCC can be rapidly and safely switched on and off. What behaviors might such zombie rodents be capable of? Clinical benefits will flow from this discovery as well, such as a better understanding of mental diseases and the design of new and powerful anesthetics, with few side effects.

Eventually, a theory that bridges the explanatory gap, that explains why activity in a subset of neurons is the basis of (or, perhaps, is identical to) some particular feeling, is required. This theory needs to make comprehensible why that activity means something for the organism (e.g., why does it hurt?) and why qualia feel the way they do (e.g., why does red look one way, quite different from blue?).[31]

Along the way, the great debate that swirls around the question of the exact relationship between neuronal and mental events needs to be resolved. *Physicalism* asserts that the two are identical; that the NCC for the percept of purple *is* the percept. Nothing else is needed. While the former is measured by microelectrodes, the latter is experienced by brains. A favorite analogy is with temperature of a gas and the average kinetic energy of the gas molecules. Temperature is a macroscopic variable that is recorded by a thermometer, while the kinetic energy is a microscopic variable that requires quite a different set of tools to study. Yet the two are identical. Even though, superficially, they appear quite distinct, temperature is equivalent to the average kinetic energy of molecules. The faster the molecules move, the higher the temperature. It does

---

[31] The term "explanatory gap" was introduced by Levine (1983). There is no guarantee that science will discover a final, objective theory of consciousness. As Chalmers (1996) and others have argued, one might have to settle for some sort of nonreductive physicalist account of consciousness or for an ontological dualism with rigorous, quantitative bridging principles linking the domain of subjective experiences with objective reality. Only time will tell.

not make sense to talk of the rapid molecular motion causing temperature as if one is the cause and the other the effect. One is sufficient and necessary for the other.[32]

At this point, I am not sure whether this sort of strong identity holds for the NCC and the associated percept. Are they really one and the same thing, viewed from different perspectives? The characters of brain states and of phenomenal states appear too different to be completely reducible to each other. I suspect that their relationship is more complex than traditionally envisioned. For now, it is best to keep an open mind on this matter and to concentrate on identifying the correlates of consciousness in the brain.

1.5 | RECAPITULATION

Consciousness resides at the nexus of the mind-body problem. It appears as mysterious to 21st-century scholars as when humans first started to wonder about their minds several millennia ago. Nevertheless, scientists today are better positioned than ever to investigate the physical basis of consciousness.

My approach is a direct one that many of my colleagues consider naive or ill-advised. I take subjective experience as given and assume that brain activity is both necessary and sufficient for biological creatures to experience something. Nothing else is needed. I seek the physical basis of phenomenal states within brain cells, their arrangements and activities. My goal is to identify the specific nature of this activity, the neuronal correlates of consciousness, and to determine to what extent the NCC differ from activity that influences behavior without engaging consciousness.

The focus of this book is on sensory forms of consciousness—and on vision in particular. More than other aspects of sensation, visual awareness is amenable to empirical investigation. Emotions, language, and a sense of the self and of others are critical to daily life, but these facets of consciousness are left for later, when their neural bases will be better understood. Similar to the quest to understand life, discovering and characterizing the molecular, biophysical, and neurophysiological operations that constitute the NCC will likely help solve the central enigma, how events in certain privileged systems can be the physical basis of, or even be, feelings.

It would be contrary to evolutionary continuity to believe that consciousness is unique to humans. I assume that the human mind shares some basic properties with animal minds—in particular, with mammals such as monkeys

---

[32]There is an extensive philosophical literature on this topic, with many, many variants. I refer the curious reader to Patricia Churchland's books, which deal extensively with this topic (1986, 2002).

and mice. I ignore niggling debates about the exact definition of consciousness and whether or not my spinal cord is conscious but is not telling me. These questions must be answered eventually, but today they only impede progress. You don't win a war by fighting the most arduous battle first.

Blunders will be committed and oversimplifications will be made in the course of this sustained, empirical, long-term undertaking, but these will only become apparent as time passes. For now, science should rise to the challenge and explore the basis of consciousness in the brain. Like the partially occluded view of a snow-covered mountain summit during a first ascent, the lure of understanding this puzzle is irresistible. As Lao Tsu remarked many years ago, "A journey of a thousand miles begins with a single step."

Now that we have started, let me acquaint you with some key concepts that will guide our quest. In particular, I need to flesh out the notions of explicit and implicit neuronal representations, essential nodes, and the various forms of nervous activity.

CHAPTER TWO

Neurons, the Atoms of Perception

The idea seemed so obvious to me and so elegant that I fell deeply in love with it. And, like falling in love with a woman, it's only possible if you do not know much about her, so you cannot see her faults. The faults will become apparent later, but only after the love is strong enough to hold you to her.

Richard P. Feynman

Scientists observe the world in a perfectly cold and objective manner. Each fact is registered, its significance weighed and, if found sound, incorporated into one of the theoretical edifices that describes the cosmos and everything in it, such as quantum mechanics, general relativity, or natural selection.

This cliché is a far cry from the actual working habits of researchers. This idealized view is particularly inappropriate for neuroscience, a young endeavor whose object of study is, for its size, the most complex entity in the known universe. In order to make some sense out of the observations flooding in from biology and psychology laboratories around the world, researchers must have some preliminary idea of what to look for. It is impossible to absorb all the existing facts about the brain without some sort of filter that separates the wheat from the chaff. There is just too much data, much of it conflicting, for any other strategy to prevail.[1] Scientists must always keep an open mind about these biases, constantly reexamining them in the light of new evidence or insights.

The problem this book tackles is that the brain, a physical organ, can give rise to feelings, to specific conscious percepts. How does this happen? Much

---

[1] These conflicts arise because conditions are difficult to precisely replicate when dealing with intricate organisms. Even seemingly minute differences in "identical" protocols, such as the background level of the light, whether the animal was fixating or free-viewing, whether it was juvenile or adult, the conditions under which it was reared, and so on, can significantly affect the experimental outcome. Undoubtedly, some of the observed variability is due to the distinct genetic heritage of subjects. Yet even genetically identical animals, clones, kept on the same feeding and day-night schedule, display a surprising amount of variability in their behavior. One individual will show an effect, while the next one won't.

neural activity at any one time does not correlate with subjective states yet can still influence behavior. What is the difference between this and the activity that is sufficient for consciousness?

Neurons are the atoms of perception, memory, thought, and action, and the synaptic connections among them shape and guide how individual cells are transiently assembled into the larger coalitions that generate perception. Any theory that explains the neuronal basis of consciousness, therefore, must describe specific interactions among nerve cells on the millisecond time scale.

Let me plant two ideas here: First, explicit neural representations are essential for the NCC. Second, multiple forms of neural activity exist. Properly looked after, both ideas reap enormous benefit in terms of being able to interpret neuronal behavior.

This chapter requires some conceptual heavy lifting. Once this material is digested, however, most of the remaining ideas in the book will be easy to follow. The chapter starts off with a preamble, a terse description of the nature of cortex. You will need to become familiar with at least some of its properties, as only brainmatter, so far at least, gives rise to consciousness.

2.1 | THE MACHINERY OF THE CEREBRAL CORTEX

Even though the brain looks to the casual observer like a mushy, overcooked cauliflower, it is exceedingly differentiated. One general characteristic of its operations is the absolutely astonishing variety and specificity of the actions it performs. Sensory systems handle an almost infinite variety of images, scenes, sounds, and so on, and react to them in detail with remarkable accuracy. They are highly evolved, are considerably specified, and can learn a great deal from experience.

There is a strong selective advantage in reacting rapidly. The adage, "the best is the enemy of the good," applies here, because it is better to achieve a rapid but occasionally imperfect result than to find the perfect solution later. The organism that takes its time to figure out the optimal solution may be eaten by a faster competitor working with a so-so result. This is all the more important given the slow components that the brain has to deal with, "switching" at speeds a million times slower than transistors. Another general principle is to use several rough-and-ready methods in parallel to reach a conclusion, rather than following just one method accurately.

The main function of the sensory cortex is to construct and use highly specific feature detectors, such as those for orientation, motion, and faces.[2]

---

[2]How are feature detectors formed? In a broad sense, neurons do this by detecting common correlations in their inputs and altering their synapses (and perhaps other properties) so that they can more easily respond to them.

Animal studies with microelectrodes reveal segregated cortical neighborhoods whose neurons are specialized to carry out these different jobs. For instance, neurons in one occipital-temporal region are particularly sensitive to the color or hue of stimuli; neurons in an area called MT detect movement; neurons in part of the posterior parietal cortex program eye movements; and neurons in the auditory cortex encode timbre. Clinical observations of neurological patients reinforce the view that particular regions of the cerebral cortex subserve specific functions. If an adult loses any one such area by a stroke, bullet, or some other trauma, very specific and peculiar deficits can result.[3]

Cortical areas in the back of the brain are organized in a loosely hierarchical manner, with at least a dozen levels, each one subordinate to the one above it. When a group of neurons within one of these regions receives a strong, driving input from lower in the hierarchy, the neurons send their output to another area or group of neurons located higher in the hierarchy (neuroanatomists talk of a lower region "projecting" into a higher one). When examined in detail, however, things are less clear-cut, because feedback connections abound, so some areas have an ambiguous position within this hierarchy, and shortcuts exist.

The incoming sensory information is usually not enough to lead to an unambiguous interpretation.[4] In such cases, then, the cortical networks *fill in*. They make their best guess, given the incomplete information. Filling-in happens throughout the brain. This general principle, expressed colloquially as "jumping to conclusions," guides much of human behavior.[5]

Any visual scene gives rise to widespread activity throughout the brain. *Coalitions* of neurons, coding for different objects in the world, compete with

---

[3]I'll return to the topic of brain damage in Chapter 13. Some of the cortical regions that specialize in distinct stimulus attributes are treated in Chapter 8.

[4]This ambiguity has been formalized in mathematical terms as perception as a set of ill-posed problems (Poggio, Torre, and Koch, 1985).

[5]*Filling-in* is a catch-all term used for distinct perceptual phenomena that include illusory boundary completion (Figure 2.5), the retinal blind spot (Section 3.3), the apparent motion of a spot that disappears behind an occluding box, the shape of a partially hidden object, and other experiences where you clearly see something that isn't there (for one taxonomy of these phenomena and what they imply for the philosophy of mind, see Pessoa, Thompson, and Noë, 1998). Filling-in and reinterpretation of incomplete or contradictory data makes human speech intelligible. When comparing a videotape of Francis Crick being interviewed about our work with the exact, word-for-word transcript, I was struck by the discrepancy between what I heard and what Francis actually said. I simply didn't notice his incomplete sentences, dropped words, and repetitions. The powerful, unconscious biases that govern people's social lives in the form of gender-, racial-, or age-based prejudices, born from the sum of life's experiences, are another manifestation of filling-in operating at a cognitive level. None of these effects are a question of logically deducing the existence of something, akin to Sherlock Holmes's chain of reasoning based on minute observations. Rather, the brain automatically infers aspects of the stimulus that are missing and presents these as a fully elaborated percept.

each other; that is, one coalition strives to suppress the activity of neurons that code for other objects in the scene via inhibition and vice versa. This is particularly true in the higher echelons of the brain. Paying attention to an event or object biases this competition in favor of the attended event or object.[6]

You can experience this competition when trying to remember some acquaintance's name. It may be on the tip of your tongue but, maddeningly enough, you're unable to quite recall it. Instead, you come up with names of unrelated people. Suddenly, half an hour later, the right name pops into your mind. Speculating a bit, I predict that the brain activity associated with the distracting names suppressed the neurons responsible for the right name. As the longer-term effects (including synaptic modifications) of this suppression wear off, the right neurons eventually become active and the name suddenly, and unexpectedly at this point, materializes.

The NCC are closely related to this suppression of competing cellular assemblies, representing alternative interpretations of the scene. Usually only a single coalition survives—the one whose properties you are then conscious of. Under some conditions—when the neural representations don't overlap—two or three coalitions may coexist peacefully, at least for a while. Such winner-take-all tendencies do not imply, however, that neurons in other parts of the brain can't remain active, vestiges of the unconscious mind.

Elections as a Metaphor for Neuronal Competition

Democratic elections serve as a metaphor for these highly dynamic processes. Many candidates compete, each one backed or opposed by powerful coalitions representing environmentalists, trade unions, the military-industrial complex, churches, party organizations, and so forth. Ultimately, a single coalition and its candidate emerge as the winners. The activity associated with the winning coalition corresponds to the conscious state.

Losing coalitions don't disappear after the election, however, but continue to remain active and influence politics. And they may well win the next election. Politics in a democracy is a competitive game, with vehement changes taking place within days, akin to the interactions among excitatory and inhibitory neurons that occur within a fraction of a second. As your attention wanders from one object to the next, first one coalition wins—you become conscious

---

[6]The idea that groups of cells, *neural assemblies*, underlie percepts goes back a long way. Its best known advocate in the 20th century was Hebb (1949). See also Freeman (1975); Palm (1982 and 1990); Flohr (2000); Varela et al. (2001); and Harris et al. (2003). Coalitions imply neural assemblies plus competition among them. Desimone and Duncan (1995) advanced the idea that attention biases the fight for dominance among these coalitions. This will be taken up in Chapter 10.

of the first object—before it is suppressed by a second coalition and your mind becomes aware of the other object.

The metaphor of consciousness as a political process must not be mistaken for a mechanistic model.[7] It is intended to help familiarize you with the complexities of the events occurring among forebrain neurons in relation to consciousness.

2.2 | EXPLICIT REPRESENTATION, COLUMNAR ORGANIZATION, AND ESSENTIAL NODES

Our first guiding principle is that the NCC require *explicit* neuronal representations. Cells that encode information in an *implicit* manner are not sufficient for a conscious percept, although they may influence behavior.

The Depth of Computation

Before I explain what exactly I mean, let me introduce the concept of *logical depth of computation*. It is a measure from the theory of computation of the number of steps necessary to come to some conclusion.[8] Think of it as the amount of mathematical work that went into the computation and that the recipient is saved from having to repeat. The logical depth of retinal ganglion cells, informing their target cells outside the eye about local contrasts in their field of view, is much less than the logical depth of a population of cortical neurons whose activity unambiguously signals the presence of a leopard.

The tide-tables published in coastal newspapers are an example of reducing the logical depth of computation *the reader* has to perform. The times and heights of the high and low tides can, to a first approximation, be computed from the orbital positions of the earth, the moon, and the sun using Newton's laws (taking the local water depth into account). Alternatively, they can be extrapolated from previous tide data. Both methods, however, require a lot of data and many calculations and are expensive undertakings. Tide-tables, on the other hand, express this information precisely and unequivocally, so sailors, beachcombers, and surfers can directly access the data at minimal cost.

---

[7]It also, erroneously, suggests that there can only be a unique winner in the neuronal competition for dominance.

[8]Bennett (1988) discusses logical depth. Norretranders (1998) provides a lively and readable account of how this might apply to computers and brains.

What Is Meant by Explicit and Implicit?

An explicit representation is one that has more logical depth than an implicit one because it is, in essence, the summation of all the implicit information.

TV news provides an analogy. The pattern of colored dots on the screen contains an implicit representation of the newscaster's face, but only the brightness of each individual picture element (pixel) and its location are explicitly represented on the television screen (see also Figure 2.3). A machine vision algorithm would have to infer laboriously the presence of a face from these pixels, a nontrivial task. If the algorithm summarized its computation in the form of a light-emitting diode that flashed any time a face appeared on screen, no matter its size, tilt or facial expression, that would constitute an explicit face representation. Neurons that behave in a similar fashion have been found (Figures 2.2 and 2.4). Defined properly,[9] the implicit/explicit distinction is an absolute one, independent of the observer.

All of the visual information that the brain can access is implicitly encoded by the membrane potentials of the more than 200 million photoreceptors in the two eyes. This ocean of data is of little use, however, until higher processing stages have extracted meaningful features. The logical depth of retinal activity is quite shallow.

An explicit coding for small, twisted pieces of wires was discovered by the electrophysiologist Nikos Logothetis and his colleagues, working at Baylor College in Texas, following a proposal by the MIT theoretician Tomaso Poggio. They trained macaque monkeys over a long period to become highly adept at recognizing any one particular twisted paper clip and at distinguishing it from similar ones. The scientists then recorded action potentials from nerve cells in the inferotemporal cortex (IT), a high-level region of cortex concerned with visual objects (see the front endpages). Figure 2.1 illustrates the firing activity of one such cell.

When the paper clip was seen from one particular vantage point, the neuron fired vigorously. As the object was rotated away from the cell's preferred angle, the cellular response decreased. Paper clips bent in different ways, though similar enough to look the same to the untrained eye, evoked only a minuscule response from the cell, as did pictures of other objects. About one out of every

---

[9]Our notion of explicit and implicit can be formalized by demanding that the existence of the to-be-represented feature or object must be inferred from a suitably weighted linear or nonlinear combination of cells. Thus, an explicit face representation is one in which a single-layered neural network can detect whether or not a face is present in the firing activity of a pool of neurons. This way, an explicit representation can be defined independent of an observer. In general, any explicit representation must be grounded in an earlier, implicit stage.

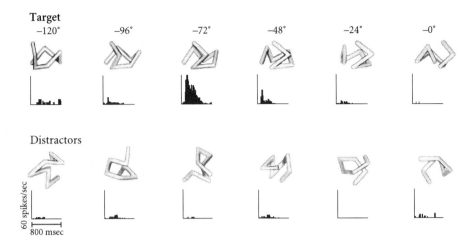

FIGURE 2.1 *Explicit Encoding at the Single Neuron Level* Firing activity of a neuron located in the inferotemporal cortex of a monkey trained to recognize wire-frame objects. The averaged response is shown below the image seen by the animal. The cell fires vigorously to one particular view of one particular paper clip. Rotate this target by 24° or more away from the preferred view, and the cellular discharge is reduced. Clips bent in different ways fail to excite the neuron. Modified from Logothetis and Pauls (1995).

ten cells that Logothetis recorded from fired in this highly selective manner. Collectively, these cells represented paper clips in an explicit manner.[10]

An explicit representation should be *invariant* to those aspects of the input that do not convey any specific information about the feature symbolized. That is, the cell should remain selective, no matter whether the room light is dim or bright, whether the paper clip is far away or close by, whether the monkey is cocking its head to the left or to the right, and so on. This level of invariance implies that information has to be thrown away (for instance, the amplitude of the background light). As a general rule, the deeper one proceeds into the cortex, the less the neurons care about the exact location, orientation, or size of the stimulus, the more information will be discarded, and the bigger the neuron's logical depth of computation.

---

[10] Of course, the monkeys were not born with paper clip cells. Rather, as the animals were trained to distinguish one bent wire frame from distracting ones, cortical synapses rearranged themselves to carry out this task (Logothetis et al., 1994; Logothetis and Pauls, 1995). The experimentalists chose paper clips because the animals had no prior exposure to them. Kobatake, Wang, and Tanaka (1998), and Sheinberg and Logothetis (2001), discuss how training affects the cellular responses.

Of all the trillions of cells found in the human body, only a tiny minority have this amazing ability to explicitly encode important aspects of the outside world. Liver, kidney, muscle, or skin cells do change in response to variations in their environment, but this information is never made explicit.

I am *not* implying that all explicit representations participate in conscious perception. Rather, an explicit representation is a necessary but not sufficient condition for the NCC.

The Columnar Organization of the Cortex

Key to the distinction between explicit and implicit is the *columnar organization* that is such a singular feature of the sensory cortex. Most neurons within a column extending perpendicular to the cortical sheet, from top to bottom, a few millimeters in thickness, have one or more features in common. For instance, cells stacked above each other in V1 code for the orientation of visual stimuli (e.g., everything that has a diagonal orientation) within a particular region of visual space, while a column of cells in area MT represent one particular direction of movement (e.g., everything that moves rightward). Neurons are not haphazardly arranged within the brain but assemble according to orderly principles that neuroscientists are uncovering bit by bit.[11]

I surmise that the feature represented in this columnar fashion is the one that is made explicit. Thus, V1 cells express visual orientation in an explicit manner, and MT neurons the direction and amplitude of movement. Explicit coding and columnar organization are distinct concepts. There is no logical reason why neurons that explicitly code for say, motion, have to be arranged in a columnar fashion. But—possibly to minimize length of axonal wiring[12]— these two architectural features appear to go hand in hand.

From Grandmother Cells to Population Coding

An extreme form of explicit representation is neurons that respond to one particular object or concept, and to that object alone. Such highly specific cells are referred to as *grandmother neurons*: They would become active every time you saw your grandmother, but not when you looked at your grandfather or some random elderly woman. The conjoint activity of a few such groups of neurons

---

[11] The vertical column of neocortical neurons, of common embryological origin, has been recognized to be a key component of brain organization since its discovery and characterization by Lorente de No and Mountcastle. A subunit is the minicolumn, encompassing about 100 neurons, with many minicolumns making up a column (Rakic, 1995; Mountcastle, 1998; and Buxhoeveden and Casanova, 2002).

[12] See footnote 17 in Chapter 4.

could conveniently represent any complex proposition, such as a smiling or dancing grandmother or grandmother's glasses.[13]

All kinds of objections have been raised to the idea that neurons respond to specific individuals, yet such cells do exist. Figure 2.2 illustrates spiking activity recorded from a neuron in the human *amygdala*, a set of subcortical nuclei of the medial temporal lobe that receive input from higher-level visual cortical areas (and elsewhere). The neurological patient viewed pictures of actors, politicians, and other celebrities, animals, buildings, and so on, while the activity of the neuron was monitored in the laboratory of the neurosurgeon Itzhak Fried at the University of California at Los Angeles.[14] The neuron responded to 3 out of 50 images: a line drawing of U.S. President Bill Clinton, his presidential portrait, and a group photograph with him. It failed to fire to images of other famous men or other presidents. At the level of individual pixels, these three images are quite different from each other; the degree of invariance displayed by the cell is therefore quite remarkable. Think of the depth of computation required for a computer algorithm to decide whether or not Bill Clinton was present in an image.

Given the celebrity status of then President Clinton, it made sense for the brain to wire up neurons responding to his constant media presence. I am not claiming, however, that this one cell constitutes the entire neuronal correlate of the percept "President Clinton." The firing of one cortical neuron is too weak to strongly activate, by itself, the cells to which it is connected. Many cells are needed. This also enhances the robustness of this coding scheme. I suspect

---

[13]The grandmother cell concept, also called *Gnostic neurons*, is set out in considerable detail in a book by the Polish neurophysiologist Jerzy Konorksi (1967). The British electrophysiologist Horace Barlow (1972) provided an early critique, proposing instead a coding scheme in which a thousand *cardinal cells* represent individual percepts. The discovery by Charles Gross and his colleagues, working at the Massachusetts Institute of Technology in Cambridge, of cells in the inferotemporal cortex that fired selectively to hands and faces, provided a boost to Konorksi's ideas (Gross, Bender, and Rocha-Miranda, 1969; Gross, Rocha-Miranda, and Bender, 1972). Barlow (1995) and Gross (2002) review the historical context. Textbooks with in-depth discussions of the various ways populations of neurons can represent information include Dayan and Abbott (2001), Rao, Olshausen, and Lewicki (2002), and Rolls and Deco (2002).

[14]It is rare to record the firing activity of single neurons in the human cortex. Almost all of these data have been gained by studying certain epileptic patients. To eliminate or reduce their frequent seizures that are not controllable by drugs, the part of the brain responsible for triggering the epileptic attacks needs to be destroyed by surgery. This affords the opportunity to record individual cell activity either during the operation itself or during the week-long monitoring period preceding it, when electrodes are directly implanted into the patient's brain to help locate the initial seizure focus. For a highly readable account of such procedures, see the popular book by Calvin and Ojemann (1994) or the more scholarly Ojemann, Ojemann, and Fried (1998). The work on visual representations in single cortical neurons in humans that I refer to was carried out by Gabriel Kreiman, at the time a graduate student in my laboratory, under the guidance of Itzhak Fried (Kreiman, Koch, and Fried, 2000a,b; Kreiman, 2001; Kreiman, Fried, and Koch, 2002).

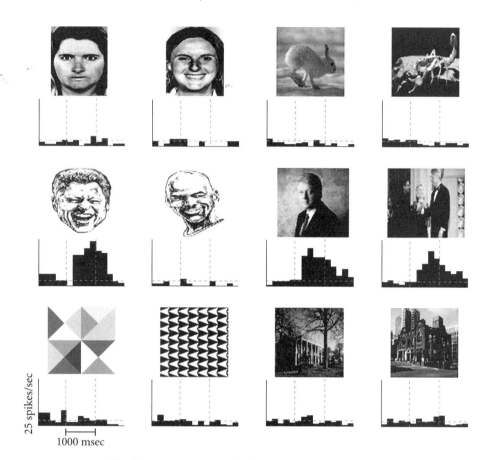

25 spikes/sec

1000 msec

FIGURE 2.2 *A Cell Selective to Pictures of Bill Clinton* The firing pattern of an amygdala neuron from a patient looking at drawings and photographs for one second each (interval between the stippled lines). The cell responded vigorously to a pencil drawing, an official portrait, and a group photo that included the former U.S. President. It remains indifferent to images of other U.S. Presidents (not shown), famous athletes, or unknown actors. Modified from Kreiman (2001).

that there will be numerous cells for frequently encountered objects, such as celebrities, grandma, your guard dog, your laptop computer, and so on. But the face of the stranger who just bagged your groceries at the supermarket is not represented in this sparse manner, but differently.

A more common form of neuronal representation is *population coding*, in which information is encoded by the spiking activity of a large group of more broadly tuned cells. Taken on its own, the firing of any one cell says little. Yet if interpreted appropriately, the firing pattern of the entire population expresses a wealth of detail. Neuroscientists speak of a *distributed representation*. In a fully

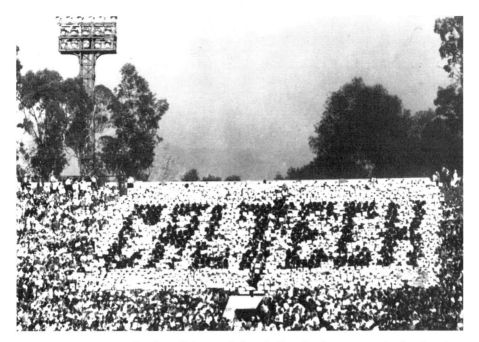

FIGURE 2.3 *An Example of Implicit Population Coding* Each spectator in the cheering section at the Rose Bowl stadium in Pasadena, California, had a single sheet of black or white cardboard. At a signal, everybody flashed their cards, spelling out CALTECH. Any one card, by itself, acts as a binary picture element—without significance to the individual holding it. The meaning inherent in the population activity relies on an external observer (the audience, in this case). In the brain, the readout has to be done by other groups of cells. Courtesy of the California Institute of Technology.

distributed code, all neurons that are part of the ensemble contribute some information (Figure 2.3 illustrates a real-life example of an implicit, coarse-coded population coding strategy). In a *sparse representation*, only a minority of neurons are active at any one time. A very sparse representation converges, in the limit, to a grandmother neuron representation.

A well-known form of retinal population coding, described in Chapter 3, is that for color. It is based on the conjoint activity in three types of photoreceptors (cones) that have distinct response profiles as a function of wavelength of the incident light. The percept of hue arises by combining information from all three classes. The unfortunate individuals who have but a single cone type can only see shades of gray.

Another example of population coding includes face neurons in the upper tier of the visual hierarchy (Section 8.5). One group encodes the identity of the face, while another set is concerned with its facial expression (angry? scared?). A third group includes neurons whose response varies in a graded manner as

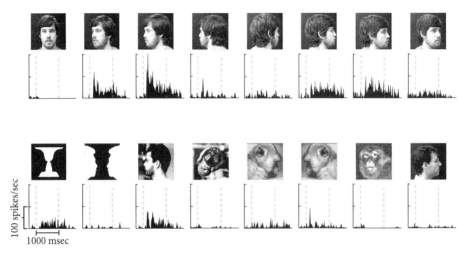

FIGURE 2.4 *A Face Cell* The firing rate of an IT neuron from a monkey looking at various mug shots (between the dashed lines). The cell's preferred stimulus is a bearded human face seen in profile. From D. Sheinberg and N. Logothetis, private communication.

the angle at which the face is seen gradually changes (Figure 2.4). A complete representation for faces may also include the highly specific neurons I've talked about (Figure 2.2), together with cells that signal the face's gender, hair, skin texture, and angle of gaze. Seeing any one face, even a completely unknown one, gives rise to widespread activity at many loci in the brain, with some cells firing vigorously but most responding in a weaker and more desultory fashion. Those attributes that are made explicit—that is, for which there exists a columnar organization—are the ones that are sufficient, under the right circumstances, for conscious perception.

Distributed representations have one principal advantage over sparse ones: they can store more data. Say that you need to encode the facial identity of everybody you can recognize by sight, perhaps a few thousand people. If each face is encoded by the firing of a single grandmother neuron, you need a few thousand cells to do that (leaving aside the fact that for reasons of robustness, several copies of each neuron would be desirable). A population code, on the other hand, makes use of combinatorics to encode a much larger number of faces. Assume that two face neurons responded either not at all or by firing vigorously. Between them, they could represent four faces (one face is encoded by both cells not firing, the second one by firing activity in one and silence in the other, and so on). Ten neurons could encode 2^{10}, or about a thousand faces. Reality is more complex than this, but the basic idea of combinatorial coding still holds: It has been calculated that less than one hundred neurons

FIGURE 2.5 *Illusory Kanizsa Triangle* Although no triangle exists on the paper itself, you clearly perceive one. For every such direct experience, there will be one or more groups of neurons explicitly representing the different aspects of the percept. This is our activity principle.

are sufficient to distinguish one out of thousands of faces in a robust manner. Considering that there are around 100,000 cells below a square millimeter of cortex, the potential representational capacity of any one cortical region is enormous.[15]

The Activity Principle

A few years ago, Francis and I postulated the following *activity principle*: underlying every direct and conscious perception is an explicit representation whose neurons fire in some special manner. A vivid example is the *Kanizsa Triangle* (Figure 2.5), named after the Italian Gestalt psychologist Gaetano Kanizsa. Everybody sees a triangle, even though no edges are present between the three Pacmen. This illusion is so compelling that I expect individual neurons to respond to it. And indeed, neurons that get "fired up" to illusory edges are found in the visual cortex (Figure 8.2).

An important corollary to the activity principle is that if no such group of cells explicitly encodes some feature, one cannot be conscious of it. That's why you don't see a black, empty region outside your field of view, behind you. You can perfectly well infer the presence of objects in this empty quarter, but only indirectly, by sound, touch, or other means. Your brain lacks an explicit representation for this part of the world; accordingly, that part of the environment is not part of your visual experience.

It is all too easy to slip into the fallacy of the *homunculus*, to implicitly assume that some agent is looking at the brain, perceiving, and making deci-

---

[15]Abbott, Rolls, and Touvee (1996) estimate that a mere 25 temporal lobe neurons can identify one out of 3,000 different faces with better than even odds. That is, such a mini-network could label each one of these faces as familiar or unfamiliar. Such capacity calculations have also been made for the ability of rat hippocampal place cells to signal the location of its body using visual and other cues. On the order of 100 place cells suffice to encode a 1×1 meter region with a spatial resolution of a few centimeters (Zhang et al., 1998; Brown et al., 1998). Likewise, about 100 cortical cells can signal the direction of a moving cloud of dots (Shadlen et al., 1996).

sions. But there isn't (at least not in the conventional sense; see Chapter 18). What there is, is a vast collection of interconnected neurons. You can be consciously aware of an object or event only if there exists an explicit, columnar organization for it. If this representation is lost, awareness for those aspects symbolized by this group of neurons is also gone. However, the loss may not be permanent, as brains have amazing powers of recuperation.

Essential Nodes in the Brain

Destruction of a specific chunk of brainmatter may render the patient unable to experience some particular aspect of the world, without a generalized loss of any one sense. The British neuroscientist Semir Zeki at University College in London, England, coined the term *essential node* to describe this damaged portion of the brain for that particular conscious attribute. For example, a region in the fusiform gyrus contains an essential node for the perception of color, a more anterior part of this gyrus includes an essential node for face perception, while part of the amygdala is needed for perceiving fearful facial expressions.[16]

The idea of essential nodes is based on careful observations of neurological patients. It does not specify which particular groups of neurons in that part of the brain are critical to the affected aspect of conscious perception. Is it all neurons, or only the excitatory ones? Alternatively, is it only those that project outside the cortical area in question? A further complication is that an essential node often has a twin in the opposite hemisphere. If so, would that aspect of the percept be lost only if both nodes were inactivated? Consider *achromatopsia*, the loss of color perception following localized trauma to the visual cortex that leaves other visual abilities intact. In some patients the damage is restricted to one cortical hemisphere, and objects in the associated field of view are devoid of color; they can only be seen in shades of gray. Given that the essential node in the other hemisphere is intact, objects appear with their normal hues in that portion of the visual field.[17]

It is plausible that the locus in the brain where a stimulus attribute, say faces, is made explicit corresponds to an essential node for that feature, thereby linking a single-cell concept (explicit coding) to a clinical one (essential node).

---

[16]Zeki (2001); Zeki and Bartels (1999); and Adolphs et al. (1999).

[17]Two classical accounts of complete or of hemi-achromatopsia are Meadows (1974) and Zeki (1990). There is a loose parallel with genes. These usually occur in cells in pairs (one from the mother, the other from the father). Mutants can be recessive or dominant (with gradations in between). A recessive mutant must occur in both copies to alter the phenotype; a dominant mutant need only occur in one of them. Some properties of the phenotype are largely controlled by a single gene. More often the phenotype is under the control of more than one gene. Conversely, a single gene can influence more than one aspect of the phenotype. In the brain, similar complications associated with the idea of an essential node are encountered.

Conscious perception is synthesized from activity at many essential nodes. In the case of faces, for instance, this would include patches encoding for eyes and the nose, the gender and identity of the face, its angle of gaze, its emotional expression, and so on. This could be termed *multi-focal* activity. The conscious percept of the entire face is built up from the activity in and between these nodes if they are active for a certain amount of time (on the order of 0.2 to 0.5 sec). Damage to any one node leads to a loss of the particular attribute that it represents, while other aspects remain.

Keep in mind that the loss must be specific to a particular aspect of perception. For example, the whole of V1 is not an essential node for motion or color because elimination of V1 effectively entails loss of all normal visual perception.

2.3 | FIRING RATES, OSCILLATIONS, AND NEURONAL SYNCHRONIZATION

This book is liberally sprinkled with statements such as "a neuron responds to a face" or "the firing activity is elevated." What exactly do I mean? This question is related to the fundamental problem of the code(s) used by neurons to communicate information to each other. As you will see, it is important to distinguish different forms of neural activity. Explicit neuronal representations may use one or several of these forms.

Action Potentials as a Universal Communication Protocol

One of the basic observations of neuroscience is that action potentials are the primary means of conveying information rapidly from one neuron to the next.[18]

Zipping along the axon at speeds ranging from one to tens of millimeters per millisecond—depending on the diameter of the axonal fiber and whether it is surrounded by insulation—spikes communicate the timing of an event in one neuron to hundreds or more target cells distributed throughout the brain, both close by and far away. Propagating information by virtue of pulses is a near universal and robust communication protocol for most animals. All-or-none pulses are more immune to noise and environmental degradations than are continuous voltage changes, which would also take longer to propagate.

Other means of communication available to the brain are either too slow or too global to be useful for rapid perception and motor action. For example,

---

[18]This is not true for some tiny animals. As predicted by theoretical arguments (Niebur and Erdős, 1993), the roundworm *C. elegans* does not possess the sodium channels necessary for the rapid action potentials prevalent in vertebrates, arthropods, and other phyla (Bargmann, 1998).

a massive release of some neurochemical would affect all neurons that carry the relevant receptors within a volume dictated by passive diffusion. Diffusion, moreover, severely limits the speed at which changes in concentration propagate beyond a few micrometers.

A more global means of communication is the *local field potential* (LFP) generated by synaptic and spiking activity that can be picked up by an electrode millimeters and even centimeters away from its origin. However, the electromagnetic field is a crude and inefficient way for neurons to share information. Except for pathological conditions (such as epileptic seizures), the extracellular potential generated by spikes is tiny (in the sub-millivolt range) and decays inversely with distance. Furthermore, the local field potential affects all points at a fixed distance equally. While I don't rule out that such *ephaptic interactions* may play some functional role (for instance, within the optic nerve where a million fibers are closely bundled together), the biophysics of neural tissue sharply limits their role.[19]

Yet another mode of action involves groups of inhibitory cortical interneurons linked by special, low-resistance organelles referred to as *electrical synapses* or *gap junctions*. Under some conditions, all these interneurons trigger action potentials at the same time, acting as a single unit. Not enough is known about this phenomenon to implicate it in conscious perception.[20]

This is the hard reality faced by any sub-neuronal or field theory of consciousness. How else but with spikes can the highly peculiar character of any one subjective experience—a subtle shade of pink or a rhapsodic waltz tune—be communicated across multiple cortical and subcortical regions? Unless some discovery dramatically changes the way neurobiologists view the way individual nerve cells work, action potentials traveling along axons and triggering synaptic events are *the* canonical means of quickly disseminating information within nervous tissue.

Let me illustrate the daunting problem faced by the intrepid neuroscientist trying to understand how neurons talk to each other, with the help of an analogy. Think of a huge, open-air soccer arena with a game in progress. Above the stadium hovers a blimp equipped with TV cameras and microphones and a bunch of researchers trying to decipher the way people down there communicate with each other. From far away, the crew can hear the roar of the crowd when a goal has been scored and the pregnant silence before a penalty kick. As the microphones are lowered on wires to the ground, sounds associated with

---

[19] Holt and Koch (1999) model the biophysics of ephaptic interactions among axons and neurons. Graded electrical potentials within neurons can communicate information over short distances, as in the retina.

[20] Networks of cortical inhibitory interneurons linked by gap junctions often show rhythmic, synchronized activity around 8 Hz (Gibson, Beierlein, and Connors, 1999; Beierlein, Gibson, and Connors, 2000; Blatow et al., 2003).

smaller and smaller groups of people can be picked up: first, the portion of the stadium where the home team is based, then one bleacher, until, ultimately, a single spectator can be heard. However, the process is random, in that each time a different spectator is overheard. Furthermore, it is not possible to identify the spectator, their age, gender, occupation, and so on. The scientists in the blimp just know that, on a fast time scale, these people communicate with sounds. But how? Some argue that the only feature that matters is how loudly the spectators talk to each other. Only the amplitude of the sound, from a soft whisper to a loud scream, encodes useful information. The rest is noise. This example is somewhat akin to the firing rate code discussed next.

Firing Rates

Brain scientists take the cardinal nature of action potentials as given. What is contentious is the nature of the neural code that is employing these spikes.

A flash of light, a picture, or the sound of a voice triggers an irregular train of action potentials. If the same stimulus is repeatedly presented, the exact time the individual spikes occur jitters from one trial to the next (relative to the stimulus onset), while the average number of spikes varies less. That is, the first time around, the neuron fires 12 spikes above and beyond its "spontaneous" rate in the 200 msec interval following the stimulus presentation, while the following three presentations evokes 11, 14, and 15 spikes, respectively; therefore, the mean response of the neuron is 13 spikes. Such widespread observations support the *firing rate* view of coding: the assumption that what is relevant is a continuously varying firing rate, obtained by averaging the spiking response over many repetitions of the stimulus presentation. A firing rate code assumes a population of neurons that all express more or less the same features, making this coding strategy expensive in terms of neurons, yet robust to damage. Almost all neurophysiological recordings are evaluated and presented in this manner.

The most rigorous link between the firing rate and behavior has been established for individual nerve cells in cortical area MT. A monkey is trained to perform a demanding perceptual motion task (explained more fully in Section 8.3), while the firing activity in MT is recorded. In one of electrophysiology's finest hours, William Newsome, Anthony Movshon, and others related the average number of spikes fired by a neuron over a two-second period in response to a moving stimulus to the probability that the animal, on that particular trial, detected the motion signal. This allowed the physiologists to predict the behavior of the animal under, admittedly, somewhat restrictive and unnatural conditions, from the response rate of the neuron.

In a rate code, only the number of spikes per unit time matters. Such a code does not carry any temporal modulation beyond those imposed by the input. When a light steadily flickers on and off, therefore, the firing rate should vary with the same rhythm. Furthermore, the exact time at which one cell generates a spike should not depend on the time at which similar neurons spike. That is, two neighboring neurons might jointly increase their spiking rate in response to a stimulus, but in a rate code, the timing of action potentials in one cell will not be correlated at the millisecond level with those in the other.

This vanilla-flavored view of rate encoding in the nervous system has much to recommend it. It is simple, robust, and compatible with decades' worth of data and models, in particular for neurons close to the sensory periphery. At its heart, it assumes that neurons are noisy, unreliable devices, and that the nervous system averages over many cells to compensate for these shoddy components.[21]

Much data suggest, however, that there is more to information coding than changes in firing rates, that the level of noise in the brain is minimal, that neurons are sophisticated computational devices, and that the exact time of occurrence of spikes is important. Interestingly, what is considered noise under the rate coding paradigm is part of the signal under this alternative view of neuronal coding. This is the situation of the spectators in the stadium analogy. They not only talk more softly or loudly, but the sound itself is highly modulated in time, giving rise to human speech! The following subsection discusses the evidence that spike discharges are patterned in a periodic manner.

Oscillations in the Brain

The brain is a gargantuan and complex assembly of nonlinear processing elements. And, as any electrical engineer knows, the challenge of designing high-gain, feedback switching circuits is in steering a careful course between the Charybdis of quiescence or "death," and the Scylla of massive excitation or "epileptic seizure." Even if these can be avoided, networks with positive feedback are prone to oscillate unless active damping measures are taken.[22]

An *electroencephalogram* (EEG) reveals the widespread occurrence of brain rhythms or waves. The electrical potential recorded outside the skull is replete with oscillatory activity in different frequency bands. The frequency of these oscillations varies from one to close to 100 cycles per second (Hz). They persist in characteristic form during various behavioral states as well as during pathology (hence the usefulness of the EEG for clinical practice).

---

[21] Single spikes can convey up to several bits of stimulus information. These rates are close to the upper bounds on information transmission in noisy, neuronal communication channels. The wonderful book by Rieke et al. (1996) introduces the information theoretical approach to neural coding.

[22] Indeed, given the ease with which transgenic mice, whose synaptic receptors have been modified, develop seizures, preventing runaway excitation must have been a major evolutionary constraint. Crick and Koch (1998a) discuss the implications for cortical neuroanatomy.

In a quietly resting individual, the dominant rhythm occurs in the *alpha band*, between 8 and 12 Hz. Opening the eyes or initiating some purposeful mental effort causes this activity to be replaced (the *alpha blockade*) by high-frequency oscillations in the *beta* (15 to 25 Hz) and *gamma* bands (30 or more Hz). The gamma band is linked to cognitive operations. During drowsiness and sleep, a family of high-amplitude and low-frequency oscillations appears in the *delta* band between 1 and 4 Hz. Specific disturbances in sleep can be diagnosed by perturbations in these slow rhythmic discharges.

Periodic electrical brain potentials reflect synchronized activity in the underlying cortical and subcortical neurons and supporting cells. It is difficult to pinpoint the cellular generators responsible for specific EEG patterns because of the low resistivity of the neuronal tissue to electrical current flow and the distorting effect of the skull.[23]

Recording the local field potential from electrodes placed below the skull confirms the existence of discrete oscillatory episodes that wax and wane, depending on the behavioral and mental state of the subject. These *intracranial EEG* recordings reveal another rhythmic discharge pattern that can be reliably observed within the hippocampus and some of its recipient structures: ongoing oscillations of 4 to 8 Hz (the *theta* band), which are linked to cognitive processes such as working memory and navigation.[24]

Since the sense of hearing is exceedingly good at picking out signals amid a noisy background, electrophysiologists often amplify the electrical activity of neurons and broadcast the resulting spike discharge over a loudspeaker. Under some conditions, a steady whoosh can be heard superimposed onto the crackling noise made by individual action potentials. Appropriate mathematical operations, such as the Fourier transform, confirm the existence of a periodic signal generated by the tendency of many cortical neurons to fire periodically (every 20 to 30 msec). Some cells have such a pronounced regularity that they discharge in an almost clock-like manner. The frequency of these rhythms is broadly distributed between 30 and 70 Hz, with a peak occurring around 40 Hz, hence their colloquial name: 40 Hz or *gamma oscillations* (Figure 2.6).

Discovered in the rabbit olfactory system by Lord Adrian in the mid-20th century, 40 Hz oscillations were considered an oddity and neglected by the mainstream. They were rediscovered within the cat visual cortex in the late

---

[23]The EEG primarily reflects the contribution of synaptic and dendritic membrane currents and only indirectly that of action potentials (Freeman, 1975; Creutzfeldt and Houchin, 1984; Creutzfeldt, 1995; and Mountcastle, 1998).

[24]Theta oscillations in humans are described by Kahana et al. (1999) and Klimesch (1999). For relevant single cell data from rodents, see O'Keefe and Recce (1993) and Buzsáki (2002).

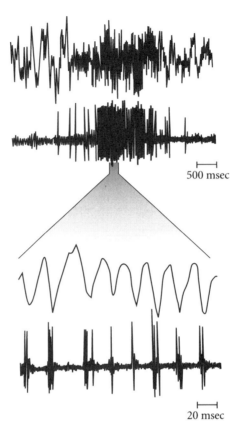

FIGURE 2.6 *Oscillations in the 40 Hz Range* The local field potential (first and third trace from the top) and spiking activity from a number of nearby neurons (second and fourth trace) recorded in the primary visual cortex of a cat while a moving bar was presented on a computer monitor. Rhythmic activity around 40 Hz can be observed in the lower two traces, which are magnifications of portions of the upper ones. Modified from Gray and Singer (1989).

1980s by Charles Gray and Wolf Singer at the Max Planck Institute for Brain Research in Frankfurt, Germany.[25]

The stimulus dependencies of these rhythms have been reasonably well characterized in both cat and monkey visual cortex. Largely absent during spontaneous activity, they strongly depend on visual stimulation, but are not

[25] Walter Freeman at the University of California at Berkeley realized early on the potential significance of these oscillations for olfactory information processing (Freeman, 1975). The original publication that triggered the modern exploration of 40 Hz oscillation is Gray and Singer (1989). Other relevant studies include Eckhorn et al. (1988); Engel et al. (1990); Kreiter and Singer (1992); and Eckhorn et al. (1993). For an overview of the relevant literature, see Ritz and Sejnowski (1997), and Friedman-Hill, Maldonado, and Gray (2000).

time-locked to the stimuli. Gamma oscillations can be routinely observed in the local field potential and, less frequently, when recording multi-neuron activity (that is, the summed spikes of neighboring cells). Detecting these rhythms in the spiking pattern of individual neurons has proven to be more problematic, with different laboratories reporting quite disparate results.

Counterparts of these oscillations can be seen in electrical scalp recordings. While the change in electrical potential on the head in response to some stimulus is tiny, the signal can be amplified by averaging hundreds of trials to yield a reliable signal, the *evoked potential*. Psychologists have measured *visually evoked potentials* while subjects undergo visual experiences, and have concluded that activity in the gamma band indicate the formation of a visual percept, based on coalitions of neurons firing away at 40 Hz. That is, it has been hypothesized that the neuronal correlates of a visual percept are cell ensembles in the cortex that have a prominent rhythmicity. While this interpretation is plausible, the limited spatial resolution of bulk electrical activity recorded outside the skull severely constrains the usefulness of EEG and related methods. Think of how little about the ocean's structure and depth can be inferred from measuring the waves crisscrossing its surface.[26]

The *auditory evoked potential* following a click delivered via headphone to the ears contains an easily visible 25 msec periodicity, corresponding to 40 cycles per second.[27] Indeed, the absence of this prominent component is taken as an index of the depth of anesthesia and predicts the transition from the awake brain to unconsciousness. The more modest the 40 Hz component, the less likely the patient will report intra-operative awakening or recall. By itself, this link between global consciousness—as defined clinically—and activity in the 40 Hz regime is not so helpful in understanding the specific function of the oscillations. After all, if the AC power adapter of your laptop fails to buzz at 50 or 60 Hz (depending on where in the world you are), the computer will be without power and will be shut down. That does not imply, however, that 50 or 60 Hz electrical activity relates in any *specific* fashion to the operations performed by the computer. An appropriate conservative interpretation of the

---

[26] Revonsuo et al. (1997); Keil et al. (1999); Rodriguez et al. (1999); Tallon-Baudry and Bertrand (1999); and Klemm, Li, and Hernandez (2000) link specific aspects of visual perception to increased power in the gamma frequency band (and often concomitant decreases in lower frequency EEG bands). Engel and Singer (2001) review this literature. What makes the interpretation of these data problematic in terms of underlying neuronal mechanisms, is that the EEG represents the cumulative electrical signature associated with activity taking place over large regions of brain tissue, tissue that contains up to 100,000 discrete neurons per cubic millimeter. Varela et al. (2001) summarize the perils and promises of EEG techniques for deciphering the dynamic brain. Recent computational advances (Makeig et al., 2002) ameliorate the deleterious effects of averaging the electrical signal over hundreds of trials.

[27] The auditory evoked potential recorded from the human scalp clearly shows two to three waves separated by 20 to 25 msec (Galambos, Makeig, and Talmachoff, 1981). For the link to anesthesiology, see Madler and Pöppel, (1987) and Sennholz (2000).

40 Hz link with anesthesia is that when the cortex is so severely affected by some drug that this signature activity disappears, consciousness ceases as well.

If spiking with a 40 Hz rhythm is important to the brain, it can be only because the neurons receiving these spikes are able to decode them. They must be able to distinguish pulses spaced 20 to 30 msec apart from those that occur randomly in time or those that occur with a different rhythm. This can't be properly assessed without considering the degree and extent of synchronization among neurons, a further significant twist in the coding story.

Temporal Synchronization among Neurons

The dominant electrophysiological paradigm probes the brain with a solitary electrode that tracks the activity of one or a few nearby neurons (as in Figures 2.1, 2.2, and 2.4). While the success of the past decades vividly demonstrates the fecundity of this method, it has severe limitations.

On general grounds, it might appear hopeless to infer anything about the brain by listening to one out of billions of nerve cells. What chance, for example, does an electrical engineer have to understand the operations of a digital computer if she could monitor but one out of the tens of millions of transistors in the machine's central processing unit? In hindsight, I can only admire the tenacity and determination of the early explorers of brains for going forward despite these appalling odds. Single cell electrophysiology has unearthed the basic processing elements of the nervous system and the way they are interconnected. To gain a deeper understanding of the dynamics of competing neuronal assemblies, however, the spiking activity of tens, hundreds, thousands, and even more neurons must be considered.

In particular, the single electrode technique neglects a potentially rich source of information, namely the exact temporal relationship between spikes from multiple neurons. If two cells code for the same feature, are they more likely to fire at the same time or not? Do they tend to fire in a synchronized or in an independent manner?

Imagine a gigantic Christmas tree, festooned with a few hundred electric lights, each of which randomly flickers on and off. Your task is to make a group of lights on the top of the tree stand out. One way to achieve this is to increase the flickering rate of that group of lights. Another way is to trigger each light in the group at the same time. Simultaneous flashing this set of lights increases its saliency considerably (this is true whether or not the lights in the group switch on and off with a fixed period or at random, as long as they all do it together). The same logic also applies to the brain, with the "observer looking at the tree" replaced by some neuronal network. The biophysics of neurons renders them more susceptible to synchronized, excitatory synaptic input than to random input. For example, 100 fast excitatory synaptic inputs, distributed over the dendritic tree of a large pyramidal neuron, are sufficient to generate an action potential if they are activated within a millisecond of each other. If the presynaptic spikes arrive smeared out over a 25 msec window, however, twice as many synapses are needed to fire the cell. Synchronized synaptic input is usually more efficient at driving its target cell than if the input is desynchronized.[28]

All of this is widely accepted. Contention revolves around whether cortical cells integrate massive numbers of inputs over tens of milliseconds or whether neurons detect the coincident arrival of a few inputs with sub-millisecond precision.

The German theoretical neuroscientist Christoph von der Malsburg recognized in the 1980s that synchronization of firing could be used by the nervous system to solve the notorious *binding problem* (which will be treated in more detail in Section 9.4). How does the brain "know" which firing activity distributed in the multifarious maps throughout the cortex corresponds to which attribute of what object? As already mentioned, a meaningful object like a face evokes spiking activity at multiple locations in the cortex and related satellite systems. How is all of this distributed activity combined into one percept? Furthermore, how can this activity be distinguished from the activity caused by another, simultaneously visible face? All the spikes surely look the same. von der Malsburg proposed that the brain could tell these neuronal assemblies apart by synchronization. Like the electric lights on the Christmas tree, neurons within one coalition expressing one percept fire in a synchronized manner, but are not synchronized with the coalition coding for another face or for objects in the background.[29]

It was with a great deal of justifiable excitement, therefore, that Gray, Singer, and their colleagues described not only 40 Hz firing patterns but also the way in which these oscillatory responses became synchronized in a stimulus-dependent manner (Figure 2.7). The scientists moved two bars across the receptive fields of the sites in the visual cortex of a cat where two electrodes were placed. This evoked appropriate spiking activity, but the exact time at which action potentials were triggered at one site was independent of the timing of action potentials at the other. The spikes were not synchronized.

---

[28]The number of synapses needed to trigger a spike can be considerably lower if the synaptic input is spatially clustered on or around the main, apical dendrite, and in the presence of even low densities of voltage-dependent sodium and calcium currents. Biophysically faithful simulations demonstrate that, in principle, pyramidal neurons with voltage-dependent currents in the dendrites can be sensitive to submillisecond coincidences in synaptic inputs (Softky, 1995). A sustained shift in the cell's resting potential can bring the neuron closer to threshold, such that a smaller number of synaptic inputs will suffice to trigger action potentials. For a textbook exposition of synaptic integration in cortical neurons, see Koch (1999).

[29]von der Malsburg's original report (1981) is rather difficult to digest. For an up-to-date review that is easier to follow, see von der Malsburg (1999).

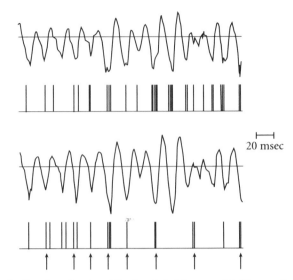

FIGURE 2.7 *Spike Synchronization* The local field potential (first and third trace) and neuronal spiking activity (second and fourth trace) at two sites in the cat visual cortex in response to a lone light bar sweeping across the visual field. Arrows indicate spike pairs from the two sites that occur within a few milliseconds of each other. The local field potential, indicative of the electrical activity in a large region, cycles about 40 times each second. Modified from Engel et al. (1990).

Synchronization increased significantly when the two bars were replaced by a single, elongated bar whose movement could be seen by cells at both sites.[30]

Spike synchronization has been reported in a variety of preparations, from the locust's olfactory system to visual, visuo-motor, somatosensory, and motor cortices in behaving cats and monkeys.[31]

The magnitude and probability of synchronous firing is inversely related to the distance between the cells (the farther apart they are, the smaller the degree of synchronization) and proportional to how similar the selectivity of the two neurons is. That is, if both cells prefer bars of the same orientation, synchronization will be stronger than if the orientation tuning of the two differ sub-

---

[30] The original publication reporting synchronization among cat V1 cells is Gray et al. (1989). Kreiter and Singer (1996) extended these results to area MT in the awake macaque monkey (but see Thiele and Stoner, 2003).

[31] For reviews, see Gray (1999), Singer (1999), and Engel and Singer (2001). A critical evaluation of these ideas is provided by Shadlen and Movshon (1999). The most compelling data about the relevance of oscillatory and synchronized activity to behavior have been obtained by Gilles Laurent and his group at the California Institute of Technology in the insect olfactory system (Stopfer et al., 1997; MacLeod, Backer, and Laurent, 1998; Laurent, 1999; and Laurent et al., 2001).

stantially. Often, coincident firing has a precision of 10 msec or less, meaning that a spike in one cell is associated with a spike in the other that occurs within 5 msec.

To return to the stadium metaphor, it will be obvious to the observers in the blimp above that the speech patterns picked up by the microphones are correlated among neighboring spectators and that this correlation falls off with distance (the farther apart the fans sit, the less likely they are to talk to each other). However, at times, even people sitting on the opposite sides of the stadium have correlated outputs, as when the crowd roars when the ball approaches the goal.

The relationship between synchronization and oscillations is a thorny one. In principle, both could occur independently. Consider, for example, the major stock indexes, such as the Nasdaq, Dow Jones Industrial, Nikkei, DAX, and so on. These are all significantly correlated on a day-to-day basis. If trading in stock increases in the U.S., the other major stock markets quickly pull apace; yet this correlation does *not* have any obvious periodic component. For the opposite case, consider menstruation. Two randomly chosen women will have their own menstrual cycles with a roughly 28-day periodicity. The chances that they share the onset of their menses is small, an example of oscillations without synchronization. In tightly coupled feedback systems such as the brain, on the other hand, oscillations and synchronization are closely related, with the latter usually implying the former. Indeed, when two neurons that are far apart become synchronized, they do so in an oscillatory fashion.[32]

In 1990, Francis and I asserted that synchronized 40-Hz oscillations within the subset of neurons that correspond to an attended object is a signature of the NCC. In other words, the content of consciousness can be identified, at that moment, with the set of forebrain neurons firing in a phase-locked manner with a 20 to 30 msec periodicity.[33]

Our claim of a link between synchronization in the gamma band and consciousness generated widespread enthusiasm, interest, and derision inside and outside the neuroscientific community. The interpretation of the relevant empirical findings is fraught with considerable difficulties. The reasons are complex, but boil down to knowing what subset of neurons to record from; picking out a faint voice from a cacophony of loud background noises is not easy. In the fullness of time, these issues will be laid to rest using multi-unit recording techniques to simultaneously and continuously monitor the spiking activity of hundreds of identified neurons in behaving animals.[34]

---

[32] Engel et al. (1991).

[33] The original publications are Crick and Koch (1990a,b); see also Crick (1994). Horgan (1996) provides an entertaining journalistic account with a 'twilight of science' twist. Metzinger (2000) and Engel and Singer (2001) review the relevant evidence in favor of our hypothesis.

[34] One problem is knowing which type of neuron is currently being recorded from. To where

Today, Francis and I no longer think that synchronized firing is a sufficient condition for the NCC. A functional role more in line with the data is that synchronization assists a nascent coalition in its competition with other nascent coalitions.[35] As explained in Chapter 9, this occurs when you attend to an object or event. A neuronal substrate of this bias could be synchronized firing in certain frequency bands (see footnote 11 in Chapter 10). Once a coalition has established itself as a winner and you are conscious of the associated attributes, the coalition may be able to maintain itself without the assistance of synchrony, at least for a time. Thus, one might expect synchronized oscillations to occur in the early stages of perception, but not necessarily in later ones. It's a bit like tenure in the academic world—once you've obtained it, you can relax a little.

I've outlined firing rate, oscillation, and synchronization coding strategies. Let me allude to one more, *ultra-sparse temporal coding*. While individual neurons in early cortical areas can generate in excess of 100 spikes within one or two seconds, a cell in the hippocampus might signal with a handful of spikes. Such meager firing can't easily be reconciled with the conventional view of rate coding unless the rate is computed over large ensembles of neurons. In other networks, an appropriate stimulus triggers a brief burst of activity, say one to four spikes within 10 msec or so. For the following seconds, the neuron is quiet, with no "spontaneous" firing at all. The observed specificity can be amazing, with the cell contributing a single note to the ongoing music and then falling silent.[36]

Alternative coding principles have been proposed.[37] So little is known about the mesoscopic scale of neural organization—encompassing anywhere from a

---

does it project? From where does it receive most of its input? Another overriding difficulty is detecting cross-correlations between two neurons that are part of a large coalition with a thousand or more members. The increase in correlation between any two neurons might be minute. Picking this up requires endless repetitions in order to attain statistical significance, and raises the specter of the subject learning to respond in an automatic, unconscious manner. Furthermore, synchronization due to the stimulus itself must be disentangled from synchronization induced by reciprocal and feedback connections (if the firing rate of two neurons increases from 2 to 20 spikes per second, the number of coincident spikes will automatically increase a hundred-fold, even if they fire completely at random). All of these problems demand advanced experimental and computational techniques. These are difficult issues to tackle, but science is up to the task!

[35] A little synchrony among inputs can go a long way to increase their postsynaptic punch (Salinas and Sejnowski, 2001).

[36] Ultra-sparse coding in time has been best characterized in the cricket's olfactory system (Perez-Orive et al., 2002) and in a songbird's motor pathway (Hahnloser, Kozhevnikov, and Fee, 2002). My nightmare is that cortical neurons of relevance to the NCC make use of the same coding principle. Without precise knowledge of the identity of the recorded neurons, it will be exceedingly difficult to detect and decipher their message over the din made by the firing of their more promiscuous neighbors.

[37] Other neuronal coding schemes include the *synfire chain* model (Abeles, 1991; and Abeles et al., 1993) and *first-time-to-spike* models (Van Rullen and Thorpe, 2001). Evidence for trav-

few to tens of thousands of neurons—that it is difficult to rule out any one coding scheme at this point in time. Oscillatory synchronization is given particular prominence in this book because there is significant evidence that it is important to our quest.

2.4 | RECAPITULATION

The NCC involve temporary coalitions of neurons, coding for particular events or objects, that are competing with other coalitions. A particular assembly—biased by attention—emerges as the winner by dint of the strength of its firing activity. The winning coalition, corresponding to the current content of consciousness, suppresses competing assemblies for some time until it either fatigues, adapts, or is superseded by a novel input and a new victor emerges. Given that at any one time one or a few such coalitions dominate, one can speak of sequential processing without implying any clock-like process. This dynamic process can be compared to politics in a democracy with voting blocs and interest groups constantly forming and dissolving.

Francis and I postulate that the NCC are built on a foundation of explicit neuronal representations. A feature is made explicit if a small set of neighboring cortical neurons directly encode this feature. The depth of computation inherent in an implicit representation is shallower than in an explicit one. Additional processing is necessary to transform an implicit into an explicit representation. Examples of explicit representations are stimulus orientation in V1 or face encoding in IT. An explicit representation is a necessary, but not sufficient, condition for the NCC.

An essential node is a part of the brain that, when destroyed, causes a specific deficit for a class of percepts, such as face, motion, color, or fear perception. We hypothesize that the location of the explicit representation for some attribute corresponds to its essential node.

The neuronal substrate for both concepts is the columnar organization of information. That is, the receptive field property common to cells below a patch of cortex corresponds to the essential node for that property and to an explicit representation.

Neural activity can take diverse forms. Key to all is the rapid propagation of information across the brain via action potentials. The firing rate code assumes

eling, standing, and rotating waves in cortical tissue is reviewed by Ermentrout and Kleinfeld (2001). The possible relevance of *bursting* to perception and memory is elaborated upon by Crick (1984), Koch and Crick (1994), and Lisman (1997). A burst is a stereotypical sequence of two to five action potentials occurring within 10 to 40 msec, followed by a profound refractory period (Koch, 1999). Rao, Olshausen and Lewicki's (2002) book provides an excellent account of these and other probabilistic coding strategies.

that the variable of interest is purely encoded by the number of spikes triggered by a neuron over some meaningful interval, that is, by how loudly it shouts. Firing rates are widely used in the nervous system, in particular in the periphery where maintained rates can exceed 100 spikes per second. What remains contentious is the extent to which additional coding strategies, such as coding via oscillations or via synchronization, are prevalent.

Francis and I had suggested earlier that conscious perception is based on synchronous firing neuronal assemblies that wax and wane rhythmically and interact with each other within a few hundred milliseconds. While little data has directly supported this conjecture, there is evidence that oscillatory firing activity around 40 cycles per second, coupled with synchronized spiking, is needed to establish a percept when more than one input vies for attention.

Equipped with this framework, I shall now outline the design of the mammalian visual system in Chapters 3 and 4. Whenever possible, I will link its neuronal and architectural attributes to specific features of conscious vision.

CHAPTER THREE

The First Steps in Seeing

Le bon Dieu est dans le détail.

Attributed to Gustave Flaubert

Others assert that the devil is in the details. No matter who is responsible for the minutiae of reality, science is undoubtedly about details, gadgets, and mechanisms. While I can wax lyrically about consciousness, qualia, and zombies, some basic facts about the brain are essential for understanding how it works. Because most of this book is concerned with seeing, I'll start by describing retinal processing and eye movements. Subsequent chapters discuss those aspects of seeing that depend on the cortex. The story that emerges often clashes with the deep-seated intuitions people have about the way they see.

3.1 | THE RETINA IS A LAYERED STRUCTURE

You see by way of light passing through the cornea and lens of your eye. These act as a camera, focusing an inverted image of the scene through the vitreous gel inside the eyeball onto the retina. Light traverses this miniature nervous system before individual photons are absorbed in the photoreceptors at the back of the retina (Figure 3.1). The optical signals are converted into electrical ones that are processed in a complex series of steps by horizontal, bipolar, amacrine, and ganglion cells. One census identified about five dozen distinct cell types, each one probably serving a distinct function. These large numbers are disconcerting for physicists and mathematicians trained to look for simple, powerful, and universal principles to explain the design and function of the brain. They also serve as a warning that the final count of distinct cellular actors for the cortex and its satellites could easily number in the many hundreds.[1]

---

[1] Mammalian retinae contain more than 50 distinct cell types, each with a different function (DeVries and Baylor, 1997; MacNeil and Masland, 1998; Masland, 2001; and Dacey et al., 2003). I will return to the theme of cell types in Section 4.3.

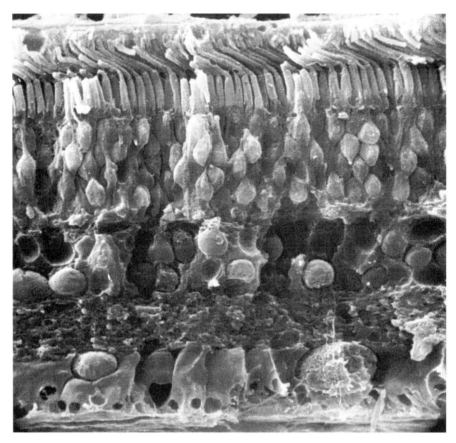

FIGURE 3.1 *A Cross-Section of the Retina* In this photo, light arrives from below and passes through the entire retina (of a rabbit) before it gives rise to a photochemical reaction in the photoreceptors (at the top). The visual information, converted into changes in the electrical potential across the membrane, percolates in the reverse direction through the various cellular layers until it gives rise to all-or-none action potentials in ganglion cells (at the bottom). More than one million ganglion cell axons make up the optic nerve along which the spikes travel to more central processing stages. Copyright by R.G. Kessel and R.H. Kardon, *Tissues and Organs: A Text-Atlas of Scanning Electron Microscopy*, W.H. Freeman & Co., 1979, all rights reserved.

Retinal neurons enhance spatial and temporal contrasts and encode wavelength information by evaluating the differential photon catch in distinct photoreceptor populations. The details of this processing are not directly relevant to my quest.[2] The sole output of the retina is the 1.5 million axons of the ganglion cells, constituting the *optic nerve*.

---

[2] For an account of the biophysical and computational processes occurring in the retina, see Dowling (1987), Wandell (1995), and the lovingly illustrated textbook by Rodieck (1998).

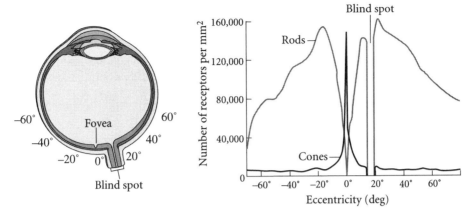

FIGURE 3.2 *Photoreceptors Are Unevenly Distributed* A schematic cross-section of the eye is on the left. The angle relative to the point of sharpest seeing, the fovea, is referred to as *eccentricity*. The density of cones drops off dramatically outside the fovea. Conversely, night vision, mediated by the much more common rods, is optimal some distance away. No receptors sample the incoming brightness at the blind spot. Here, ganglion cell axons form the optic nerve that connects the eye to the brain proper. Modified from Wandell (1995).

Inspecting a state-of-the-art video camera under a microscope reveals millions of identical circuit elements tiling the image plane. Like one of the big new housing developments in the American West, a few basic designs are endlessly replicated. Eyes follow a different design strategy.

Two classes of photoreceptors are spread unevenly across the retina. About one hundred million *rods* work best under dim light conditions, while five million *cones*, responding more rapidly than rods, mediate daylight vision. For most day-to-day activities (including reading), the output of the rods is saturated and only the cones provide a reliable signal.

The point of highest resolution is found in the central part of the fovea (Figure 3.2). Vision is sharpest here. The effective density of cone receptors drops rapidly with increasing distance from the fovea, to level off beyond 12° of visual angle, or *eccentricity*, away from the fovea. The central one degree of vision is heavily overrepresented by both photoreceptors and ganglion cells at the expense of the rest of the visual field.[3]

Because of the uneven receptor distribution—many in the center and few in the periphery—humans constantly move their eyes to bring the fovea to bear on those portions of the environment that are of interest. This movement

---

[3] The central part of the fovea, about 1° of visual angle in size—the width of your thumb at arm's length is around 1.5 to 2°—is specialized to ensure that vision there is as good as possible.

permits the retinal neurons to sample that region with the highest possible resolution. Subjectively, the uneven distribution of photoreceptors goes largely unnoticed. Vision appears everywhere sharp and clear—an illusion, but a compelling one. Even a cursory inspection reveals that you can't see all that well "out of the corner of your eyes." Fixate on the central • in the line below and try to identify as many letters as possible without moving your eyes:

txet siht fo tsom • daer t'nac uoy

You won't be able to read more than two or three characters on either side. In order to comfortably see each letter, their size needs to increase proportional to the distance from the central spot.

3.2 | COLOR VISION USES THREE TYPES OF CONES

The much-cherished sense of color is a construct of the nervous system, computed by comparing activity in the different cone classes. There are no "red" or "blue" objects in the world. Light sources, such as the sun, emit electromagnetic waves over a broad wavelength spectrum. Surfaces reflect this radiation over a continuous range and the brightness incident to the eyes is continuous as well. Nevertheless, all of us persist in labeling objects as red, blue, violet, purple, magenta, and so on. Color is not a direct physical quantity, as is depth or wavelength, but a synthetic one. Different species have fewer or more cone types, and therefore experience quite different colors for the same objects. For example, some shrimp have eleven cone classes. Their world must be a riot of colors!

Most mammals make do with two types of cone receptors. The exceptions are humans, apes, and old world monkeys, which possess three types. Distinguished by the portion of the spectrum of light to which each is most sensitive, they are referred to as *short-*, *middle-*, and *long-wavelength* cones, or, more succinctly, as S, M, and L cones. Due to the overlap in receptor sensitivity, any one photon can be absorbed by the photopigments in the different receptor types. Collectively, each cone class signals the number of photons it absorbs but nothing explicitly about the spectral composition of the light. In this early stage, color is thus implicitly encoded by three numbers, the relative activation of the three cone types, the basis for Thomas Young's and Hermann von Helmholtz's celebrated *trichromacy theory* of color vision. Now that more is understood about the genetic variation in photopigments in the general human population, trichromacy needs to be enlarged to accommodate the color perception of women with four cone photoreceptor classes and men with only two.[4]

---

[4]The retinae of some women express two forms of the L photopigment that differ by 4 to 7 nm in the long-wavelength portion of the spectrum (Nathans, 1999). Sensitive psychophysical tests

At any one eccentricity, the three classes of cones are not distributed evenly. S cones are absent from the central part of the fovea. Given that this is the point of sharpest seeing, you would think that this deficit would be obvious to anybody. It can't be seen directly, however, so it must be inferred. The way it is done is to ask observers to look at a violet annulus (think of a squashed doughnut; see the bottom row in Figure 3.4) with a central hole. As long as subjects are accurately fixating the center of the annulus, thereby placing the hole over the portion of the retina devoid of S cones, the brain assumes that the surrounding violet stimulus extends into the center. As a consequence, a complete disk, rather than an annulus, is seen. I mentioned already in Section 2.1 that inferring missing data based on information from neighboring areas is something the brain engages in all the time.[5]

Even outside the fovea, S cones are much less common than M and L cones. Furthermore, patches of retina dominated by M receptors are intermingled with patches where L cones dominate. This irregular distribution does not show up, however, when looking at evenly colored surfaces, which should appear spotty, probably because of pervasive filling-in mechanisms that operate throughout the visual field, all part of the great con job called perception.[6]

3.3 | A HOLE IN THE EYE: THE BLIND SPOT

At some distance from the fovea, the axons of all ganglion cells are bundled together and exit the eye (Figure 3.2). No photoreceptors are in this area, so there is no direct information about this part of the image, either. This is the *blind spot*.[7]

---

can evaluate the color perception of these "extraordinary" women (Jordan and Mollon, 1993; and Jameson, Highnote, and Wasserman, 2001). If the visual cortex learned to process advantageously the additional wavelength information, these *tetrachromat* women would experience subtle hue variations forever unavailable to the rest of humanity. In particular, they should be able to distinguish two colors that look identical to trichromats.

[5]The original psychophysical experiments are described in Williams, MacLeod, and Hayhoe (1981) and Williams et al. (1991). Curcio et al. (1991) directly visualizes the distribution of S cones in the human retina.

[6]The analysis of human retinae (Roorda and Williams, 1999) reveals patches of a tenth of a degree extent that contain only L or M cones, limiting people's ability to perceive fine color variations.

[7]The blind spot is located around 15° along the horizontal meridian on the nasal side of the retina. Find it by closing the left eye (you won't see much with both eyes closed) and fixating the tip of your left thumb with the right, open eye. Now slowly move the index finger of the right hand, extended at arm's length, from the outside toward the thumb, while keeping your eye glued to the stationary thumb. You will discover that at some point (when the two fingers are somewhere between 15 and 25 cm apart) the tip of the index finger disappears. When the finger

Normally, input from one eye makes up for the blind spot in the other eye. Yet even if you close one eye, you still won't see a hole in your visual field. A single bad pixel in your home video camera, however, manifests itself as an ugly black spot in each image frame. What, then, is the difference?

Unlike electronic imaging systems, the brain does not simply neglect the blind spot; it paints in properties at this location using one or more *active processes* such as completion (as in Figure 2.5), interpolation (as just encountered on the previous page), and filling-in (Section 2.1). Cortical neurons fill-in on the basis of the usually sensible assumption that the visual properties of one patch in the world are similar to those of neighboring locations (in terms of their color, motion, orientation of edges, and so on). Accordingly, if you place a pencil across the blind spot, you'll see a single, uninterrupted pencil with no hole in its middle. Neurons above and below the blind spot signal the vertical edge; thus, the neurons responsible for the visual representation of the blind spot *assume* that the edge was also present at the blind spot.[8]

The psychologist Vilayanur Ramachandran at the University of California in San Diego carried out numerous ingenious experiments to study filling-in. As in the foveal experiment just described, he placed a yellow annulus over the blind spot such that the center—devoid of yellow—falls entirely within the blind spot. Observers perceived an intact and complete yellow disk, even though they could vividly see the annulus when looking a little bit off to one side. The brain goes beyond the information given at the retina by making an "educated" guess about what might be at the blind spot. As no retinal neurons respond to light patterns falling onto the blind spot, the NCC can't be in the retina. Otherwise you would see two holes when looking at the world.[9]

---

is farther out, however, you can still see it. You just discovered that you don't see anything in a patch of about 5° diameter. Remarkably enough, this simple observation, known to most school-aged children today, was not made until the second part of the 17th century by l'Abbé Edme Mariotte in France. He inferred the existence of the blind spot by careful anatomical examination of the retina (Finger, 1994, provides an historical account). The Greeks, Romans, and other ancient civilizations, despite their vast intellectual, artistic, and organizational achievements, failed to appreciate this basic fact of human vision.

[8]The activity of the V1 neurons that represent the blind spot in the monkey have been recorded. These cells have large binocular receptive fields that extend outside the blind spot and inform the rest of the brain of the presence of large surfaces covering the blind spot (Fiorani et al., 1992; Komatsu and Murakami, 1994; and Komatsu, Kinoshita, and Murakami, 2000). For related physiological experiments probing interpolation using artificial blind spots, see Murakami, Komatso, and Kinoshita (1997) and DeWeerd et al. (1995).

[9]Ramachandran and Gregory (1991) and Ramachandran (1992). Kamitani and Shimojo (1999) induced artificial blind spots using transcranial magnetic stimulation. For an exhaustive compendium on filling-in, see Pessoa and DeWeerd (2003). Dennett (1991; see also Churchland and Ramachandran, 1993) has rightly emphasized that this does not imply a pixel-by-pixel rendering of the missing information on an internal screen. Instead, active neuronal mechanisms perpetrate the deceit that information is present where none should be visible.

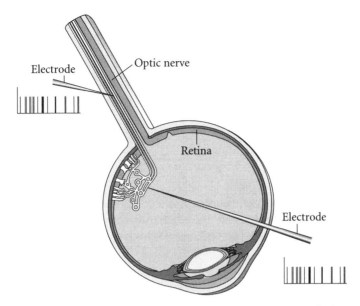

FIGURE 3.3 *Recording the Activity of Ganglion Cells* Action potentials from ganglion cells can be picked up by either placing a microelectrode near their cell bodies in the retina or in the optic nerve outside the eye. Modified from Enroth-Cugell and Robson (1984).

3.4 | RECEPTIVE FIELD: A KEY CONCEPT FOR VISION

The all-or-none spiking activity of ganglion cells, the sole conduit for information leaving the retina, is relatively easy to detect with microelectrodes (Figure 3.3). Pioneered by Stephen Kuffler, at the time working at Johns Hopkins University in Baltimore, such experiments led to a refinement of the concept of the *receptive field*, introduced by Keffer Hartline at the Rockefeller University during his investigations of the visual system of the horseshoe crab, *Limulus*. Operationally, the receptive field of a neuron is defined as the region in the visual field in which an appropriate stimulus, here a flashing spot of light, modulates the cell's response.[10]

Electrophysiologists frequently connect the amplified output of their electrode to a loudspeaker to more easily locate the receptive field of a neuron by listening to its discharge. In the absence of any stimulus, many cells spontaneously generate one or a few spikes per second. If a small spot of light is placed in the cell's receptive field, however, the speaker erupts with a crackling that sounds like a machine gun firing away. This sound is the hallmark of an

---

[10]Kuffler (1952); and Ratliff and Hartline (1959).

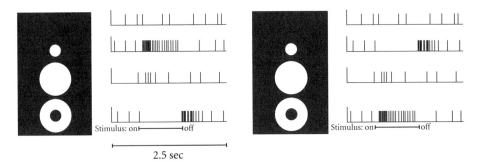

FIGURE 3.4 *On-Center and Off-Center Cells* Firing response of an *on-center* (left) and an *off-center* ganglion cell (right) in the cat's retina in the dark (top row), to a small spot of light covering the receptive field (second row), a much larger spot of light (third row) and an annulus (bottom row). These neurons respond best to round patches of light or darkness. Modified from Hubel (1988).

on-center cell (Figure 3.4, left). When the spot of light is moved a bit outside the *center* of the receptive field, it has a suppressive effect. This is true for a light stimulus anywhere within a small region surrounding the central area. Removing the light from this inhibitory *surround*, by turning it off, provokes the cell into an off-response. Thus, for an on-center cell, a spot of light surrounded by a ring of darkness yields the strongest response.

Off-center cells show the same concentric *center-surround* organization, but with an inverted sign (Figure 3.4, right); that is, a central region of darkness surrounded by an annulus of light maximally excites the neuron.

The receptive field of most retinal ganglion cells possesses a spatial antagonistic structure, with responses from the central patch opposing the responses from the peripheral region. This can best be demonstrated by a large spot of light that covers both center and surround; typically, cells will respond only weakly (Figure 3.4).[11]

As emphasized in Section 2.1, the notion of a neuron's receptive field constitutes the cornerstone of perceptual neuroscience and is not restricted to its spatial layout (that is, its center-surround organization). It includes the wavelength of the light to which the cell is maximally sensitive, the direction of motion of the stimulus the neuron prefers, and so on. This concept has been extended to other sensory modalities as well. For instance, the receptive field of an auditory neuron includes the pitch to which it is optimally sensitive and whether it is excited by sound delivered to one or the other ear.

---

[11]Formally, on- and off-center cells encode the positive and negative half-wave rectified local image contrast. If the contrast is positive, on-cells respond and off-cells are silent; the converse is true if the contrast is negative.

Two, usually unarticulated, assumptions underlie this concept. Foremost is the belief that the analysis of a complex scene by the entire organism can be broken down, in a highly atomistic fashion, into the response of individual nerve cells. This is, of course, oversimplified and groups of two or more cells, firing in concert, are likely to encode stimulus attributes that are not represented at the level of individual neurons.[12] Furthermore, any quantitative receptive field analysis relies on a choice of what feature of the neuronal response is critical to the rest of the brain. Is it simply the number of spikes or the peak discharge rate, two commonly used measures that assume a rate code (Section 2.3), or is there something about the temporal patterning of spikes that conveys information? For reasons of biological robustness and methodological convenience, most neuroscientists simply count spikes within some meaningful interval.

I am now in a position to succinctly summarize one research strategy for discovering the NCC. It is to quantitatively correlate the receptive field properties of individual neurons with the subject's perception. If the structure of conscious perception does not map to the receptive field properties of the cell population under consideration, it is unlikely that these neurons are sufficient for that conscious percept. In the presence of a correlation between perceptual experience and receptive field properties, the next step is to determine whether the cells are, by themselves, sufficient for that conscious percept or whether they are only incidentally linked to perception. To prove causation, many additional experiments are needed to untangle the exact relationship between neurons and perception.

A simple example will have to suffice at this point. Rather surprisingly, people don't know whether they see an image with their left or their right eye! If a small light is projected from dead-ahead into either one of the eyes, an observer can only guess which eye was stimulated (provided cheating, by blinking or moving the head, is prevented). The neurons that underlie visual consciousness do not encode *eye-of-origin* information in an explicit manner.[13]

3.5 | MULTIPLE PARALLEL PATHWAYS EXIT THE EYE

Let me return to a more mundane, but critical, aspect of the eye—the axons of ganglion cells. It was the patron saint of neuroscience, the Spaniard Santiago

---

[12] For the conflicting claims on how much information is found in correlated retinal ganglion cells spikes see Meister (1996); Warland, Reinagel, and Meister (1997); and Nirenberg et al. (2001).

[13] This does not imply that eye-of-origin information isn't exploited in binocular stereo or vergence eye movements. Humans usually don't have conscious access to this information (von Helmholtz, 1962; Ono and Barbeito, 1985; and Kolb and Braun, 1995). See Section 6.5.

Midget cells

Parasol cells

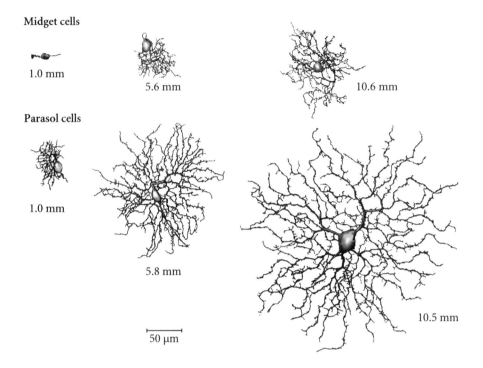

1.0 mm

5.6 mm

10.6 mm

1.0 mm

5.8 mm

10.5 mm

50 μm

FIGURE 3.5 *Retinal Ganglion Cells* Two cell classes dominate retinal output to the thalamus. At a given distance from the fovea, *midget cells* have small, compact dendritic
trees and are much more common than *parasol neurons*, which possess larger dendritic trees. Their size increases steadily when moving away from the fovea (that is, with
eccentricity, indicated in millimeter distance from the fovea). Modified from Watanabe
and Rodieck (1989).

Ramòn y Cajal who, at the end of the 19th century, first stained and identified
the basic cell types of the vertebrate retina. Neurons are commonly classified
like postage stamps—by their looks; that is, by the morphology, position, and
size of their cell bodies, dendrites, and axonal terminations. Today, this information is often supplemented by identifying unique molecular constitutive
elements, for instance, the presence of particular calcium-binding proteins.[14]

By far the most numerous ganglion cells are midget neurons (Figure 3.5). In
the fovea, a single cone provides, via an intermediary, the only input to a pair of
on- and off-midget cells. While the on-cell increases its firing rate when stimu-

[14]For a translation of Ramòn y Cajal's best-known work, including extensive comments, see
Ramòn y Cajal (1991). The modern study of the primate retina was inaugurated by Stephen
Polyak (Polyak, 1941; Zrenner, 1983; Kaplan, 1991). For a masterful summary of today's knowl-
edge of retinal anatomy and physiology, consult Rodieck (1998).

lated by a spot of light, the off-cell does the opposite. It will, instead, fire more vigorously when light is turned off inside the central region of its receptive field. Given the one-to-two connectivity between individual cone photoreceptors and midget cells, they serve as the conduit for signaling fine image details.

About one in ten ganglion cells is of the parasol type. At any fixed distance from the fovea, parasol cells have larger dendritic trees than midget cells (Figure 3.5). A parasol neuron collects information from many cones and expresses this as either an increase (on) or a decrease (off) in firing rate when a light is turned on within its receptive field's center. The spatial extent of its dendritic tree increases with retinal eccentricity, as does the size of the associated receptive field.

The Lateral Geniculate Nucleus: Midway between the Retina and Cortex

When injecting a cell body with a chemical tracer, the substance is transported all the way to the axon terminals, staining the entire axonal process on the way, allowing neuroanatomists to visualize the projection patterns of a cell population. Conversely, in retrograde transport the tracer moves back along the axon toward the cell body.

Applied to ganglion cells, these techniques reveal that at least nine out of ten project to a central, thalamic structure, the *lateral geniculate nucleus* or LGN (Figure 3.6). It is the best known of several thalamic nuclei that process visual information.

The LGN is strategically positioned between the retina and the cortex. Incoming retinal information is switched over onto a geniculate relay neuron that sends this data onward to the primary visual cortex. The receptive field of the projection cell is nearly identical to that of its input fibers, so much so that it is usually assumed that no significant transformation of the retinal input occurs in the LGN.

Yet that assumption is unlikely to be true. The forward projection from the LGN to the primary visual cortex (V1) is paralleled by a massive cortical feedback. In the cat, about ten times more fibers project back from V1 to LGN than project forward. Think of a video camera hooked up to a computer with a much thicker cable snaking back from the computer to the camera. About half of all synapses in the LGN originate in the cortex and many other synapses come from diffuse projections in the brainstem. What are they doing? It is likely that the cortex selectively enhances or suppresses retinal input passing through the LGN. Yet the function of this massive feedback pathway, characteristic of all thalamic nuclei, remains baffling.[15]

---

[15]For the anatomy of the forward and feedback pathways, see Sherman and Koch (1998), the monograph by Sherman and Guillery (2001), and Section 7.3. Many investigators believe that the cortico-geniculate or, more generally, the cortical feedback to all thalamic nuclei, helps to

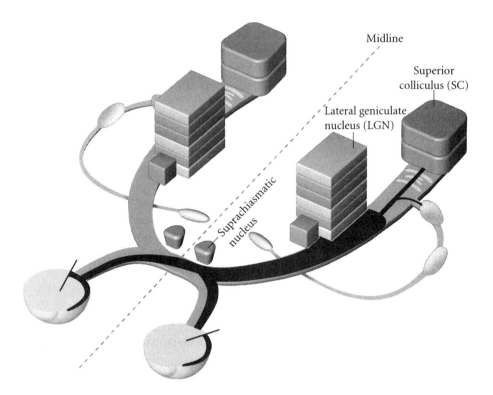

FIGURE 3.6 *What Happens to the Retinal Output?* About 90% of fibers in the optic nerve project to the *lateral geniculate nucleus* (LGN) of the thalamus and from there onto the primary visual cortex. This pathway dominates conscious visual perception. About 100,000 ganglion cells project to the *superior colliculus* (SC) at the top of the midbrain. These cells mediate relatively automatic opto-motor behaviors. Smaller sub-populations project to minor nuclei involved in housekeeping tasks outside the pale of consciousness. This is a schematic drawing. Panel **C** in the front endpages provides absolute scale. Modified from Rodieck (1998).

The LGN resembles a six-layered, warped cake. The lower two layers contain large cell bodies, called *magnocellular* neurons, while the upper four layers are characterized by small cell bodies termed *parvocellular* neurons. Closer inspection reveals a further substructure sandwiched between these layers: small,

---

predict the presence of stimuli. This is known as *predictive coding* (Koch, 1987; Mumford, 1991, 1994; and Rao and Ballard, 1999). Przybyszewski et al. (2000) cooled V1 in the cat, thereby turning it off, and showed that this affected the visual contrast-response curve of geniculate neurons.

cone-shaped *koniocellular neurons*. The visual environment is mapped in a continuous manner onto all geniculate layers.

The Geniculo-Cortical Pathway Dominates Retinal Output

Each midget ganglion cell in the retina sends its output to one of the four parvocellular layers in the LGN. There, relay cells project into a sharply defined sublayer in V1, cryptically labeled $4c\beta$, a fraction of a millimeter thick (see Figure 4.1). The entire population of midget ganglion cells at all eccentricities, their geniculate targets, and their cortical recipients are known as the *parvocellular stream, channel*, or *pathway*. Similarly, each parasol ganglion cell projects to one of two magnocellular layers. Geniculate cells located there innervate layers $4c\alpha$ and 6 of the primary visual cortex. Collectively, this brotherhood of cells is referred to as the *magnocellular pathway*. The koniocellular neurons have their own distinct termination zone in V1.

In biology, function and structure are tightly linked. Thus, the distinct anatomy of retinal ganglion cells and their separate termination patterns in the LGN and V1 are associated with profound differences in their behavior and function (Table 3.1).

Parvocellular neurons respond in a *sustained* manner to the on- or offset of light—that is, they keep on firing (albeit at a reduced rate) for as long as the stimulating light pattern is present, while magnocellular neurons respond in a much more *transient* manner. In general, magnocellular neurons prefer rapidly changing stimuli, as occur during motion, while parvocellular neurons prefer sustained or slowly changing input.

There are many more parvocellular cells than magnocellular ones. Parvocellular cells represent the world at a fine grain. They also care about color. A subcategory is *red-green opponent cells* that receive inputs from L cones in the central, excitatory part of their receptive field, and opposing input from M cones in their surround. Complementary cells are driven by a greenish spot of

TABLE 3.1 Conscious Vision is Mediated to a Significant Extent by Two Pathways that Originate in the Retina and Reach into V1

Property	Parvocellular neurons	Magnocellular neurons
Color opponency	Yes	No
Receptive field size	Smaller	Larger
Response to light step	Sustained	Transient
Low-contrast, moving stimuli	Weak response	Strong response
High-acuity vision	Yes	No
Percentage of ganglion cells	70%	10%

light directed at their center and are inhibited by a reddish annulus. These populations correspond to the *red-green opponency channel* that had been inferred from sensory measurements as early as the 18th century. Magnocellular neurons are much less sensitive to wavelength and have no color opponency organization to speak of. They carry a signal related to the intensity or luminosity (with L, M, and S cone contributions).

A striking feature of these pathways is their anatomical independence. This makes it possible to selectively and deliberately destroy one or the other pathway by multiple injections of a chemical poison that destroys all the cell bodies in the appropriate layers of the LGN of monkeys. After complete interruption of either channel, the animal is trained to recognize color or patterns that require low or high acuity to properly resolve, similar to the way your optometrist tests your vision.

Eliminating the parvocellular layers profoundly affects color and high fidelity spatial vision. The monkey has great trouble detecting either fine details or faint patterns and completely loses its ability to find a target purely on the basis of color. The animal's sensitivity to patterns that change rapidly with time remains intact. Destruction of the magnocellular pathway has no discernible effect on the monkey's sensitivity to fine details, but does limit its ability to detect rapid temporal changes.[16]

A third pathway, parallel to the magno- and the parvocellular stream, is the koniocellular one. Koniocellular neurons lack a pronounced, spatial center-surround organization, signaling instead chromatic opponency. That is, they respond to the difference between S cones and the sum of L and M cones. They are thought to be involved in the *blue-yellow opponency channel* inferred by Ewald Hering on the basis of perceptual color experiments.[17]

As long as the eyes are open, these pathways, with over one million fibers, carry more than 10 million bits per second of visual information. This is a lot. Yet, as you shall learn in Chapter 9, the vast majority of this data stream is discarded by the conscious mind.

Although the magno-, parvo-, and koniocellular neurons dominate retinal output, they are not the only ones. Besides a large projection to the superior colliculus, discussed next, numerous minor classes of ganglion cells relay visual information to a motley collection of small nuclei that mediate blinking, gaze and pupilary control, diurnal rhythms, and other regulatory functions (Figure 3.6). None of these contain a map of the visual world. They are unlikely to play a role in conscious vision.

---

[16]The system has redundancy: The sense of visual motion partially survives destruction of the magnocellular layers; likewise, depth perception can be subserved by either system (Schiller and Logothetis, 1990; and Merigan and Maunsell, 1993).

[17]Koniocellular geniculate neurons are driven by specific types of retinal ganglion cells. For their properties, see (Dacey, 1996; Nathans, 1999; Calkins, 2000; and Chatterjee and Callaway, 2002).

3.6 | THE SUPERIOR COLLICULUS: ANOTHER VISUAL BRAIN

About 100,000 ganglion cell axons run from the retina to the *superior colliculus* (SC) on top of the midbrain. The SC is the most important visual processing center in fish, amphibians, and reptiles. In primates, much of its function has been taken over and extended by the cortex. Nevertheless, the superior colliculus remains important for orienting responses as well as eye and head movements.

Patients who have lost part or all of V1 and adjacent cortical regions are blind in their affected visual field, even though their retino-collicular pathways are intact.[18] Thus, SC activity probably is insufficient for conscious vision.

The colliculus is critically involved in the fast eye movements called *saccades* that primates incessantly engage in (more on these in the next few pages). The SC signals the difference between where the eyes are pointed to now and where they will go next. This information is relayed directly to brainstem oculomotor areas controlling eye muscles as well as to the pulvinar nuclei of the thalamus.

The SC can be divided conveniently into superficial, intermediate, and deep layers. The superficial layer receives direct input from retinal ganglion cells in a topographic manner. Neurons in the deeper layers have been linked to behavior by direct injection of electric current. If the amplitude is strong enough, a saccade is triggered.

3.7 | EYE MOVEMENTS: VISUAL SACCADES ARE UBIQUITOUS

The eyes and their distinct patterns of movements are a fascinating source of information—not only for poets but also for scientists. Six eye muscles are responsible for rotating the eyeball in several distinct patterns.

A *saccade* is a rapid movement of both eyes yoked together. Evolution minimized the duration for which the eyes are in transit to less than a tenth of a second. The brain aims to reach a particular spot; once the eyeball is launched, no visual control is exerted until the eye comes to rest again. When the eye movement is off-target, a *corrective* saccade of small amplitude brings the target right onto the fovea.

You move your eyes all the time. You read by skipping with a series of small saccades across the text. You look at a face by constantly glancing at its eyes, mouth, ears, and so on. At a couple of saccades per second, your eyes move more than 100,000 times a day, about as often as your heart beats. Still, almost

---

[18]The clinical evidence is documented by Brindley, Gautier-Smith, and Lewin (1969); Aldrich et al. (1987); and Celesia et al. (1991).

none of this tireless motion makes it into consciousness (this claim will be buttressed in Section 12.1).

The intervals between saccades are brief, as short as 120–130 msec. This corresponds to the minimum time needed to process visual information during the fixation periods.

Rapidly displacing the eyes appears effortless, but requires fine coordination among a large cast of players dispersed throughout the brain. Drawn in bold strokes, two parallel pathways mediate saccades. Generating reflexive, orienting eye movements (as when something appears off to one side) is the job of the superior colliculus. Planned, voluntary saccades are the responsibility of posterior parietal and prefrontal cortical regions. If one system is impaired, the other one compensates to a limited extent.[19]

When you track a target, say a bird in flight, your eyes move in a pattern known as *smooth pursuit*. This movement involves quite distinct parts of the brain.

Vision Fades When the Image Is Stabilized

If eye movements are prevented (for instance, by artificially stabilizing an image at the same retinal location), vision rapidly fades. If you are ever a subject in a visual functional brain imaging experiment, you will be instructed to keep your eyes as still as possible to minimize motion artifacts that cause a reduction in the signal-to-noise amplitude. You will lie in the magnet and studiously stare at the fixation mark. This can lead to a gradual fading of the entire visual field—a sort of blackout—that can be counteracted by blinking.[20]

It is often assumed that fading is a purely retinal phenomenon, caused by a temporal derivative-like operation implemented by retinal neurons. They follow the motto: If nothing changes, don't bother to report anything. This cannot be the complete story, however, because experiments carried out in the late 1950s showed that the fading of line drawings depended on a variety of global figural qualities not expressed in the retina.

Unfortunately, little is known about the neuronal basis of fading. The excitability of the neurons expressing visual consciousness should mirror the perceptual fading. That is, as an image fades from consciousness, so should the relevant activity of the NCC.

---

[19]The neurophysiology of eye movements is summarized by Schall (1991); Corbetta (1998); and Schiller and Chou (1998).

[20]It can take anywhere from a fraction of a second to a minute or more for an image to fade (Tulunay-Keesey, 1982; and Coppola and Purves, 1996). Fading depends on whether the subject attends to the figure, whether the figure is meaningful, and so on (Pritchard, Heron, and Hebb, 1960).

Saccadic Suppression, or Why You Can't See Your Eyes Move

What effects do eye movements have on the rest of the system? When playing around for the first time with a video camera, you quickly discover that filming your toddler by following her around the house is likely to induce nausea when viewing the result. Sudden camera movements and turns give rise to an uncomfortable sense of induced motion. Why, then, don't you experience such feelings each and every time you move your eyes? Subjectively, the outside world looks remarkably steady. How come?[21]

Another expected detrimental effect of rapid eye movements is image blurring, as would occur, for instance, while trying to capture a moving car on a photograph using a slow shutter speed. During the 30- to 70-msec duration of the saccade, the visual field should be horribly smeared out, yet it continues to look sharp. What is going on?

The stability and sharpness of the visual world during eye movements is a consequence of numerous processes, including *saccadic suppression*, a mechanism that interferes with vision during eye movements. You can experience saccadic suppression by looking in a mirror and fixating first your left and then your right eye, back and forth. You will never catch your eyes in transition. Your eyes are not moving too fast, because you can see perfectly well the saccades a friend is making. During the time your eye is in transition, vision is partially shut down. This eliminates blur and the feeling that the world out there is jerked around every fraction of a second.[22]

Why, then, isn't everyday vision characterized by annoying blank periods? This must be prevented by some clever, *trans-saccadic integration* mechanism that fills in these intervals with a "fictive" movie, a composite of the image just before and just after the saccade. The mechanisms and neuronal sites of this integration remain largely unknown.[23]

---

[21]The world doesn't have to appear stable, as the neurological patient R.W. knows only too well (Haarmeier et al., 1997). His world spins in the opposite direction if he tracks something with his eyes or head. His visual acuity and ability to judge motion are normal. Bilateral lesions in his parieto-occipital cortex destroyed motion compensation.

[22]How this occurs remains a hotly debated question. One school asserts that eye movements actively suppress intrasaccadic motion processing, while the opposing camp asserts that visual factors such as forward and backward masking cause the suppression (Burr, Morrone, and Ross, 1994; and Castet and Masson, 2000). More likely than not, multiple processes contribute. Note that saccades don't completely prevent vision (Bridgeman, Hendry, and Stark, 1975). That something can be seen during saccades can be ascertained by looking at the crossties of railroad tracks from a moving train while making a saccade against the direction of motion of the railroad car. The artist Bill Bell has exploited this in his "Lightsticks" art pieces. Viewed on a dark background, these vertical bars of blinking LEDs paint a picture of an animal, flag, or face onto the retina of the viewer who rapidly saccades across them. When fixating them directly, however, only a flickering bar of red light is seen.

[23]McConkie and Currie (1996).

Blinks

The eye cleans itself by blinking the lids and lubricating the front of the cornea with fluids from the tear glands. Typically, you'll make a few blinks while reading this paragraph. Each one briefly blocks the pupil, causing an almost complete loss of vision for a tenth of a second or so. Yet, while you are exquisitely sensitive to a brief flickering of the room lights, you are almost totally oblivious to blinks.[24]

Accordingly, I expect the NCC neurons to be indifferent to blinks. That is, while retinal neurons should stop firing during a blink, the NCC neurons should remain active during this temporary shutdown of vision.

Adding up all of the little snippets of the running movie that constitutes daily life that are "lost" due to saccadic and blink suppression amounts to a staggering 60 to 90 minutes each day! An hour or more during which sight should be compromised, yet is not. And, until scientists began to study this in the 19th century, no one was aware of this.

3.8 | RECAPITULATION

The retina is an amazing tissue of highly laminated neural processors, thinner than a credit card, with more than fifty specialist cell types. Ganglion cell axons make up the optic nerve that leaves the eye. Think of them as wires that convey messages encoded as a temporal sequence of electrical pulses, organized along multiple parallel channels. A loose analogy can be made with a set of dozens of cameras, one transmitting black-and-white information, one red-green, and another one blue-yellow color opponency information, one channel emphasizing locations whose intensity is changing in time, and so on.

The best-studied of these are the magno-, parvo- and koniocellular pathways that project, via the lateral geniculate nucleus, into the primary visual cortex. Magnocellular neurons signal luminosity and temporal change, as occur during motion, while parvocellular neurons transmit red-green information and fine spatial details. The koniocellular pathway cares about blue-yellow opponency and less well understood image features. All of these underpin conscious, visual experience.

The second largest tract leaving the eye projects to the superior colliculus and is involved in automatic forms of rapid eye movements. A great deal of further machinery is dedicated to subserving saccades and other eye movements that are rapid, accurate, and adaptive. Minor sets of ganglion cells project to odd places in the brainstem. These control gaze, the pupilary diameter, and

---

[24]Volkmann, Riggs, and Morre (1980); and Skoyles (1997).

other important household functions. Most of this information is likely to be inaccessible to consciousness.

You do *not* see with the eyes but with the brain proper. Discrepancies between what ganglion cells encode and what you consciously perceive include the dramatic decrease in spatial acuity away from the fovea, the existence of a mere two photoreceptor types at the point of sharpest seeing, the paucity of color representation in the periphery, the blind spot, image blur during eye movements, and transient loss of visual input during blinks.

Neuronal structures in the thalamus and cortex read out the optic nerve signals and generate a stable, homogeneous, and compelling view of the world. While the eyes are necessary for normal forms of seeing, the NCC are most certainly not to be found in the retinae. So let me now come to the visual cortex.

CHAPTER FOUR

The Primary Visual Cortex as a Prototypical Neocortical Area

This must be taken as a general principle, that the cortical
substance…imparts life, that is, sensation, perception, understanding
and will; and it imparts motion, that is the power of acting in agreement
with will and nature.

From Emanuel Swedenborg

Y[ou] can survive without the cortex, but only in a vegetative state, without awareness. The Swedish polymath and mystic who penned the chapter quote in 1740 was among the first to elaborate on the importance of the cortex to mental life. The cortex is the ultimate substrate of perception, memory, speech, and consciousness.

The cerebral cortex can be subdivided into the phylogenetically old olfactory and hippocampus cortex, and the more recent *neocortex*. This multilayered structure crowning the brain is only found in mammals; in fact, the neocortex is as much a defining feature of mammals as are the mammary glands. Given the importance of the neocortex to conscious perception, it behooves us to study its anatomy and physiology in detail.

This chapter highlights the general properties of the neocortex (or cortex, for short), as well as the peculiarities associated with the primary visual cortex—the destination of the retino-geniculate input. The primary visual cortex is by far the best explored cortical area.[1] I'll survey other cortical regions in Chapters 7 and 8.

---

[1] For details on the neocortex, its constitutive elements, architecture, and evolutionary lineage, consult White (1989); Abeles (1991); Braitenberg and Schüz (1991); Zeki (1993); Peters and Rockland (1994); Mountcastle (1998); and the lucid evolutionary account by Allman (1999).

4.1 | MONKEY VISION AS A MODEL FOR HUMAN VISION

Any plausible theory of consciousness must be based on neurons. Studying them necessitates the use of microelectrodes, anatomical dyes, and other invasive and often irreversible actions. Human brains, therefore, are for the most part off-limits.

The species of choice to explore the neuronal basis of perception is the macaque, which, except for people, is the most wide-ranging primate genus (for the classification of humans and monkeys, see footnote 21 in Chapter 1). Macaques include the rhesus monkey, *Macaca mulatta*, and the crab-eating macaque, *Macaca fascicularis*. These animals, evolving independently of humans for the past 30 million years, are not endangered, and adapt well to captivity.

During the course of evolution, the *amount* of cortex has increased several hundredfold from simple primates (such as prosimians) to humans, but the *types* of cortical cells have not changed commensurately. In fact, small and large excitatory pyramidal neurons and spiny stellate cells, as well as inhibitory basket, nonspiny stellate cells, double bouquet neurons, and other members of the diverse menagerie of inhibitory neurons, are found in all mammals.[2]

The sole exception, so far, are *spindle* neurons, a class of giant cells restricted to two neocortical regions in the frontal lobe. Found in high densities in humans, they are much sparser in the great apes and altogether absent in monkeys, cats, and rodents. A few tantalizing hints point toward their possible involvement in self monitoring and self awareness.[3]

Monkeys are naturally curious and can be trained over months to carry out quite complex visual-motor behaviors. When their performance on a multitude of visual tasks is compared in an appropriate manner to humans, the similarities exceed the differences. The many experiments reported in this book are a testament to the fact that monkeys share with humans motion, depth, form, and color perception, and respond to the same visual illusions as people do. Like humans, macaques have forward placed eyes, three classes of cone photoreceptors, an emphasis on the fovea compared to the visual periphery, the same types of eye movements and similar cortical regions subserving vision.

---

[2]Not all cortical regions expanded equally during evolution. For instance, V1 constitutes 12% of the cortical area in monkeys, but only 3% in humans, while the prefrontal cortex increased from 10% in monkeys to 30% in humans (Allman, 1999).

[3]Spindle neurons, the *Korkzieher* cells of von Economo and Koskinas (1925), are characterized by elongated and large cell bodies in the lower part of layer 5, the output layer of the cortex (Nimchinsky et al., 1999). Absent in newborn infants, their numbers stabilize in adults at about 40,000 neurons in the anterior cingulate cortex and 100,000 or so in FI, another frontal area. These regions are involved in self-evaluation, monitoring, and attentional control.

As one moves from simpler to more elaborate behaviors, differences between species inevitably emerge. This book is primarily concerned with conscious sensory perception, rather than with the self, abstract reasoning, or language. At that level, the distinctions between monkey and human vision are more likely to be quantitative than qualitative.[4]

4.2 | THE NEOCORTEX IS A LAYERED, SHEET-LIKE STRUCTURE

The human neocortex and its connections occupy about 80% of the volume of the brain. Different from other brain structures, such as the thalami, basal ganglia, or brainstem, the neocortex is a sheet whose extent vastly exceeds its thickness. It is highly convoluted and has a laminated substructure (see the back endpages). The size of one cortical sheet varies across species, ranging from around 1 cm^2 in the shrew, to 100 cm^2 in the macaque monkey, 1000 cm^2 in humans, and several times this area for some whales. Think of your cerebral cortex as two 2-3 mm thick pancakes, 35 cm in diameter, crumpled up and stuffed into your skull.

The overall density of neurons is relatively constant, independent of area (with the sole exception of V1), about 100,000 cells below one square millimeter of cortex.[5]

The gray matter of the neocortical sheet, the mass of neuronal cell bodies, dendrites, synapses, and supporting cells, is subdivided into layers based on the densities and types of cell bodies and fibers (as is apparent when looking at the back endpages). Traditionally, six layers have been recognized in the neocortex, but finer subdivisions have been made. Neurons can be tagged by their *laminar position*. The layer in which a cell body is located is indicative of the overall role of the neuron within the cortical architecture. These kinds of anatomical rules, alluded to in the following, are expanded upon in Chapter 7.

The topmost layer 1, directly below the membranes enclosing the brain, is conspicuous for its dearth of cell bodies (Figure 4.1). This layer is a recip-

---

[4]Brewer et al. (2002) emphasizes the similarities and Vanduffel et al. (2002) the differences between the two species in the organization of visual cortical areas as assayed using fMRI. Preuss, Qi, and Kaas (1999) document minor differences in the microanatomy of V1 between apes and humans. Preuss (2000) addresses the question of what is unique, if anything, about human brain architecture.

[5]For quantitative references regarding size, density, and thickness of the neocortex, see Passingham (1993) and Felleman and Van Essen (1991). The anatomical reference for the constant cell number below 1 mm^2 of cortex comes from Rockel, Hiorns, and Powell (1980). Given a packing density of 50,000 cells per mm^3, a total surface area of 2 × 100,000 mm^2, and a thickness of about 2 mm, the average human cortex contains on the order of 20 billion neurons and 200 trillion synapses (2 × 10^{14}).

ient zone of feedback pathways from other cortical regions and for some unspecific thalamic inputs. Think of it as providing the larger context for the neurons lying below it. The next two layers 2 and 3, part of the *superficial* or *upper layers*, are, in contrast, densely populated with neurons. Cortico-cortical forward projections that remain within the cortex originate, as a rule of thumb, in superficial layers. Layer 4 is richest in cell bodies—in the case of V1, small, nonpyramidal neurons called *spiny stellate cells*. It is often subdivided into sublayers and is the input zone of the cortex; as discussed in Chapter 3, most of the geniculate input terminates in two distinct laminae within layer 4. The bottom two layers 5 and 6, the *deep or lower layers*, are the home of many tall pyramidal neurons. Whenever the cortex needs to talk to the rest of the nervous system, spikes are sent via the axons of deep layer pyramidal neurons. If information needs to be conveyed from V1 to the superior colliculus, for example, it must be shipped to a layer 5 pyramidal neuron. Likewise for the output of the motor cortex. The brain's white matter, consisting entirely of axonal bundles and their fatty coverings (which assures rapid pulse conduction), starts just below layer 6.

On the whole, the cortex is remarkably homogeneous. This universal or "unitary" viewpoint assumes that most of the differences between, say, visual and auditory cortex, arise due to the distinct nature of the input—a stream of images versus sounds. That is not to deny regional specializations. Layer 4 in the motor cortex, for instance, is poorly developed, whereas layer 4 in the primary visual cortex is particularly thick. Specializations make sense, because the main job of the motor cortex is to control muscles (an output function) while V1 requires high-resolution visual input.

4.3 | A PLETHORA OF CORTICAL CELL TYPES

Morphological, pharmacological, and molecular criteria are used to differentiate types of neurons. Even if two neurons look alike, they may be situated in different layers and send their axons to distinct target zones, and their spikes may convey different messages. A smorgasbord of cell types found in human V1 is illustrated in Figure 4.1 and in monkey V1 in the back endpages.

Based on the immediate effect that cells have on the membrane potential of their target cell, they are divided into excitatory and inhibitory neurons. About four-fifths of all neurons in the cortex are excitatory. Synaptic output from such a cell causes a brief, positive elevation of the membrane potential in its target cell, toward the threshold for generating an action potential, enhancing the probability that a spike will be triggered.

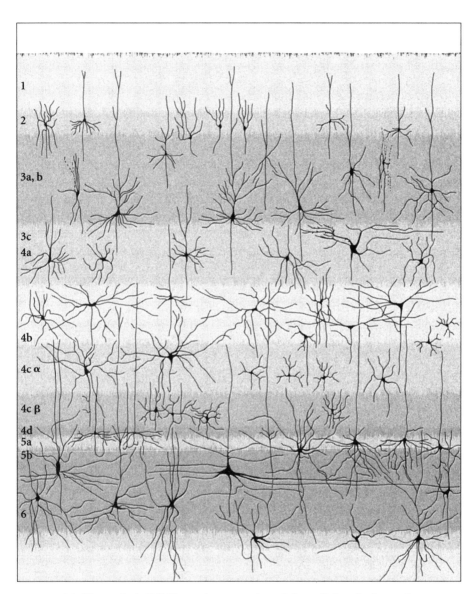

FIGURE 4.1 *Neocortical Cell Types* A composite of the cellular denizens that populate the human primary visual cortex. Notice their predominant vertical organization. Neurons are usually referenced with respect to the layer from which their cell body originates (see label on the left). The same cell types are found throughout the neocortex. Only a miniscule fraction of all cells present in this region are shown. Modified from Braak (1976).

Pyramidal Cells: The Workhorse of the Cortex

Cortical neurons have a predominantly vertical organization, perpendicular to the surface. When looking at a suitably stained section of the cortex (as in Figure 4.1), one is reminded of a forest whose branches and roots stretch somewhat horizontally, but whose main thrust is upward.

This orientation is most obvious for *pyramidal cells*, which account for three out of every four cortical neurons. Their defining feature is an *apical dendrite* that rises straight from the pyramidal-shaped cell body toward the surface. Dozens of *basal dendrites* emanate from the cell body, radiating outward in all directions, like fuzzy hair.

The axons of many pyramidal neurons leave their home base to communicate with other cortical areas or with subcortical targets in the thalami, basal ganglia, and elsewhere. Before leaving for their distant targets, the axons give off local branches, called *collaterals*. Axonal collaterals provide to their neighborhood a carbon copy of the message sent to distant parts of the brain. Synapses at the business end of these axons excite their targets by releasing the messenger molecule *glutamate*.

Pyramidal cells are responsible for almost all inter-areal communication and are the only means of rapidly conveying a message outside the cortex proper. The 200 million-strong *corpus callosum* fiber bundle connecting the two cortical hemispheres (Figure 17.1), the feedback pathways between different cortical regions and from the cortex to the thalamus (Chapter 7), and the *corticospinal tract*, by which the motor cortex influences the voluntary musculature, all originate from pyramidal cells. These wide-ranging projections usually do not involve branching axons (except toward the end, when the axon makes a profusion of synaptic contacts within the target zone). That is, it is uncommon for a pyramidal neuron to send one branch to cortical area *A* and another to cortical area *B*. Instead, two sets of neurons with slightly different layers of origin, morphology, and so on are used, one for conveying the information to *A* and one to *B*. It is as if the information needs to be specially prepared for its recipient and this requires different neurons.

The situation is quite different for the multiple projection systems originating in the brainstem, which release noradrenaline, serotonin, dopamine, or acetylcholine at many locations in the forebrain. As discussed in Chapter 5, these ascending pathways seem to implement a widespread *broadcast*, in the nature of "Hello, wake up, an important event is happening," whereas a cortical cell conveys a specific message to a specific address.

The apical dendrite of the large pyramidal cells whose cell bodies are located in layer 5 can reach all the way to the surface, like an antenna. Smaller pyramidal cells have an ascending apical dendrite that may terminate in the layer just above them.

The dendrites of excitatory neurons are covered with *dendritic spines*, 1 µm long thorn-like structures. Much of the cortical traffic involves spines, because each one carries at least one excitatory synapse. A large neuron might be covered with 10,000 spines, indicating that *at least* that number of excitatory synaptic inputs converge onto it (but not necessarily from as many neurons, since one axon can form multiple synapses with one neuron).

Although pyramidal neurons are found throughout the cortex, their micro-anatomy can differ substantially from one region to the next. Guy Elston at the University of Queensland in Australia stained and reconstructed layer 3 pyramidal cells in many cortical areas in the macaque monkey. He and his colleagues found a systematic increase in the complexity of the basal dendrites of this one cell type (in terms of the extent of its dendritic tree, the number of branch points, and the number of excitatory synapses) as they sampled cells from progressively more anterior regions. Thus, the dendritic trees of pyramidal neurons in the front of the brain are substantially more elaborate and larger than those found at the opposite pole, in V1, being the target for up to 16 times more excitatory synapses. Neurons in higher cortical regions are more complex, and presumably computationally more powerful, than those in sensory regions.[6]

Spiny stellate cells form a subclass of excitatory neurons. Confined to layer 4 of the primary visual cortex, they are extremely densely packed (with an effective density of up to 180,000 cells per cubic millimeter) and can be thought of as pyramidal neurons that have lost their apical dendrite. Stellate cells are predominantly local; their axons rarely venture outside their neighborhood.

Like many people, the cortex overwhelmingly talks to itself. Only a small fraction of the 300 to 800 million synapses per cubic millimeter of cortical tissue are made by axons from outside this cortical region. The rest are made by and onto nearby neurons. In V1, less than 5% of excitatory synapses originate from geniculate axons. A similar fraction derives from higher cortical areas feeding back to V1. Most of the other synapses—the vast majority—derive from intrinsic neurons. By and large, these percentages are probably representative of other cortical areas, too. It is imperative for the well-being of the cortex that this massive positive feedback is controlled; otherwise, the entire tissue would explode into a paroxysm of firing.[7]

---

[6]Elston, Tweedale, and Rosa (1999); Elston (2000); and Elston and Rosa (1997, 1998).

[7]The minute percentage of geniculate synapses on V1 cells is surprising, given the ease with which these neurons can be excited by visual input (LeVay and Gilbert, 1976; White, 1989; Ahmed et al., 1994; and Douglas et al., 1995). Budd (1998) echoes this view for feedback from V2 into V1; only a minority of synapses belong to axons originating in other cortical areas (V2, MT, and so on).

Inhibitory Cells Are a Diverse Bunch

Neurons whose dendrites are devoid of dendritic spines have a smooth appearance, so they are classified as *smooth neurons*. Their synaptic terminals release the inhibitory neurotransmitter gamma-amino butyric acid (GABA). Activation of a GABAergic synapse lowers the firing probability of the postsynaptic cell by briefly moving the membrane potential away from the spike threshold. Strong inhibition can completely shut down a cell, preventing any spiking.

Smooth cells are interneurons, making synapses in the vicinity of their cell body or in layers directly above or below them, but not in distant cortical regions. About two dozen types of inhibitory interneurons have been described, collectively accounting for about 20% of all cortical neurons. They are highly heterogeneous in form and function. Some primarily target the soma or axon hillock, regulating the initiation and discharge of fast action potentials. Others innervate dendrites, where they assist with local computations or with determining the timing of action potentials.[8]

The most numerous inhibitory interneurons are *basket cells*. They are found in all layers, have dendrites that radiate a few hundred micrometers away from their plump cell body, and possess a nest-like array of synapses that ensheath the cell bodies and proximal dendrites of excitatory neurons. Other inhibitory cell classes include chandelier and double-bouquet cells.

How Many Cell Types Are There?

How many distinct neuronal elements are there likely to be? Neural network theory demands just two—excitatory and inhibitory cells—but hundreds of types is the more likely answer. In the retina alone, more than fifty cell types are recognized. If any one cortical area had the same diversity, and there is no reason not to expect this, the number of distinct cell classes could number in the hundreds.[9]

Retinal neurons *tile* visual space; each point is covered by the dendrites of each cell type at least once. Collectively, each cell type has access to the entire visual field. The same tiling principle, applied to the visual cortex, yields esti-

---

[8]These computations include, but are not limited to, subtraction, veto operations, delays, logarithms, and so on (Koch, 1999) as well as controlling the onset and extent of synchronization and oscillations (Lytton and Sejnowski, 1991). McBain and Fisahn (2001) review the literature on cortical interneurons.

[9]In the hippocampus, several dozen inhibitory cell types have been identified by Freund and Buzsáki (1996) and by Parra, Gulyas, and Miles (1998). For an estimate of the number of neurons in a superficial layer of V1, see Dantzker and Callaway (2000) and Sawatari and Callaway (2000). Cell type counts in *any one cortical area* easily exceed 100 if factors such as the laminar position of the cell's body, the shape and extent of its dendritic morphology, where its axon projects to, the laminar specificity of its synaptic input, and whether it is excitatory or inhibitory, are considered.

mates of a thousand cell types.[10] If each of these had its own, idiosyncratic pattern of synaptic connectivity with every other cell type, a staggering number of specific cell-to-cell interactions could be realized. This enormous potential for specificity should not be surprising, considering the molecular realm, with its lock-and-key interactions among proteins and enzymes. Why should neurons be any less complex and specific than molecules?

4.4 | V1: THE MAIN ENTRY POINT FOR VISION

Now that the principal cortical actors have been introduced, let's turn toward the part of the stage where they first appear within the visual system, namely, the primary visual cortex (V1) or *Brodmann's area 17*. In humans, much of V1 is buried within the *calcarine fissure* on the medial wall of the brain (see the front endpages).[11]

The size and thickness of V1 in one hemisphere is comparable to that of a credit card. The location and orientation of such landmark features as the calcarine fissure vary from one individual to the next and even between the two hemispheres of a single subject. The exact pattern of cortical indentations and gyrations is as unique as a fingerprint.

The output of the LGN, the few million strong *geniculate axons*, projects into distinct sublayers of V1, depending on which type of retinal ganglion cells the LGN relay cells receive input from (Section 3.5).

The World Is Mapped onto V1 in a Topographic Manner

If an engineer had designed the visual system, it is likely that the retinal output would directly connect to V1 on the same side of the brain. Evolution, however, chose to do the job in a slightly different manner. It not only interposed the LGN between the retina and cortex but also devised a semi-crossed projection pattern. As a consequence, the entire left half of the visual field is mapped onto the right V1 and the right hemifield is represented by the left V1 (Figure 3.6).[12]

---

[10]The *tiling hypothesis*, which states that each cell type must be able to sample each point in visual space at least once, was proposed by Francis Crick in 1983 (unpublished manuscript). If the average radius of the basal dendrites of pyramidal neurons is 100 μm, for example, then about 32 pyramidal neurons of one type are needed to evenly cover one mm^2 of the cortex once. For a discussion of tiling, see Stevens (1998).

[11]Toward the end of the 18th century, the Italian Francesco Gennari reported seeing a line or stria situated about midway through the cortical gray matter at the back of the head. This band, consisting of myelinated axons from the LGN that terminate in layer 4, ends abruptly at the boundary with the secondary visual area (V2). Because this striation is visible to the naked eye, V1 is also referred to as *striate cortex*.

[12]Anatomists call this a *contralateral* projection, while a projection to a structure on the same side of the head is called an *ipsilateral* projection.

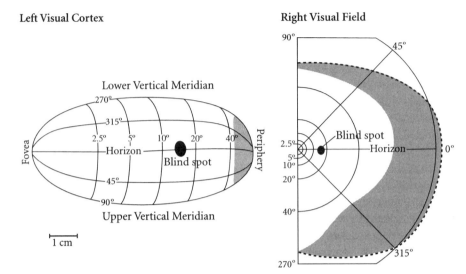

FIGURE 4.2 *The View of the World from V1* The left primary visual cortex, unfolded and spread out, receives input from the right visual field. The fovea maps onto the most posterior pole of the cortex, while the horizon runs along the bottom of the calcarine fissure. (Near) vertical lines in the cortex correspond to half circles of constant eccentricity in visual space. The gray region encompasses the crescent-shaped region that is only visible to the right eye. Nothing is seen outside the dashed lines. Modified from Horton and Hoyt (1991a).

The visual pathways are organized in a maplike manner, with neighboring locations in the visual field projecting onto nearby locations in the cortex. This is known as a *topographic organization*. Following the retinal overrepresentation of the fovea (Figure 3.2), the central parts of the visual field are given much more importance than the periphery (Figure 4.2). Indeed, the central 1° takes up as much cortical real estate in V1 as that part of the visual periphery that can only be seen by one eye.[13] Physiologists refer to this spatial organization as a *retinotopic map*.

Despite the overall orderly representation of these maps, significant scatter does exist. At a fraction of a millimeter scale, there are large fluctuations between adjacent receptive field locations and, occasionally, abrupt jumps. In other words, the projection of the world onto V1 is smooth and continuous on the macroscopic level, but jittery and occasionally discontinuous on the microscopic scale.

---

[13]The central 10° occupy slightly more than half of V1. For references about the map properties of V1, see Horton and Hoyt (1991a); DeYoe et al. (1996); Tootell et al. (1998b); and Van Essen et al. (2001).

A Dramatic Transformation of Receptive Field Properties in V1

David Hubel and Torsten Wiesel at Harvard Medical School discovered in the late 1950s that a profound change in the receptive field organization occurs in V1. Until then, researchers had tried—rather unsuccessfully—to get cortical cells to respond vigorously to spots, annuli, and other circular stimuli. What Hubel and Wiesel found, by following up a chance observation, was that most cells in V1 were turned on by edges, bars, or gratings—anything that had a particular orientation. Some cells preferred a bright slit of a particular orientation, some a dark bar on a bright background with the same slant, and some a sharp boundary between light and dark. These neurons are the building blocks for form perception.[14]

The orientation of the visual input is not the only stimulus attribute that is computed from the geniculate input. Many cells like moving stimuli, and many of those fire only when an appropriately oriented bar is moving in one particular direction, its *preferred direction* (Figure 4.3). Motion in other directions does not excite the neuron. In some cases, motion in the cell's *null direction* evokes inhibition that suppresses even spontaneous firing. The cell's firing also varies with the speed of the stimulus.

Looking more closely at all orientation-selective cells, Hubel and Wiesel found two discrete types. The minority, called *simple* cells, are fussy about the exact location of the oriented bar in visual space. Move the bar over by a fraction of a degree, and their response is much reduced. Simple cells are often linear, because the response to two small stimuli presented simultaneously can be predicted by the sum of the responses to the individual stimuli. At any given visual eccentricity, simple cells with small, medium, and large receptive fields are found. Cells with small receptive fields pick up fine, spatial details, while those with large fields respond best to coarse, elongated blobs. Students of artificial intelligence and machine vision consider this as evidence that V1 transforms the visual scene through a bank of orientation-dependent filters operating at multiple spatial scales.[15]

The majority of neurons are called *complex* cells and care less about the exact location of the edge, as long as it has the appropriate orientation and

---

[14]The original description of oriented cells in V1, the paper that launched a thousand electrodes, is Hubel and Wiesel (1959). See also Hubel and Wiesel (1962); and Livingstone (1998).

[15]Human visual psychophysical techniques—in particular, adaptation and masking—have inferred the existence of orientation-selective filters that have a similar shape to those recorded electrophysiologically and that exist at different spatial scales (Wilson et al., 1990). A reasonably good approximation of the receptive field profiles of simple cells are *Gabor* filter functions, the product of a Gaussian with a sinusoidal waveform (Palmer, Jones, and Stepnoski, 1991). Wandell's (1995) textbook links psychophysics, electrophysiology, fMRI imaging, and computational modeling of the early visual system.

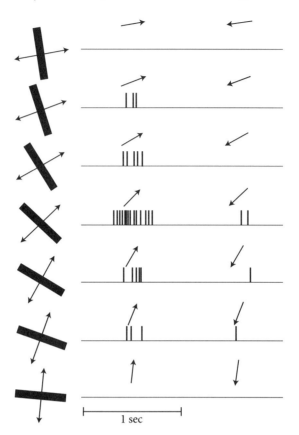

FIGURE 4.3 *A Direction Selective Cell* The response of a single neuron in monkey V1 as the orientation of a bar and its direction of motion is varied. The cell fires most strongly if the bar moves toward the upper right. Modified from Hubel and Wiesel (1968).

direction of motion. It is as if the complex cell receives input from a number of simple cells with the same orientation-selectivity but whose receptive fields are slightly offset with respect to each other. Or, put differently, complex cells are less sensitive to the exact position of the stimulus than simple cells.

Most cortical areas probably include this kind of transition from simple to complex cells. For instance, a simple-like cell for faces might respond to its preferred face only if it is located in the upper visual quadrant, while a complex-like cell will fire to the face with far less concern for where it is located within the visual field.

Neurons in V1 show selectivity for other stimulus features, as well. Some are famously known as *end-stopped* neurons, because their response to a long bar is much less than that to a shorter one. Such cells might represent the substrate for signaling the curvature of line segments or contours. Others respond to a complex spatial mixture of opponency colors.

Cortical neurons possess a large area outside their classically defined receptive field from which their response can be modulated. Stimuli in this *nonclassical* portion of the receptive field don't, by themselves, generate spikes but can profoundly alter the cell's response within the classical receptive field. Many of these effects develop over time, depending on the visual experience of the animal. This sort of plasticity has not been found in the retina.

Imagine, for example, that a single, optimally oriented bar sits smack in the middle of a cell's receptive field. The neuron, therefore, fires vigorously. If this bar is embedded into a field of similarly oriented bars, creating a homogeneous textured pattern, the response will be reduced. Conversely, if the orientation of the central bar is different from the orientation of the surrounding field of bars, the cell's activity can be larger than the response to the central bar by itself. The more salient the stimulus in the cell's classical receptive field relative to its surround, the more vigorous the cell's response. These effects can be thought of as putting the central stimulus into its proper *context* within the overall visual scene.[16]

Contextual modulations also depend on whether the bar lines up with other line elements in its neighborhood. A line element that is part of an extended contour snaking across the visual field causes a bigger response than an isolated one. All of these influences, many of which are probably mediated by feedback from higher cortical regions, occur later. They usually kick in after a 80–100 msec delay following the cell's initial response.

Nonclassical receptive field effects can be quite elaborate, a testimony to the fact that perception of any one stimulus is inexorably bound up with other elements in the display and can't be fully understood in isolation. This was, of course, the central dogma of the *Gestalt* movement that arose in Germany between the two World Wars.

Cortical Architectures and the Columnar Principle

A key principle of neuronal architecture is that nearby neurons encode similar information. This widespread feature of the cortex and other nervous tissues economizes on total wiring length (because neurons that need to be interconnected for functional reasons are next to each other).[17] Spatial clustering shows up in different ways.

---

[16]The literature on nonclassical receptive field effects and contextual modulations is vast and growing. Important papers are Allman (1985); Gallant, Connor, and Van Essen (1997); Shapley and Ringach (2000); and Lamme and Spekreijse (2000).

[17]It has been hypothesized that a *minimal wiring length constraint* operates at the level of the entire nervous system of the most extensively studied multicellular organism, the nematode worm *C. elegans*, which has 302 neurons (Cherniak, 1995). For a similar approach to the pri-

Cells in the input layer tend to be *monocular*, primarily driven by input from either the left or the right eye. The majority of cells outside this layer are *binocular*; that is, their response is influenced by both left and right eye input. Binocular cells constitute the first stage along the visual pathways where this convergence occurs. These cells can, in principle, judge the depth of features in their receptive fields by evaluating the small differences that result from viewing the same scene from slightly different points.

When traversing layer 4c with an electrode in an oblique way, cells predominantly driven by input from one eye cluster together, giving way to representations from the other eye. Visualized on the basis of radioactive tracer injected into one eye, very pretty, zebra-striped images result, with bands of labeled cells alternating with unstained ones. These *ocular dominance* strips are restricted to the input layer.[18]

When clustering extends across most layers, neuroscientists talk about a *columnar representation* of information. Neurons in a column of the cortex, reaching from superficial to deep layers, share one or more properties. As treated at length in Section 2.2, the columnar principle is closely related to explicit coding of information. Indeed, Francis and I surmise that whatever is represented in a columnar fashion is made explicit there.

In V1, at least two separate columnar representations intersect, one for orientation and one for selected aspects of color.

Columns for Stimulus Orientation

Hubel and Wiesel noted early on in their exploration of the cortex that whenever they simultaneously recorded the activity of two or more neurons from one electrode, the optimal spatial orientation of both was similar. Furthermore, whenever the electrode was moved perpendicular to the surface through the various layers, neurons had (nearly) the same orientation selectivity. Their receptive fields, moreover, covered the same location in space. This key point is worth repeating: neurons within a vertical column code for one particular region in visual space and a narrow range of orientations.

If the electrode is moved at an angle through the cortex, the orientation selectivity of the neurons changes in an orderly and generally continuous manner (Figure 4.4). Neuroscientists call these *orientation columns*. These columns can be visualized directly using high-resolution optical imaging. A full range of

---

mary visual cortex, see Koulakov and Chklovskii (2001). Electrical engineers are bound by similar constraints when they consider where to place millions of transistors, capacitors, and other components on a highly integrated silicon circuit to minimize total wire length.

[18] Ocular dominance columns in the macaque were discovered by Hubel and Wiesel (1968), and visualized by LeVay et al. (1985). In humans, these columns are approximately 800 μm wide (Horton and Hedley-Whyte, 1984).

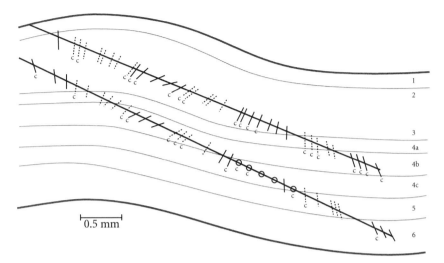

FIGURE 4.4 *Neighborhood Relationships in the Cortex* The orientation preference, color sensitivity, and ocular dominance of cells recorded along two oblique penetrations of an electrode in monkey visual cortex. Nearby neurons share stimulus selectivities. The short lines symbolize the preferred orientation of the cell, with unfilled circles indicating neurons with circular receptive fields. Dashed versus solid lines indicate whether the neuron is predominantly driven by input from the left or the right eye. The c stands for a color-sensitive cell. Modified from Michael (1981).

orientations occurs in a band of cortical tissue spanning around one millimeter.[19]

While orientation is generally mapped in a continuous manner onto the cortex, abrupt discontinuities or fractures in the orientation map exist. These appear to correlate with inhomogeneities in the receptive field topography. The map of visual space is likely distorted at the microscopic level. Careful measurements should reveal these inaccuracies, which are akin to the distortions introduced by early map makers due to faulty information (such as placing two locations next to each other that were not).[20]

What this implies for the conscious perception of space is unclear. How would such wrinkles manifest themselves? One might correlate the smooth progression of an object across space with its perceived location. The subject should note the location and the rate of change of location of a point of light flashed at consecutive displaced positions while fixating. None but other

---

[19]With the exception of patches of nonoriented cells in layers 2 and 3 and the gap in orientation selectivity among neurons in the input layer 4c, orientation columns extend through all layers (LeVay and Nelson, 1991).
[20]Blasdel (1992); and Das and Gilbert (1997).

cells are looking at the topographic map of space, however, so local inhomogeneities could well be compensated for by postsynaptic circuitry that interpolates across space. Such spatial distortions might never show up in either behavior or conscious perception.

The Blob System

In the late 1970s, Margaret Wong-Riley at the University of Wisconsin serendipitously discovered that if a monkey cortex is stained for the enzyme cytochrome oxidase (CO), a unique architecture reveals itself. A polka-dot array of patches shows up in the superficial layers 2 and 3, and much more faintly in layer 6. These *blobs* are in register with ocular dominance columns; that is, each blob falls within a single eye column. They can be looked upon as a separate compartment within V1, because blobs preferentially make synaptic connections to other blobs, while the interblob region connects to other interblob regions. Cross-correlation studies confirm these observations. Indeed, the blob system can be tracked well outside V1.[21]

Cells within the CO blobs differ from surrounding cells in that they have little or no orientation selectivity and that they care about color. *Double-opponent* neurons make their first appearance within blobs. These cells are so named because they have both spatially structured and chromatically opponent receptive fields. The most common double-opponent cell type is excited by red and inhibited by green in the central part of its classical receptive field, and inhibited by red and excited by green in its surround.[22]

Multiple Maps and Parallel Streams in V1

The visual cortex contains multiple, superimposed charts for the position, orientation, and direction of motion of stimuli, for ocular dominance, and for color. What is the relationship among these maps? Are they randomly arranged with respect to each other? Is there a regular mosaic—a *unit cell* in the language of crystallography—within which all these variables are represented? Each tile in this mosaic should encode information pertaining to all possible values of the appropriate dimensions. Theoretical arguments have been advanced that at most nine or ten attributes can reasonably be represented in a continuous manner. Yet for most areas, only one or two mappings have been reported

---

[21] Wong-Riley (1994).

[22] Evidence for spatially- and chromatically-opponent cells in monkey V1 is described by Michael (1978); Livingstone and Hubel (1984); and Conway, Hubel, and Livingstone (2002). The existence of double-opponent cells as a discrete class continues to be doubted by some (Lennie, 2000).

(Chapter 8), implying either that many other feature dimensions may yet be discovered or that they are not represented in this explicit manner in V1. At this point, neuroscience has not converged on any final picture.[23]

Whatever happened to the magno-, parvo- and koniocellular pathways last seen in the input layers to V1 (Section 3.5)? What is their subsequent fate? At least one tributary of the magnocellular pathway projects from layer 4cα into layer 4b, from whence axons are sent to the motion processing area MT. Yet the parvocellular pathway contributes as well. In general, massive intra- and interareal processing obfuscates the dichotomy between these streams. Despite earlier suggestions of an ongoing anatomical segregation between magno- and parvocellular inputs deep into cortex, they are intermixed.

Instead, two new pathways emerge from V1—the *vision-for-perception* and the *vision-for-action* streams—and flow on toward the prefrontal cortex. Their characterizing features and destinations are described in Section 7.5.

4.5 | RECAPITULATION

This chapter summarizes the mountains of data pertaining to the structure and function of the primary visual cortex and, by proxy, most cortical areas. Measured by my polestar—the quest for the NCC—what parts of this material are directly relevant to the study of consciousness?

There are many types of cortical neurons. On the basis of the laminar position of the cell body, dendritic morphology, and axonal target zones, about 100 cell types can be distinguished (possibly many more exist). Pyramidal cells dominate; a subset of them communicates the information computed within local circuits to other nodes, both inside and outside the cortex.

While the receptive field structure of retinal and geniculate cells is relatively stereotypical, cortical cells display a dizzying variety of selective responses to motion, color, orientation, depth, and other stimulus features. Their nonclassical receptive field extends far beyond the confines of the region in space that directly excites the cell. It provides the context within which any single visual stimulus is placed. Thus, the neuronal response to an isolated bar can change substantially if the bar is embedded in a field of lines.

Neurons encountered by an electrode penetrating the cortex perpendicular to its surface respond similarly in terms of receptive field location and preferred orientation. As the instrument samples from neurons that are laterally displaced, their receptive field properties change gradually. In short, like goes

---

[23]Hübener et al. (1997) provide one answer to the question of how many discrete maps there could be within the cortex, and Swindale (2000) addresses this topic from the perspective of cortical development. See also Dow (2002).

with like. This shows up in orientation and ocular dominance columns as well as in color blobs.

Following my general reasoning in Chapter 2, the existence of a columnar representation for the location and the orientation of stimuli implies that these variables are represented explicitly in V1 (remember that this is a necessary, though not sufficient, condition for the NCC). This sensitivity to oriented lines is not yet integrated into elaborate constructs, such as faces, body parts, or objects. That is, faces are implicitly encoded by V1 cells. Their explicit representation doesn't come until later.

In the next chapter, I will try to clarify some of the conflicting claims surrounding the concept of the NCC, before arguing in Chapter 6 that neurons in V1 are not part of the NCC for seeing.

CHAPTER FIVE

What Are the Neuronal Correlates of Consciousness?

Many people want to achieve what they call "higher consciousness."
What's remarkable is that, for them, a higher consciousness is not a
metaphorical state but, rather, a literal, physical, vibrational condition. It
has a reality to it that could theoretically be measured by careful use of a
consciousness-ometer.

From *Captured by Aliens* by Joel Achenbach

The concept of the neuronal correlates of consciousness is appealing because of its simplicity. What could be more elegant than a special set of neurons, engaging in some particular type of activity, that are the physical basis of a specific conscious percept or feeling? A popular hypothesis, introduced in Section 2.3, is that the NCC are a temporary subset of particular neurons in the cortico-thalamic system whose firing is synchronized) Upon closer inspection, though, many subtleties and complexities become apparent.

The entire brain is sufficient for consciousness—it determines conscious sensations day in and day out. Identifying all of the brain with the NCC, however, is not helpful, because likely a subset of brainmatter will do. I am interested in the *smallest* set of neurons responsible for a particular percept.

What are the required background conditions for any conscious content to be expressible by the brain? Will the study of emotion or of anesthesia be helpful in discovering the NCC? Will there be commonalities among the NCC for seeing a face, for hearing a high C tone, and for agonizing over a dull toothache? How much overlap will there be among the NCC for seeing something, recall-

[margin handwriting: Entire brain not minimal]

ing it, or dreaming about it? How specific are the NCC going to be? These thorny questions are addressed in this chapter.[1]

5.1 | ENABLING FACTORS NECESSARY FOR CONSCIOUSNESS

Myriad biological processes must be in place for consciousness to occur. In considering the NCC, it is important to distinguish between *enabling factors* and *specific factors*.

Enabling factors are tonic conditions and systems that are needed for any form of consciousness to occur at all, while specific factors are required for any one particular conscious percept, such as seeing the glorious, star-studded alpine night sky. Some neuronal events might defy such a dichotomy, *modulating* instead the degree of consciousness. For now, however, this simple scheme is sufficient.

Some authorities argue for the need to distinguish between the *content* of consciousness, on the one hand, and the "quality of being conscious" or "consciousness as such" on the other.[2] This distinction maps straightforwardly onto my classification.

The ability to be conscious of anything requires enabling neuronal conditions, which I call NCC_e. The mode of action of NCC_e should be more global and sustained than the local, highly idiosyncratic, and much more rapid onset and disappearance of the NCC for any one percept. Without the relevant NCC_e in place, the organism might still behave in a crude fashion, but it would do so without any awareness (a few pathological conditions where this might occur are discussed in Chapter 13). By definition, no NCC can form without the NCC_e.

Is it possible to be conscious without being conscious of anything in particular? That is, can the NCC_e be present without any NCC? Some types of

---

[1] An account of current thinking about the NCC can be found in the collection edited by the philosopher Thomas Metzinger (2000). In particular, Chalmers (2000) dissects the difficulties in precisely defining the NCC. See also the essays in the special 2001 issue on "Consciousness" in the journal *Cognition*. Teller and Pugh (1983) and Teller (1984) called the neural substrate of experience the *bridge locus*, a concept not too dissimilar from the NCC. Not everybody believes, however, that for every conscious experience there will be an NCC whose activity is sufficient to produce that experience. For arguments against this type of *isomorphism*, see Pessoa, Thompson, and Noë (1998); and O'Regan and Noë (2001).

[2] Pertinent references includes Moore (1922); Grossman (1980); Baars (1988, 1995); Bogen (1995a); and Searle (2000).

meditation

meditation aim for this kind of content-less form of consciousness.[3] For now, however, this seems difficult to study in a rigorous manner.

What are some enabling factors? A proper blood supply is needed because unconsciousness follows within seconds without it.[4] This does not imply that consciousness arises from the heart. Likewise, the myriad of glia cells in the brain play a supporting, metabolic role for the organ but do not possess the required specificity and celerity to subserve perception directly.

In a series of landmark studies in the late 1940s, Giuseppe Moruzzi and Horace Magoun demonstrated that a large region in the brainstem known as the *midbrain* or *mesencephalic reticular formation* (MRF) controls the level of arousal or wakefulness in animals.[5] It has also been called an *ascending activation system*. Direct electrical stimulation of this multifaceted and complex structure arouses the forebrain. The cortical EEG changes abruptly from the slow, high amplitude, synchronized waveforms characteristic of deep sleep to the fast, low voltage, desynchronized activity typical of the wakened brain. Arousal occurs in the absence of any sensory stimulation. Bilateral lesions of the MRF—destruction of one side is typically insufficient—cause the animal to be unresponsive to even intense sensory stimulation. In patients, damage to this area of the brainstem is associated with stupor or coma.

The notion of a monolithic activating system has given way to the realization that 40 or more highly heterogeneous nuclei with idiosyncratic cell structures are housed within the brainstem (that is, the medulla, the pons, and the midbrain). The architecture of these *nuclei*, three-dimensional collections of neurons, each of which has a prevailing neurochemical identity, is profoundly different from the layered organization of the cortex. Cells in different nuclei manufacture, store, and release at their synaptic terminals different neuro-

---

[3]Meditation techniques emphasize emptying the mind of everything by focusing on a single thought, idea, or percept. It takes years of practice to suppress the constant shifts of attention (Chapter 9) and focus for an extended period on one thing without falling asleep. Due to the ever-present neuronal adaptation, awareness for this one thing can gradually ebb away and fade, leaving the brain without any dominant coalition and the subject without any content of consciousness, yet still awake.

[4]For healthy young men, unconsciousness occurs in 6.8 sec! This was established by abruptly blocking the internal carotid artery via a cervical pressure cuff in volunteers (Rossen, Kabat, and Anderson, 1943). The general course of events from consciousness to abrupt unconsciousness and back—which often includes intense visual dreams and euphoric feelings upon awakening—was confirmed by acceleration-induced fainting of pilots and other volunteers spun in centrifuges at high g's (Forster and Whinnery, 1988; and Whinnery and Whinnery, 1990). The neurobiology of *loss of consciousness* is a fascinating but little explored area of relevance to near-death experiences, absence seizures, and other unusual phenomena.

[5]Their original experiments, carried out on cats, are described in Moruzzi and Magoun (1949) and Magoun (1952). See also Hunter and Jasper (1949). The books by Hobson (1989) and Steriade and McCarley (1990) provide a more modern view on brainstem control of wakefulness and sleep.

transmitters, such as acetylcholine, serotonin, dopamine, noradrenaline, histamine, and others. Individual neurons within these cellular aggregates project widely—though not indiscriminately—throughout much of the central nervous system.[6] Many of the brainstem nuclei monitor and modulate the state of the organism, including wake-sleep transitions. Collectively, they process signals relating to the internal milieu, to pain and temperature, and to the musculoskeletal frame.

The *locus coeruleus*, a compact mass of 10,000 or so neurons on each side of the pons, contains more than half of all *noradrenaline*-releasing cells in the brain. To make up for their small number, coeruleus neurons broadcast their information widely. A single axon branches profusely and might reach many areas, including the frontal cortex, thalamus, and visual cortex. During the rapid-eye-movement (REM) part of the sleep cycle, the time when most dreams occur, these noradrenergic cells are silent, or almost so. Their level of activity increases as the animal wakes up and becomes especially prominent during situations that demand extreme vigilance and fight-or-flight reactions.[7] Nevertheless, because the intense dreams that are so characteristic of REM sleep are consciously experienced—though usually not consciously remembered—the lack of noradrenergic input to the cortex during dreams would rule out noradrenaline[8] as part of the NCC_e.

If a single neurotransmitter is critical for consciousness, then it must be *acetylcholine*. To rigorously establish this claim is difficult, however, because the synaptic release of acetylcholine, called *cholinergic transmission*, is widespread, occurring in the distal periphery, where motorneurons contact muscles, and centrally, deep in the cortex. Depending on which receptors are inserted into the membrane of the receiving, *postsynaptic*, target cell, the release of acetylcholine can cause either a rapid but short-lived increase in the membrane potential, bringing it closer to the threshold for firing an action potential, or a more sluggish but longer lasting up- or down-regulation of the excitability of the cell.[9]

Two major cholinergic pathways originate in the brainstem and in the basal forebrain (Figure 5.1). Brainstem cells send an ascending projection to the

---

[6]To learn more about brainstem nuclei and their relationship to consciousness, consult the excellent papers by Parvizi and Damasio (2001); and Zeman (2001).

[7]Foote, Aston-Jones, and Bloom (1980); Foote and Morrison (1987); and Hobson (1999). When locus coeruleus neurons shut down, firing activity in the hippocampus and elsewhere is severely reduced. This might explain why you can't remember what you dreamed, because the transfer from short-term memory into long-term memory is impaired. Will biotechnology develop a drug that releases noradrenaline in the hippocampus during REM sleep, permitting recall of dream events? Will this open a Pandora's box of repressed obsessions, memories, and thoughts?

[8]Likewise, the locus coeruleus neurons are silent during cataplexy attacks, when the subject typically retains full awareness (Wu et al., 1999). See also footnote 16 in Chapter 1.

[9]Hille (2001) comprehensively surveys neurotransmitter action on ionic channels.

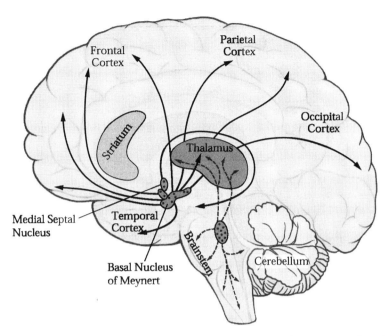

FIGURE 5.1 *The Cholinergic Enabling System* Activity in a discrete set of nuclei that release the neuromodulator acetylcholine is an enabling factor for consciousness, part of the NCC$_e$. These cells are positioned to influence processing throughout the cortex, the thalamus, and the basal ganglia (what is called the forebrain). There is no evidence, however, that their activity is sufficient for any one specific percept. Modified from Perry and Young (2002).

thalamus, where release of acetylcholine facilitates the relay of information from the sensory periphery to the cortex. Cholinergic cells are therefore well-positioned to influence all of the cortex by controlling the thalamus. In contrast, cholinergic basal forebrain neurons send their axons to a much wider array of target structures, innervating the thalamus, hippocampus, amygdala, and cerebral cortex.[10]

Cholinergic mechanisms fluctuate with the sleep-wake cycle. In general, increasing levels of spiking activity in cholinergic neurons are associated with wakefulness or REM sleep, while decreasing levels occur during non-REM or slow-wave sleep. Lastly, many neurological pathologies whose symptoms include disturbances of consciousness, such as Parkinson's disease, Alzheimer's disease, and other forms of dementia, are associated with a selective loss of cholinergic neurons.[11]

[10] Steriade and McCarley (1990); and Woolf (2002).

[11] The case for acetylcholine as subserving consciousness is made most emphatically by Perry et al. (1999). See also Hobson (1999); and Perry, Ashton, and Young (2002).

I conclude from these sundry data that activity in cholinergic neurons is an enabling factor for consciousness, a part of the NCC_e. Insufficient levels of this neurotransmitter prevent the formation of the neuronal coalitions that underlie the NCC proper.

Another enabling factor is sufficient activity in the so-called *nonspecific thalamic nuclei*—that is, regions in the thalamus that do not subserve any one sensory modality and that project to the superficial layers of many cortical regions. Best known are the five or more *intralaminar nuclei* (ILN). The ILN are targeted by the cholinergic brainstem neurons and are part of an ascending activation system as well.

People can lose large chunks of their cerebral cortex without a generalized loss of consciousness. In fact, a few hundred patients live reasonably well with but a single cerebral hemisphere. Comparatively small, bilateral lesions in the thalamic ILN or parts of the brainstem, however, can completely knock out all awareness.[12] The unfortunate victim of such a calamity is unresponsive to any stimuli, with no evidence of any mental life.[13]

Depending on the size and exact location of the destruction within the multitude of brainstem nuclei, global aspects of consciousness are impaired to a variable extent. Incrementally increasing damage moves the patient from a state of wakefulness through a series of clinical syndromes with ever more severe cognitive disabilities. These range from the *minimally conscious state* to a *(persistent) vegetative state* to *coma*, where neither purposeful movements and reactions nor any sleep-wake cycle remain, and only rudimentary reflexes can be elicited. In terms of subjective experience, coma is a close cousin of death.[14]

Neurons in the brainstem or in the ILN do not exhibit any explicit representations nor do they encode stimulus orientation, shape, color, or other specific

---

[12]Hunter and Jasper (1949); Llinás and Paré (1991); Bogen (1995b); Baars (1995); Newman (1997); Purpura and Schiff (1997); and Cotterill (1998) all emphasize the pivotal role of the thalamic intralaminar nuclei in enabling consciousness. The ILN project strongly to the basal ganglia and, in a more distributed manner, to much of the neocortex. The ILN receives little, if any, input from the sensory neocortex (e.g., from V1, MT, or IT). I have argued (Koch, 1995) that activity within the ILN cannot mediate specific sensory states, because ILN cells lack the necessary explicit representations.

[13]A legal case that made headlines in the 1970s was that of Karen Ann Quinlan. At age 21, she imbibed a mixture of alcohol and prescription sedatives and went into cardiac arrest followed by ischemic brain damage. Quinlan never woke up but slipped into a persistent vegetative state characterized by an intact sleep-wake cycle, and occasional nongoal directed movements, but no apparent cognition or awareness. Her parents won permission from the court to remove her from her mechanical ventilator. She nevertheless survived another nine years until she died from opportunistic infections. A postmortem analysis (Kinney et al., 1994) revealed that Quinlan's two thalami, including the ILN, were massively damaged, while her cerebral cortices and brainstem were relatively intact

[14]The neuronal correlates of the progressive diminution of arousal in a clinical setting are discussed in Plum and Posner (1983); Giacino (1997); Schiff and Plum (2000); Zeman (2001); Zafonte and Zasler (2002); and Schiff (2004).

sensory attributes. These nuclei therefore lack the basic infrastructure to support the content of stimulus awareness.[15]

Without the ascending influence of the brainstem and thalamic nuclei, an organism cannot be conscious of anything. Collectively, they bathe the forebrain in a life-sustaining elixir, a finely adjusted brew of acetylcholine and other substances crucial to homeostasis, arousal, and the sleep-wake cycle. They are enablers but not content-providers. That is the job of the cortex and the thalamus.

5.2 | EMOTIONS AND THE MODULATION OF CONSCIOUSNESS

Antonio Damasio has made the case that *extended consciousness*—those aspects of consciousness that generate the sense that there is an owner and observer inside the brain—must, of necessity, be matrixed within a critical background of information from the body that it inhabits. Damasio suggests that extended consciousness ceases without the propioceptive, visceral, and other bodily sensations that continually inform the brain about the state of its body. Likewise for emotions. He argues that a sense of the self requires emotions; disregard them, and the study of awareness becomes futile and empty.[16]

There is no question that moods dramatically affect human lives and behavior, as when you are angry or sad. Mood disorders are responsible for untold suffering in the form of depression, sleeplessness, angst, alienation, and other ill conditions to which humans are prey. Moods and emotions are critical to survival and color the way you view the world.

More general, *evaluative* responses, as in "Hmmh, that looks good," "Yuck, how disgusting," "Uh-oh, that is threatening," permeate everyday thinking. A complete science of consciousness therefore needs to account for these evaluative factors and how they affect conscious perception and the underlying NCC.

Francis and I chose to limit the scope of our quest by focusing on experimentally accessible aspects of consciousness that can be easily manipulated in the laboratory. Given today's technology, it is rather difficult to study moods and emotions—with the singular exception of fear—at the single neuron level. For example, poets and songwriters believe that colors look brighter and more

---

[15] Schlag and Schlag-Rey (1984) report that cells in the ILN of monkeys have large visual receptive fields and are quite insensitive to stimulus dimensions or brightness. Minamimoto and Kimura (2002) conclude that ILN regions play an essential role in orienting the animal to visual events that require it to act.

[16] Damasio's (1999) monograph, *The Feeling of What Happens*, largely inspired by clinical data, is enjoyable to read. LeDoux's (1996) book documents the neurobiology of emotions, while Dolan (2002) reviews the contributions that functional brain imaging have made toward the emerging understanding of emotion and behavior.

vibrant when in love. Even if this could be empirically verified in lovesick college students, it seems rather tricky—but not impossible—to come up with an animal model to investigate how moods regulate the thalamo-cortical responses to sensory stimuli.

When you are sad, happy, or angry, events and percepts can take on different meanings. But the movie-in-your-brain persists; you continue to see the world in motion, color, depth, and so on. Under laboratory conditions, when a slightly bored undergraduate student views images flashed on a monitor, she can be perfectly conscious of these in the absence of any strong emotion. Similarly, patients who—due to frontal lobe damage—lose much of their emotional expression and affect, and display supreme indifference to their often dire medical predicament, are still conscious. They can see colors or hear tones and, in general, have remarkably few deficits in the way they sense the world.

A complete account of the neuronal basis of consciousness will have to explain how emotions, moods and evaluations help form and shape the dynamics of the neuronal coalition(s) that are sufficient for conscious perception. I have purposefully ignored these important considerations for now because of my focus on experimentally more tractable aspects of consciousness.

5.3 | ANESTHESIA AND CONSCIOUSNESS

Each year, millions of people have their consciousness safely, painlessly, and reversibly switched off and on again when they are anesthetized for surgical intervention.[17] Anesthetics have been around for about 150 years. Surely something can be learned about the NCC by studying them.

General anesthetics are a diverse collection of chemicals, ranging from inert gases like xenon, to nitrous oxide ("laughing gas"), chloroform, diethyl ether, phencyclidine, barbiturates, cholinergic agents, and opioids. Today's anesthesiologists administer a cocktail of drugs to achieve desired results. These include curare-like paralyzing substances to provide muscle relaxation for optimal surgical access and to block patient movement; agents to control autonomic responses (e.g., stabilization of blood pressure), and to eliminate anguish and memories; and benzodiazepines to tranquilize the patient and induce amnesia. With such a mixture, patients are routinely and safely put to sleep, are operated on, and recover without recalling anything.

---

[17] At least this is the intention. However, anesthesia may often be incomplete. On rare occasions, patients wake up during the surgical operation, terrified to discover that they can't move at all, unable to communicate to the medical personnel (Rosen and Lunn, 1987). Such episodes could be prevented if the degree of intraoperative awareness could be assessed. Surprisingly, no reliable *consciousness-ometer* exists, although EEG-based tools that evaluate power in various frequency bands show promise (Madler and Pöppel, 1987; Kulli and Koch, 1991; and Drummond, 2000).

It used to be believed that general anesthetics interfered systemically with the bilipid components of cellular membranes. However, experiments with optical isomers of these molecules—compounds that have the same chemical composition but a mirror-symmetric three-dimensional structure—strongly suggest that general anesthetics bind directly to proteins. Their most common targets are neurotransmitter-gated ionic channels at synapses. The majority of anesthetics boost the potency of inhibitory synapses. Given that these are widely distributed throughout the nervous system, it has been difficult to isolate a specific brain area that is "knocked out" by the anesthetics.

Two intravenous dissociative drugs, *ketamine* and *phencyclidine* (PCP), do not bind to inhibitory synapses, targeting instead *N*-methyl-D-aspartate (NMDA) receptors associated with excitatory synapses that use glutamate as a neuron-to-neuron messenger. NMDA *synapses* are implicated in the long-term modification of synaptic connections among neurons that underlie learning and memory. At low doses, both ketamine and PCP induce hallucinations, distortions of body image, and disorganized thought. At high doses, they cause anesthesia. The German pharmacologist Hans Flohr postulated that the peculiar properties of NMDA synapses, particularly their propensity to strengthen links among simultaneously active neurons, play a pivotal role in assembling the coalitions of neurons necessary for consciousness. Flohr postulates that complete inhibition of NMDA-dependent processes would prevent formation of large-scale assemblies of cortical neurons, causing a loss of consciousness, as in anesthesia, while partial inhibition leads to altered states of consciousness, as in psychotic states.

Flohr may well be right that consciousness ceases without NMDA receptor activation. The same can also be said, however, of the other excitatory synapses sensitive to glutamate. Furthermore, NMDA synapses are found throughout the brain, so blocking them affects myriad processes, including the communication of sensory information to the upper echelons of the cortical hierarchy. Functioning NMDA synapses are one of the many NCC_e's needed for a winning coalition to emerge and to be consciously represented.[18]

It is often forgotten that the electrophysiological characterization of nerve cells relied almost exclusively for many years on anesthetized animals. Indeed, selective visual neurons in the primary visual cortex—such as those responding to moving edges (Figure 4.3)—were first described in anesthetized monkeys. Only in the 1960s and 1970s did neuroscientists perfect the techniques necessary to routinely monitor neurons in awake animals trained to fixate, to pull a

---

[18] The molecular basis of general anesthesia is summarized by Franks and Lieb (1994 and 1998); and Antkowiak (2001). Flohr's theory is presented in Flohr, Glade, and Motzko (1998) and Flohr (2000), and reviewed critically by Franks and Lieb (2000). The edited volume by Watkins and Collingridge (1989) provides background information on the NMDA receptor. Miller, Chapman, and Stryker (1989) induced NMDA receptor blockage in V1 of cats and observed a major loss of stimulus-induced cellular responses.

lever, or to push a button.[19] That neurons respond under anesthesia belies the naive supposition that brain activity is completely shut down when the animal or patient is put under.

So, what difference does anesthesia make to the brain? How do the receptive field properties of neurons recorded in an anesthetized monkey (whose eyes are propped open) differ from those in an awake and attentive animal?[20] The handful of relevant experiments suggest that cortical cells in anesthetized animals fire less vigorously and less selectively, and that they lack some of their contextual, nonclassical receptive field properties. These effects are compounded when ascending the cortical hierarchy, leading to weaker, delayed, and less specific neuronal responses in the upper stages of the cortex.[21]

I was initially enthusiastic about the prospect that being able to safely, rapidly, and reversibly turn consciousness on and off would provide some critical insight into the NCC. This hope has not been borne out. Anesthetics bind to receptor and channel proteins throughout much of the brain. So far, they have proven to be too blunt a tool to help in our quest, though that may change in the future.[22]

5.4 | A GENERAL STRATEGY FOR CIRCUMSCRIBING THE NCC

Let me classify the different categories of neural activity with regard to their relationship to consciousness (Table 5.1). The five forms listed are nonexclusive. For example, action potentials in the retina do not directly contribute to consciousness (first row), yet also precede the NCC for visual perception (third row). And while neurons in the inferotemporal cortex are among the most promising candidates for the NCC for seeing objects (Chapter 16), in deep sleep their spiking discharge is not sufficient for consciousness.

---

[19]Nervous tissue itself has no pain receptors, even though, paradoxically, the cortex is the ultimate basis of pain sensation. This makes the long-term monitoring of individual neurons possible.

[20]Because anesthetized animals are also paralyzed, their brains are deprived of feedback from their joints and muscles. Paralysis probably explains some of the sluggish responses in regions of the cortex concerned with planning and executing movement.

[21]The direct comparison of neuronal responses between awake and anesthetized states is technically demanding because the monkey must be rapidly and safely put to sleep and awakened again without perturbing the electrophysiological setup (Lamme, Zipser, and Spekreijse, 1998; and Tamura and Tanaka, 2001). Functional imaging provides an alternative to chart differences between the awake and the anesthetized brain (Alkire et al., 1997, 1999; and Logothetis et al., 1999, 2001).

[22]My fascination with anesthesia was expressed in a joint review of the field with an anesthesiologist (Kulli and Koch, 1991). Once the NCC have been identified, drugs that interfere with them should lead to safer anesthetic procedures with fewer side effects than those used today.

TABLE 5.1 Different Forms of Neural Activity
and Their Corresponding Phenomenological States

Neural Activity	Example	Mental State
Entirely nonconscious activity	Deep stages of slow-wave sleep	Not conscious
Feed-forward activity that subserves stereotyped sensory-motor behaviors	Activity that underlies eye movements, posture adjustments	Not conscious
Activities that precede and follow the NCC	Retinal and spinal cord activity	Not conscious
Transient coalition	Cortical activity associated with nonattended events	Fleeting consciousness
Maintained coalition of cells in high-level sensory areas and frontal regions (NCC proper)	Synchronized activity between inferior temporal and prefrontal cortex	Focused, perceptual consciousness

Only two forms support phenomenal content (bottom two rows). Both are based on coalitions of neurons; if the stimulus is too short-lived or does not benefit from attentional selection, the coalition quickly dissipates and awareness is only fleeting (Chapter 9). The primary focus of this book is on the more maintained forms of perceptual awareness or consciousness, since these are easiest to study and manipulate in the laboratory.[23]

Let me now address some of the specific neuronal factors responsible for a particular percept, the NCC. What is important is the notion of the *minimal* set of neural events jointly *sufficient* for a specific conscious experience (given the appropriate enabling conditions).[24]

My basic assumption is that the NCC at any moment correspond to activity of a coalition of neurons in the cortex and thalamus and closely allied structures. What is the exact nature of this "activity?" What leads up to the production of it? How long does it last? What effect does it have on other parts of the brain?[25] Additionally, what neurons (at that particular time) form this coalition? Are they only of certain neuronal types? Does the group consist of subgroups? If so, about how many subgroups are there and how many neurons are there in any particular subgroup? What do members of one subgroup have in common? How are the different subgroups connected?

---

[23]The table leaves out pathological or altered states of consciousness.

[24]I do not stress "necessary" conditions because of the great redundancy found in biological networks. While activity in some population may underpin a percept in one case, an individual who had lost those cells might compensate with a different neuronal population.

[25]The neuronal equivalent of Dennett's persistent line of "And then what happens ..." questioning.

A different strategy is to ask how this active coalition changes as the percept changes. In particular, are there types of neurons that never form part of such a group? Or, alternatively, can every type of neuron in the brain—or, more plausibly, every type of neuron in the cerebral cortex and the associated thalamic nuclei—form part of the NCC?

Some of our working hypotheses are outlined in Chapter 2. Francis and I assume that the NCC are based on an explicit neuronal representation and that the smallest group of neurons one can usefully consider for such a representation consists of cells (probably pyramidal cells) of one type—so that they all project in a similar manner to roughly the same area—located fairly close together in a cortical column and any corresponding locations in sub-cortical structures. Most cells in the column share some common property, such as the orientation of the local contour, direction of motion, depth tuning, and so on, but express it in somewhat different ways, depending on the use to which this information is put at their target sites.

This is not to suggest that the NCC are expressed in any one column by only a single type of neuron. On the contrary, it is likely that in any one cortical patch several types of projection cells express the NCC at the moment, stacked crudely one on top of the other. Different types of cells broadcast their information to many other areas in the cortical system. As the cognitive scientist Bernard Baars emphasizes in his *global workspace* model of consciousness, the information in the NCC tends to be dispersed across the cortex.[26] That is, the NCC disseminate information widely. As one type of pyramidal cell usually does not project to many separate places, the NCC probably involve, in one place, more than one type of neuron.

Will the NCC Be the Same for Different Classes of Percepts?

Given the regional specialization of the cortex, the NCC for color differ from the NCC for motion or faces. The coalition of neurons that mediates these percepts will not have the same membership (for instance, seeing color will

---

[26]As argued in Chapters 12, 13, and 14, many behaviors are mediated by highly specialized and efficient sensory-motor agents that bypass consciousness and have their own private sources of information, such as the exact limb or eye positions. Contrast this with information that is made conscious. Once you are aware of a stimulus, you can talk about it, you can remember it later on, you can look away from it and/or perform any number of other actions. Baars (1988, 1997, 2002; see also Dennett, 1991) uses a blackboard metaphor to emphasize this difference, where information can be freely written and retrieved by the specialists that compete or cooperate for access. The data posted corresponds, at any given point in time, to the content of consciousness, and is broadcast to the rest of the community. Much action occurs behind the scenes, shaping the state of the blackboard, but all of this remains outside the pale of consciousness. Dehaene, Changeux and their collaborators in Paris have extended and refined the idea of a global workspace within a neuronal framework (Changeux, 1983; Dehaene and Naccache, 2001; and Dehaene, Sergent, and Changeux, 2003).

involve V4 cells, discussed further in Chapter 8, whereas motion perception will involve cells in different cortical regions). Zeki invented the memorable term *microconsciousness* to emphasize that the NCC at an essential node for one particular attribute, say color, can be independent of the NCC at another essential node for a different attribute, say motion.[27]

Yet there may also be overlap in the membership, for instance in the front of the brain. That is, the coalitions mediating the different forms of microconsciousness may all share some neurons. In particular, as I shall argue in Chapters 14 and 15, these shared neurons are probably located in the front of the brain. Furthermore, the NCC neurons at the various essential nodes for color, motion, faces, and so on, will have one or more properties in common, such as their axonal projection patterns, or their tendency to fire in bursts of action potentials.

How does the NCC for a face percept relate to the NCC for recalling that face? Single cell recordings in patients unearthed cortical neurons that fire selectively to the sight of specific pictures, say of animals, and to the mental image of the same pictures recalled from memory. One such cell fired to a photo of the singer Paul McCartney, but remained indifferent to pictures of other people, houses, animals, and the like. The same selectivity was observed during imagery. The amplitude of the neuron's response to the real stimulus predicted well its behavior during recall. It is therefore conceivable that the NCC for imagery either overlap with or are a subset of the NCC for normal visual perception (see Section 18.3).

What are the NCC for dreaming going to be like? Dreams seem real while they last— as real as life itself. Does this suggest that the coalition of neurons that mediates the percept of 'mom' when she's standing in front of you is closely related to the coalition that is active when you dream of her? This seems quite plausible, with the exception of earlier cortical areas, such as the primary visual cortex, that are less active during dreaming.[28]

Scientists are seeking to influence the NCC by directly, and artificially, triggering brain activity with the help of *transcranial magnetic stimulation* (TMS). This is a harmless way to tickle nervous tissue by delivering a brief but powerful magnetic field by a coil just outside the skull.[29]

---

[27] Zeki (1998); and Zeki and Bartels (1999). I'll return to microconsciousness in Chapter 15.

[28] I'll return to the neurology of dreams in the context of V1 in the following chapter. Louie and Wilson (2001) directly tackle this question by studying rats dreaming of running through mazes.

[29] The applications of TMS to transiently interfere with parts of the cortex close to the surface in normal subjects are soaring, even though the physiological basis of this technique is not understood. Its principal advantage is high temporal precision; its biggest drawback is poor spatial localization. Cowey and Walsh (2001) review the literature. Kamitani and Shimojo (1999) elegantly demonstrate how TMS can provide insight into the architecture of V1.

The interpretation of the wide range of conditions under which conscious perception is possible is made more difficult by the propensity of neurons to be associated with different assemblies. Members of a coalition for generating one percept might, under different circumstances, be members of another coalition responsible for a different percept. Or, they might serve to support rapid visuo-motor behavior not associated with any conscious percept at all (see Chapter 12). Eventually, all such complications will have to be taken into account.

Linking Single Cell Properties to the NCC

The goal of my research program is to link the molecular and biophysical properties of coalitions of neurons to stimulus awareness. Ultimately, their firing activity must be correlated with the subject's behavior on a trial-to-trial basis. Suppose, for example, that I'm monitoring the above-mentioned "McCartney" neuron. I would expect the failure of the patient to see the briefly flashed picture of the former Beatle on some trial to be reflected in a reduced firing rate or a diminished spike synchrony with other such cells *during that trial*. Of course, the firing of this neuron will be quite literally "meaningless" to the rest of the system unless it is connected to many other essential nodes (Section 14.5).

Once the NCC for some class of percepts have been located, they can be genetically manipulated in rodents, they can be tracked in infants to study the onset of different phases of consciousness, they can be observed in autistic or schizophrenic patients, and so on.

More refined experiments are needed to move beyond *correlation* to *causation*. If event A causes event B, then A should precede B and preventing A should eliminate B (unless there is another cause for B). Knowing the exact timing of events leading up to the NCC will be helpful here, as will selective interference with such precursor mechanisms. Many other experiments are possible to clarify the causal relationship between neuronal happenings and conscious percepts. Artificially exciting the candidate NCC neurons should induce a percept similar to that induced by natural stimulation. If the NCC neurons are silenced, for instance by blocking their synaptic receptors, the percept should cease. The same silencing procedure could be repeated downstream from the NCC, and so on.

Untangling cause and effect in tightly integrated feedback networks will often be difficult. An analogy can be made to crowd behavior. Who is to say what specific event or persons in a mob of angry people precipitated the ensuing riot? The protester who threw the first stone? But wasn't he encouraged by the shouting of his neighbors? And was the stone-throwing incident responsible for the shooting that followed? Is this an instance of the self-organized behavior of an entire community that can't readily be analyzed at the single person level? Perhaps. But what if the riot was instigated by a small number of *agent provocateurs* that systematically encouraged violence?

5.5 | NEURONAL SPECIFICITY AND THE NCC

Francis and I are guided in our quest for the NCC by a hunch that the NCC involve specific biological mechanisms.[30] Let me explain what I mean.

An extreme counterpoint to neuronal specificity is the hypothesis that every neuron participates to some extent in the NCC. According to this assumption, consciousness is an emergent property of the entire nervous system that cannot be localized to specific subsets of neurons. This holistic approach derives from the belief that acute, intense percepts—the deep red of a sunset and its associated meaning—cannot derive from neuroactivity of a specific and smallish group of cells. Instead, the collective, Gestalt-like interactions of millions and millions of neurons is needed for any one conscious percept. There is a deep-felt aversion to the idea that specific mechanisms could be responsible for the richness and crispness of consciousness.[31]

The molecular- and neurobiologist Gerald Edelman at the Scripps Research Institute in La Jolla, California, and his colleague, the psychiatrist and neuroscientist Giulio Tononi, now at the University of Wisconsin, stress this global aspect of consciousness. They argue that the large number of potential states

---

[30]Antecedents for the idea of neuronal specificity can be found in the literature. Historically, one of the most prescient formulations of the hypothesis that a particular subset of neurons is responsible for generating conscious experience is the concept of ω neurons introduced by Freud in 1895 in his unpublished *Project for a Scientific Psychology*. In this brief yet insightful essay, Freud attempted to derive a psychology on the basis of the newly formulated neuron theory (to which he contributed in his thesis work on the neuroanatomy of the stomatogastric ganglion in the crayfish; Shepherd, 1991). Freud introduced three classes of neurons: ϕ, ψ, and ω. The first class mediates perception and the second memory; indeed, Freud postulated that memory was represented by the facilitations existing between the ψ neurons at their contact-barriers (i.e., the synapses). The third class of neurons is responsible for mediating consciousness and qualia, even though Freud admitted, "No attempt, of course, can be made to explain how it is that excitatory processes in the ω neurons bring consciousness along with them. It is only a question of establishing a coincidence between the characteristics of consciousness that are known to us and processes in the ω neurons which vary in parallel with them." When reading the remainder of the essay, it becomes patently obvious why Freud was dissatisfied with his attempt to link the mind to the brain. At the time, almost nothing was known about the biophysics of neurons and the manner in which they communicate, the existence of Broca's speech area had barely been established, and the localization of visual function to the occipital lobe was still controversial. Subsequently, Freud abandoned neurology in favor of pure psychology (Freud, 1966; for discussion, see Kitcher, 1992).

[31]For two examples of neuroscientists advocating holistic accounts of consciousness, see Popper and Eccles (1977), and Libet (1993). Some (e.g., Dennett, 1978, 1991) claim that to attribute the percept of red to the working of a specific group of neurons constitutes what Ryle (1949) called a category error.

accessible to a conscious mind necessitates the tight interaction of very big neuronal assemblies reaching clear across the brain. These ideas may be on the right track.[32] This skepticism suggests that my quest may be quixotic—doomed to failure.

Holistic approaches to consciousness fail to explain, however, why some kinds of widespread activity within the brain generate behaviors associated with consciousness while others don't. Where is the difference between the two? Take motion-induced blindness, mentioned in Chapter 1. How can a global approach explain why you sometimes see the yellow spots, while a fraction of a second later they are gone? How can such global theories account for the fact that vigorous activity in some cortical regions is no guarantee for conscious accessibility (Chapter 16)?

It would be convenient from a methodological and practical point of view if the NCC neurons shared a unique set of traits, such as a strong synaptic interconnection, a unique cellular morphology, or a particular complement of ionic channels, conferring some privileged cellular property. This specificity would provide experimentalists—molecular biologists, in particular—with strategies for deliberately and delicately interfering with stimulus awareness by transiently and reversibly switching these NCC neurons on or off.

Of course, there is no guarantee that nature is simple; such local approaches may fail. However, it makes sense to first pursue the straightforward hypotheses advocated in this book.

One universal lesson from biology is that organisms evolve specific gadgets—machinery of such a fancy and outlandish nature—that they could be rejected on a priori grounds of smacking of an intelligent designer. This has been borne out spectacularly in the development of molecular biology. Long-chained macromolecules such as proteins owe their functional diversity to their particular one-dimensional molecular configurations. This linear representation determines their function. Their bulk properties or behavior when suspended in colloidal solutions are not particularly helpful to understand the processes occurring inside living organisms.[33]

---

[32] Edelman (1989); and Edelman and Tononi (2000). For a short summary of their *dynamic core* hypothesis, see Tononi and Edelman (1998).

[33] The thesis that specificity is the major theme of modern biology is defended in Judson (1979). Molecular specificity can also be found at the level of individual voltage-dependent channels that underlie all processing in the nervous system. A typical membrane-spanning potassium channel distinguishes a potassium ion with a 1.33 Å radius from other alkaline ions, such as the sodium ion with a 0.95 Å radius, by a factor of ten thousand. And it accomplishes this feat at a rate of up to one hundred million ions per second (Doyle et al., 1998; and Hille, 2001). These channel proteins evolved under such demanding conditions, moreover, that substituting one amino acid with another—at one of two strategic locations along a chain that consists of several thousand amino acids—turns a sodium-selective channel into a calcium-selective one (Heinemann et al., 1992).

The amazing molecular specificity of proteins reveals itself even at the behavioral level. A bit more than half of all men possess a gene for the visual pigment in their long-wavelength sensitive cone photoreceptors that codes for serine in the 180th position, while the other men express the amino acid alanine at that location. This tiny difference at the molecular level shows up in hue perception when screening men on the basis of their performance when matching reddish colors.[34]

Why should neurons be any less specific than proteins? Nerve cells, like biomolecules, have been shaped by the blind forces of natural selection over hundreds of millions of years, giving rise to as yet unfathomable heterogeneity in their shape, form, and function. This is likely to be reflected in the specificity of the NCC. I therefore look for particular mechanisms that confer onto coalitions of neurons properties that correspond to attributes of conscious percepts. One possibility might be small sets of cortical pyramidal cells that receive strong excitatory synaptic input from another set of pyramidal cells directly onto their cell bodies in a reciprocal manner. Such an arrangement might instantiate a loop, a set of neurons that, once triggered, would keep on firing until actively inhibited by another coalition of neurons. The firing dynamics of such a group might be close to that of consciousness, acting over a fraction of a second, rather than the millisecond time-scale of single action potentials.[35]

There is a loose parallel, suggested to me by the molecular biologist David Anderson, between the NCC and the function of any one protein. Its functional specificity is dictated by its three-dimensional configuration. The molecule's shape emerges out of the way that the one-dimensional sequence of amino acids coils and folds (in aqueous solution) in a way that largely defies any local analysis. Yet not every one of the hundreds of amino acids that constitutes a typical protein contributes equally. Replacing a single amino acid or a small, contiguous sequence of amino acids at some strategic location along the sequence might radically affect the protein's shape and therefore destroy its function. Short stretches of amino acids that give rise to a structural motif—such as alpha helices or beta sheets—have a critical influence on the final three-dimensional structure, while stretches of more loosely organized intervening sequences may influence the final shape only in subtle or relatively inconsequential ways. Local properties are key to explaining much of the protein's function. The same lesson may also hold for the NCC.

---

[34] The difference in the two pigments expressed in photoreceptors shifts the peak sensitivity by around 4 nm (Asenjo, Rim, and Oprian, 1994; and Nathans, 1999).

[35] Cell bodies of neocortical pyramidal cells are typically devoid of excitatory synapses, presumably because they would be too powerful. However, a small population of neurons with such a property could easily escape detection among the billions of cortical cells, unless you searched for them.

5.6 | RECAPITULATION

This chapter elaborates upon my definition of the NCC as the minimal neuronal events jointly sufficient for a specific conscious percept.

The ability to experience anything at all depends on the ongoing regulation of the cortex and its satellites by a collection of nuclei in the brainstem, the basal forebrain, and the thalamus. The axons of these cells project widely and release acetylcholine and other elixirs vital to wakefulness, arousal, and sleep. Collectively, these ascending fibers create the necessary conditions for any conscious content to occur. They enable consciousness (and are called NCC_e) but are not specific, local, and rapid enough to provide perceptual content. Only coalitions of forebrain neurons have the required properties to form NCC.

Moods, emotions, and valuations are prominent examples of factors that can modulate and bias perception. For now, I neglect these in favor of a research program exploring the cellular roots of conscious perception.

General anesthetics safely and reversibly turn off sensation during surgical intervention with its associated pain and distress. Because of their widespread effects, they have so far uncovered little of direct relevance to the quest for the NCC.

Francis and I seek the neuronal correlates of consciousness, the minimal set of neural events that are the physical substrate for a specific percept under a range of conditions (e.g., during seeing and during imagery, in patients, in monkeys, and so on). I described some of the research strategies employed for tracking down the location and properties of the NCC. They boil down to, first, carefully correlating the receptive field properties of neurons and their firing patterns with stimulus awareness on a trial-by-trial basis and, second, influencing the percept by manipulating the underlying NCC.

The specificity that is a hallmark of molecular and cellular biology suggests that the correlates of consciousness are based on equally particular biological mechanisms and gadgets, involving identifiable types of neurons, interconnected in some special way and firing in some pertinent manner. But the NCC might also encompass large cell assemblies.

Because the ideas raised in this chapter may seem rather dry, I flesh them out in the next pages, where I will argue that the NCC are not to be found among V1 neurons.

CHAPTER SIX

The Neuronal Correlates of Consciousness Are Not in the Primary Visual Cortex

The question is not what you look at, but what you see.

Henry David Thoreau

In the last chapter, I refined the notion of the NCC and described experimental means to search for such correlates. I here apply these notions to the primary visual cortex and come to the surprising conclusion that, although V1 is intimately involved in vision, many—if not all—V1 cells do not directly contribute to the content of visual consciousness.

So what? With a hundred or more cortical regions in the human brain, who cares if one of them isn't part of the NCC? The short answer is that you should care, at least if you are concerned about the neurology of consciousness. You should care because this finding implies that not just any cortical activity is automatically associated with consciousness, and also for the methods used to establish this claim.

There are good reasons why V1 cells may only indirectly contribute to conscious vision. As discussed in Chapter 14, one of the principal functions of consciousness is planning. This suggests that the NCC neurons themselves are intimately linked to the planning and executive centers of the brain. These are located, roughly speaking, in the prefrontal cortex. Because V1 neurons do not send their output to the front part of the cortex, Francis and I predicted in 1995 that V1 cells can't be directly responsible for conscious vision. While V1 is necessary for normal seeing—as are the eyes—V1 neurons do not contribute to phenomenal experience.[1] The next four sections focus on evidence for our thesis from observing humans, while the following section describes pertinent single neuron investigations in monkeys.

---

[1] We stated this hypothesis (Crick and Koch, 1995a) before most of the data presented here were known. Block (1996) casts a philosopher's eye on our claim.

6.1 | YOU DON'T SEE WITHOUT V1

Patients whose V1 is completely destroyed by a stroke or other focal lesion do not see anything. They suffer from *hemianopia* for the opposite field of view, unable to detect targets in this region (destruction of the left V1 results in loss of vision in the right field of view and vice versa).[2] This observation seems to suggest that V1 is essential for the NCC. Yet by the same logic, the electrical potential across the membrane of photoreceptors would be part of the NCC. Recall, however, that while retinal neurons are necessary for seeing, their activity differs substantially from visual experience.

I will here defend the thesis that V1 activity precedes perception of visual stimuli. Spiking V1 neurons are thus an example of pre-NCC activity (Table 5.1).

More compelling is the clinical observation that patients with an intact V1 but without the belt of cortical areas surrounding V1 on the upper (resp. lower) bank of the calcarine fissure can't see in the lower (resp. upper) quarter of the visual field.[3] In other words, a functioning early visual system, including V1, is insufficient for conscious vision.

6.2 | EVEN IF YOU CAN'T SEE IT, V1 STILL ADAPTS TO IT

On occasion, the outcome of a psychological experiment can help pinpoint where in the processing stream, from image acquisition to conscious perception, a particular process is situated. A case in point is the demonstration by Sheng He, Patrick Cavanagh, and James Intriligator from Harvard University, that an invisible stimulus can give rise to a visible *aftereffect*.[4]

Their experimental design was based on a common visual aftereffect (related in kind to the waterfall illusion treated in Section 8.3). If a subject stares for a

---

[2] For an overview of hemianopia, see Celesia et al. (1991). A few hemianopic patients retain residual visuo-motor behaviors without any visual experience in the affected field. This fascinating syndrome, known as *blindsight*, is treated more fully in Section 13.2. Some reorganization might occur in blindsight patients with long-term damage to the primary visual cortex, allowing for a minimal degree of phenomenal vision without V1 (Ffytche, Guy, and Zeki, 1996; and Stoerig and Barth, 2001).

[3] The resultant *quadrantanopia* is a consequence of the layout of the early visual areas (Horton and Hoyt, 1991b).

[4] He, Cavanagh, and Intriligator (1996). See also the commentary by Koch and Tootell (1996). The experiment by He and his colleagues was a variant of an earlier one performed by Blake and Fox (1974), which concluded that invisible stimuli can lead to measurable effects (see Chapter 16). Hofstötter et al. (2003) demonstrated the same for negative *afterimages*; whether a colored patch is consciously seen or not makes no difference to the persistence or intensity of the associated afterimage. That depends only on how long the visual brain was exposed to the colored patch.

minute at horizontal fringes and then looks at a faint, horizontal test grating, her ability to detect it will be reduced. This form of *adaptation* is orientation specific—sensitivity for vertical gratings remains (almost) unchanged—and disappears quickly. Because horizontally oriented cells fire for a prolonged period while the subject stares at the gratings, they are thought to "fatigue" and to recalibrate. Under these conditions, a much stronger input than usual is required to get the cells to respond vigorously.

He and his colleagues projected a single grating, as seen through a circular aperture, onto a computer screen. Even though this inducing grating was located in the periphery, it was clearly visible and led to a predictable *orientation-dependent aftereffect*. In a variant of the experiment, they added four similar gratings close to the original one (Figure 6.1). This *masked* the orientation of the inducing grating—subjects saw that something was there, but couldn't perceive its orientation, even when given unlimited viewing time (the masking only worked because the grating was viewed out of the corner of the eyes). Nevertheless, the aftereffect was as strong and as specific to the tilt of the invisible grating as when it was clearly visible.

What the experiment by He and colleagues shows is that visual awareness occurs at a stage beyond the site of orientation-specific adaptation, thought to be mediated by oriented cells in V1 and beyond.[5] Or, in my terms, the NCC are beyond V1.

Sheng He and Don MacLeod devised another experiment that reinforced this conclusion. Using laser interferometry to bypass the eye's optics (which otherwise blur out the fine details), they projected very thin gratings onto the retinae. These gratings induce an orientation-dependent aftereffect that could only be explained by invoking orientation-dependent neurons in V1 or beyond. Observers, however, did not see these fine fringes and could not distinguish them from a uniform field. This experiment implied that high fidelity spatial information, too fine to be seen, penetrated the visual system as far as the cortex, where it caused some effect without giving rise to a conscious sensation.[6]

Not all aftereffects are independent of seeing. Some species of motion aftereffects (Section 8.3) are considerably weakened if the inducing motion is invisible.[7]

---

[5]Dragoi, Sharma, and Sur (2000).

[6]He and MacLeod (2001).

[7]The relationship between aftereffects and visual awareness is being actively explored by a combination of psychophysical and imaging methods (Blake, 1998; Hofstötter et al., 2003; and Montaser-Kouhsari et al., 2004).

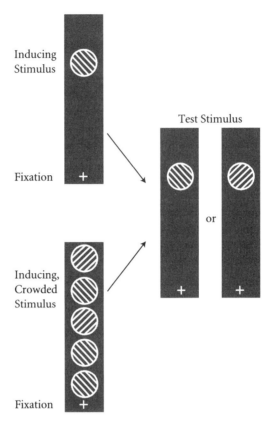

FIGURE 6.1 *Stimulating the Brain, but not the Mind* Subjects fixated the cross in either one of the two images on the left for a few minutes until a robust orientation-dependent aftereffect was obtained. Its strength was assessed by briefly flashing a faint version of one of the two test images on the right. The contrast of the leftward leaning patch had to be larger for subjects to see it compared with the rightward leaning grating. This was true even though subjects couldn't see which way the inducing grating was tilted, as it was obscured by the nearby patches (for the image on the lower left). Modified from He, Cavanagh, and Intriligator (1996).

6.3 │ YOU DON'T DREAM WITH V1

Evidence that V1 neurons are not part of the NCC comes from dreaming, too. From an experiential point of view, dreams are full of the sights and sounds of life. While dream consciousness differs from consciousness in the waking state (for instance, dreams lack introspection and insight), it certainly feels like something to dream. It is likely that the neuronal coalitions that mediate the NCC for visual dreams partially overlap with those for seeing while awake.

It used to be thought that brain activity during REM sleep was similar to activity in the waking brain. Hence, REM sleep is also called paradoxical sleep because it can't readily be distinguished from the awake state using standard EEG criteria. This contrasts with non-REM or slow-wave sleep, characterized by large and slow oscillations in the EEG.

When volunteers are deprived of sleep for one night and their cerebral blood flow is monitored using positron emission tomography while they catch up on their sleep the next night, a more nuanced picture emerges. The activity pattern of the dreaming brain has a unique signature, quite distinct from the awake brain. In particular, V1 and directly adjacent regions are suppressed (compared to slow-wave sleep), while higher-level visual areas in the fusiform gyrus and the medial temporal lobe are highly activated. These latter structures can thus be assumed to mediate the sensation of *seeing* events unfold during dreaming.[8]

Patients who lose their primary visual cortex to strokes continue to experience visual dreams, providing additional evidence that activity in V1 is unnecessary for dreaming.[9]

6.4 | DIRECTLY STIMULATING V1

It has been known since antiquity that a sufficiently strong mechanical shock to the back of the brain causes the unfortunate recipient to perceive flashes of light, called *phosphenes* (hence the stars and lightning bolts drawn above cartoon characters beaten on their head). This does not demonstrate, however, that V1 neurons are part of the NCC.

Today, somewhat more sophisticated stimulation tools are used. The Canadian neurosurgeon Wilder Penfield and his colleagues at the Montreal Neurological Institute assembled a vast catalogue of information on the local topography of brain function from thousands of open skull brain surgeries on patients treated for severe epileptic seizures. Sufficiently strong excitation of portions of the occipital lobe via electrodes sitting on the exposed cortical surface, induces elementary visual sensations such as flickering lights, blue-green and red colored discs, stars, wheels, whirling colored balls, and the like.[10]

---

[8]The imaging study of the dreaming brain was reported by Braun et al. (1998) and commented upon by Hobson, Stickgold, and Pace-Schott (1998). Regional cerebral blood flow in V1 during REM sleep was not different from that in the restful state with eyes closed. The extent to which extrastriate and medial temporal cortices are active during REM sleep while they are functionally isolated from visual input is quite remarkable. Incidentally, given the detailed visual map in V1, it is possible that its inactivity during REM sleep implies that spatial resolution during visual dreaming is lower than during normal seeing. Is this why I never read in my dreams?

[9]For the neurology of dreaming in brain-damaged patients, see Solms (1997); and Kaplan-Solms and Solms (2000).

[10]Penfield (1975). Penfield and Perot (1963) exhaustively list all relevant cases.

These findings suggest that normally sighted adults who lose their eyesight can be helped by an artificial device. Such a *neuroprosthetic* would acquire the image via a miniaturized camera, bypassing the defective retina, and would directly stimulate the visual cortex. Teams of doctors, scientists, and engineers are tackling the formidable problems associated with implanting such an electronic artifact into the brain.[11]

What can be learned from this prosthetic technology is that the NCC do not require retinal or geniculate activity. Elementary visual percepts—expressing position, brightness, and color—can be seen by directly stimulating V1. The excitation won't stop there, however. Instead, it will spread to V2 and higher areas where the NCC are located. Stimulating the primary visual cortex in a patient whose higher visual areas are destroyed could, in principle, disprove our V1 hypothesis if the patient experienced some visual percepts (mediated, perhaps, by V1's preserved subcortical output pathways). I do not think, however, that such a patient will ever be found.

6.5 | MONKEY V1 NEURONS DON'T FOLLOW PERCEPTION

The best, most direct, evidence that V1 cells don't correlate with phenomenal visual content comes from recording the spiking activity of neurons in the behaving monkey.

V1 Cells Are Responsive to Local Depth but Don't Generate Depth Perception

Chapter 4 introduced binocular cells that receive input from both eyes. They can use the small differences in perspective between the left and the right eye to extract the *binocular disparity* that make it possible to judge depth. Extend your finger some distance away and fixate it first with your left eye only and then with your right eye only. The position of your finger moves with respect to the distant background between these two views. This shift corresponds to

---

[11]A promising case of one such prosthetic device was reported by Schmidt et al. (1996). A 42-year old woman who had been totally blind for 22 years volunteered to have a hair brush-like array of 38 microelectrodes inserted into her V1 for a four-month trial period (it was subsequently removed). If individual electrodes were stimulated, she saw spot-like phosphenes. The intensity of the electrical stimulation had to exceed a threshold value for her to see anything at all. Paradoxically, the phosphene's size decreased as stimulation current was increased, possibly due to activation of long-range inhibition. At low current levels, the phosphenes were often colored. When the stimulation duration was increased beyond one second, the phosphenes commonly disappeared before the end of the stimulus. The patient almost never reported oriented lines or highly elongated blobs. Indeed, in the entire cortical stimulation literature, oriented or moving visual percepts are a rare occurrence, possibly because the domain of excitation needs to be restricted to a column coding for the same orientation or direction of motion. Other artificial vision programs are described by Norman et al. (1996) and Dobelle (2000).

the binocular disparity and encodes depth. The farther the finger is away from the eyes, the smaller the shift. Based on the firing rate of binocular cells in V1, electrophysiologists can characterize the cells' abilities to encode depth.

Through a series of ingenious image manipulations, Bruce Cumming and Andrew Parker at the Laboratory of Physiology in Oxford got disparity-selective V1 cells in the awake monkey to respond meaningfully to local depth cues (local to a patch of the image) that did not give rise to an overall depth percept. That is, these cells encoded local disparity information without an associated depth percept.

Other cells responded in an identical manner to two depth cues that yielded quite different global depth percepts. Cumming and Parker concluded that these cells represented a first critical stage for the generation of disparity-based stereo cues but that depth perception occurred further upstream.[12]

Which Eye Saw the Image?

While the vast majority of neurons beyond V1 respond to images projected into either eye, a significant fraction of V1 cells are monocular; that is, they respond only to input from one eye. An astute neuronal network could, in principle, determine which eye received the input by monitoring the activity of 'left eye' and 'right eye' cells.

This observation is pertinent when considering whether you and I have access to *eye-of-origin* information. Suppose the image of a small light is projected, via a tube, into either the left or the right eye. Do you know whether you are seeing the light with your left or your right eye? The surprising answer is no, unless you wink or turn your head. Under the appropriate conditions and with strict controls, people don't know with which eye they see.[13]

Because monocular cortical cells are restricted to V1, it is tempting to conclude that V1 cells are not part of the NCC. However, just because V1 cells

---

[12]Cumming and Parker recorded from disparity-selective V1 cells using three different paradigms designed to differentiate the response of these cells from depth perception (Cumming and Parker, 1997, 1999, and 2000). Poggio and Poggio (1984) offer a good, but somewhat dated, summary of the neuronal basis of depth perception. By directly comparing the discharges of V1 and MT cells in a behaving monkey, Grunewald, Bradley, and Andersen (2002) conclude that V1 is not directly involved in the generation of structure-from-motion (shape) percepts.

[13]You can catch a glimpse of this for yourself. Look with both eyes at an upright pencil in your outstretched hand, directly in front of you. Now close one or the other eye. The position of the pencil changes a lot when you close one eye, but hardly at all when you close the other, because most, but not all, people have a *dominant eye* (usually the right one). Thus, when you see something, it's often only one eye that does most of the seeing, although you're unaware of this fact. The study of eye-of-origin goes back to the middle of the 20th century (Smith, 1945; Pickersgill, 1961; Blake and Cormack, 1979; and Porac and Coren, 1986).

have access to eye-of-origin data does not mean that this information is necessarily made accessible to the rest of the brain.[14] It might not be important enough to behavior for evolution to have favored an explicit representation of eye-of-origin in the visual cortex beyond V1.

V1 Cells Are Affected by Blinks and Eye Movements

Recall from Section 3.7 that people are usually oblivious to blinks—those brief periods during which their eyes are covered up. One search strategy for the NCC, therefore, is to track down neurons whose activity is impervious to blinks. Timothy Gawne and Julie Martin from the University of Alabama at Birmingham showed that the cells in the upper layers of macaque V1 essentially shut down during reflex blinks. The reduction in activity was more pronounced than when there was an equally long gap in the input or the entire image was darkened. If this holds true for all cells in V1 it would be safe to conclude that V1 cells do not correspond to visual perception, because vision does not cease during blinks.[15]

As emphasized in Chapter 3, the brain automatically and nonconsciously compensates for the incessant motion of the eyes. The external world looks stable, both when your eyes abruptly dart around the room and when you smoothly track a bird flying past. This perceptual stability can be exploited to test for NCC neurons.

The neuronal responses to motion of the eye over a stationary scene can be compared to responses when the eye is resting and the scene is moved in the opposite direction. If the internally generated eye motion is carefully matched to the external image motion, they look exactly the same (e.g., moving the eyes to the left is the same as shifting the image to the right). You would need extra-retinal information to tell these two situations apart. Indeed, V1 cells respond equally to motion induced by smoothly pursuing a target with the eyes and to movement of the image in the opposite direction with the eyes fixed. Likewise, V1 cells can't tell the difference between the animal rapidly shifting its eyes and when the scene jerks in a way mimicking this saccade. In that sense, V1 behaves like the retina. Only cells in cortical area MT and beyond can distinguish between eye movement and movement of the scene.[16]

---

[14]This last point was made to Francis and me in private correspondence with Dr. Charles Q. Wu.

[15]Gawne and Martin (2000).

[16]These neurons rely either on signals from motor centers that control eye movements or on feedback signals from the eye muscles themselves to distinguish self-induced from externally generated motion. Ilg and Thier (1996) carried out the relevant electrophysiology for smooth pursuit and Thiele et al. (2002) for saccades.

In other words, as the monkey's eyes move about, the projected view of the outside world shifts across the surface of V1, in stark contrast to the way the world is experienced.

Equally compelling are experiments in which the link between the retinal image and the animal's behavior—and, presumably, the monkey's percept— is ambiguous. Recordings demonstrate quite clearly that the vast majority of V1 neurons blindly follow the visual stimulus rather than the percept. Tens if not hundreds of thousands of V1 cells generate millions of action potentials without any of this furious activity being reflected in awareness.[17] This topic is important enough to warrant separate treatment in Chapter 16.

Is Feedback to V1 Critical for Consciousness?

Are fibers carrying activity from higher cortical areas back to V1 critical to the genesis of awareness? This feedback—preferentially terminating in the super-ficial layers—might boost the firing activity of V1 cells above a threshold. A number of eminent neuroscientists have suggested that it is in the meeting of forward activity with cortico-cortical feedback that some threshold is exceeded and consciousness is generated. I return to this theme in Chapter 15.

Evidence for the role of feedback has been inferred from the late compo-nent of the summed activity of multiple V1 cells that correlate with the percept of the stimulus, rather than with the animal's response. Unfortunately, in the absence of a pharmacological blocker that selectively turns off feedback into V1 without interfering with the forward stream of information, these ideas are enormously difficult to test.[18]

---

[17] A further hint that V1 cells don't represent phenomenal vision is contained in Gur and Snod-derly's (1997) report of V1 color-opponent neurons whose cellular discharge is rapidly up- and down-modulated as the color of a grating flickers from red to green and back. This is surpris-ing, because humans can't resolve the individual colors at high rates of switching, seeing a fused yellow rather than discrete reds and greens (see also Engel, Zhang and Wandell, 1997).

[18] Physiological experiments that implicate cortico-cortical feedback connections in visual awareness are described in Pollen (1995, 1999, and 2003); Lamme and Roelfsema (2000); Lamme and Spekreijse (2000); Kosslyn (2001); and Bullier (2001). The data that I only tangentially allude to here come from a brilliant experiment by Supèr, Spekreijse, and Lamme (2001). They trained monkeys to exploit textural cues to detect a figure on a random background while measuring electrical activity in V1. Comparing trials when the figure was correctly identified with those when the figure was present but the animals failed to detect it, the experimentalists observed that, starting 60 msec after the onset of the spiking response, the activity increased when the ani-mal detected, and presumably saw, the figure. The neurophysiologists argued that this enhanced and delayed activity most likely reflected feedback from higher areas.

TABLE 6.1 Some of the Necessary Conditions for the NCC
for Any One Stimulus Attribute

1. **Explicit Representation.** The attribute should be explicitly represented on the basis of a columnar organization.
2. **Essential Node.** The attribute can't be perceived when the brain region containing the NCC is destroyed or inactivated.
3. **Artificial Stimulation.** Appropriate electrical or magnetic stimulation should lead to perception of the attribute.
4. **Correlation between Perception and Neuronal Activity.** The onset, duration, and strength of the relevant neural "activity" should correlate on a trial-by-trial basis with awareness of the attribute.
5. **Stability of Perception.** The NCC should be invariant to blinks and eye movements that disrupt sensory input but not perception.
6. **Direct Access to Planning Stages.** The NCC neurons should project to the planning and executive stages.

6.6 | RECAPITULATION

This chapter considers the extent to which activity in V1 neurons correlates with visual consciousness. Table 6.1 lists some of the necessary conditions for the neuronal correlates of consciousness that, together with the necessary background conditions (the NCC$_e$), need to be jointly satisfied for some neural activity to be part of the NCC. As discussed in Chapter 4, the first three criteria in the table are met for the primary visual cortex: V1 contains an explicit representation for the location and orientation of visual stimuli; without V1, patients can't see; and electrical stimulation of V1 gives rise to visual phosphenes. On the other hand, as you just read in this chapter, criteria 4, 5, and 6 are not met by V1 cells.

There is no doubt that under both normal and pathological conditions, V1 contains information that is not expressed in consciousness at that time. It is a much more difficult matter to prove that no V1 activity is sufficient for the current content of visual consciousness. A cautionary reading of the extant psychophysical and single-cell data is compatible with the hypothesis that V1 neurons are not part of the NCC.[19] Activities in V1, as in the retina, are nec-

---

[19]Some human fMRI data appear to contradict this position. However, as I argue in footnote 2 to Chapter 8 and in Section 16.2, methodological uncertainties about the relationship between the magnetic resonance response and neuronal spiking cast doubts on the standard interpretation of these imaging studies.

essary but not sufficient for normal conscious vision (dreaming and imagery, likewise, probably do not depend on an intact V1).

Unlike "exclusion" principles in physics—that nothing material can exceed the speed of light, or that a perpetual motion machine cannot be built—our proposal that visual consciousness does not arise in V1 is not an absolute law but is contingent on neuroanatomy. Thus, there is no assurance that the same reasoning holds for other primary sensory areas, such as primary auditory or somatosensory cortices. The case for each region has to be argued on its own merit, depending on its pattern of connectivity and on the response profile of its constitutive neuronal populations.[20]

In subsequent chapters, I give more examples of the relationship between neuronal responses and perception. Before doing so, however, I need to explain next how anatomists define distinct regions in the cortex and the relationships among them. Despite having the look and feel of an overcooked cauliflower, the cortex turns out to be a remarkably ordered structure.

---

[20]Brain imaging of patients in a persistent vegetative state unequivocally demonstrates strong but localized primary auditory and somatosensory activation following appropriate stimulation without any evidence for consciousness (Laureys et al., 2000, 2002). Thus, it *may* be true that no primary sensory center is sufficient for conscious perception of that modality.

CHAPTER SEVEN

The Architecture of the Cerebral Cortex

Thus my central theme is that complexity frequently takes the form of hierarchy and that hierarchic systems have some common properties independent of their specific content. Hierarchy, I shall argue, is one of the central structural schemes that the architect of complexity uses.

From *The Sciences of the Artificial* by Herbert Simon

Confronted with a structure as complex as the cortex, scientists divide it into smaller and smaller parts and analyze those, hoping that such a reduction will ultimately lead to an understanding of the whole. This strategy proved difficult to accomplish initially, because the gray matter of the brain looks pretty much the same everywhere. The comprehensive exploration of the cortex had to await the advent of modern microscopy, chemical stains, and dyes that selectively bind to cellular components, such as to the myelin sheet that winds around axons or to the ribonucleic acid at the cell body. With this increasing ability to target specific molecular constituents of neurons, the study of brain architecture based on subtle but marked local variations has blossomed.

7.1 | IF YOU WANT TO UNDERSTAND FUNCTION, SEEK TO UNDERSTAND STRUCTURE

Based on these staining techniques, every nook and cranny of the cortex has been catalogued and cartographed. The best-known map is that of the German neurologist Korbinian Brodmann who, in the years before the first World War, defined geographic regions in the human cerebral cortex, numbering them from 1 through 52, according to the sequence in which he studied them (Figure 7.1). Some of these divisions are still used today, though most of them, like political boundaries of yore, have shifted or fissioned, based on physiological criteria unavailable at his time and corroborated by metabolic stains (that is,

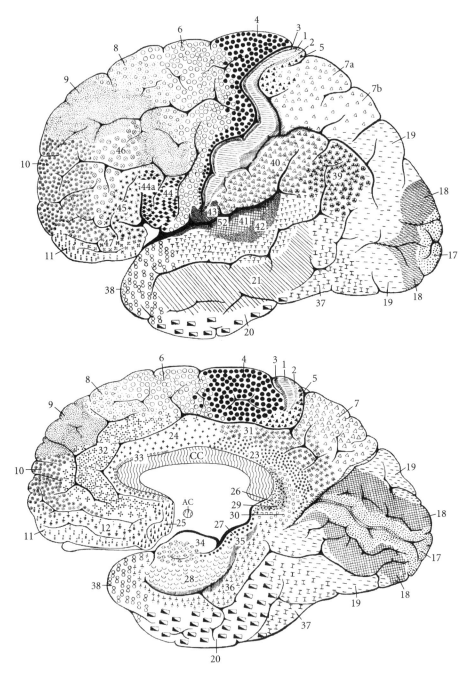

FIGURE 7.1 *Brodmann's Division of the Human Neocortex* On the basis of often minute differences in the packing density, appearance, and texture of cells in the gray matter, Brodmann divided the cortex into discrete areas, assigning a number to each. Modified from Brodmann (1914).

chemical agents that are differentially taken up by groups of cells based on their activity). Yet they retain their usefulness as geographical landmarks, much like the label "theater district" stands for a particular neighborhood in town.[1]

This ongoing process of balkanizing brain tissue is exemplified by the visual areas at the back, which surround Brodmann's area 17 (corresponding to the physiologically defined primary visual cortex). Brodmann's area 18, part of a region referred to as the *extrastriate cortex*, contains at least four separate visual areas. Such partitioning, if true for all of Brodmann's regions, implies the existence of more than one hundred cortical fields.

Do these subdivisions relate to the working of the cortex, or are they irrelevant details, like the coloring of patches on a quilt? A deeply held belief among biologists is that structure and function are intimately related. That is, differences in structure are reflected in differences in function and vice versa. Body parts that look consistently different have distinct functions. Likewise for nervous tissue. If the cellular packing density increases, or the degree of myelination changes, or some enzyme begins to appear, then it is likely that a functional border has been crossed.

The link between structure and function is very apparent in computers. The trained eye of a circuit designer can distinguish input and output pads, primary and secondary cache memories, the bus architecture, the arithmetic-logical unit, registers and other structures on the processor chip, all of which have distinct functions.

7.2 | THE CORTEX CONTAINS A HIERARCHICAL STRUCTURE

Until the 1970s, it was widely believed that the visual cortex had but a few subdivisions linked in a serial ascending manner. Propelled forward by the seminal research of John Allman and Jon Kaas on New World monkeys, and Zeki's exploration of the extrastriate cortex in Old World monkeys,[2] this straightforward picture evolved into something much more complex. Whereas the terra incognita outside primary sensory areas used to be simply labeled the *association cortex* (because little was known about its function), this ongoing research effort—whose fruits are detailed in the following chapter—identified its physiological properties and divided it up into fields of common functionality.

The question that arises is, what is the exact relationship among all of these areas? Do the interconnections among different regions reveal anything about

---

[1]I recommend the thin monograph by Braak (1980) as background material on charting the neuroanatomy of the human cerebral cortex. One should not be seduced by Figures 7.1 and 7.2 into believing that the borders between cortical areas are sharply demarcated. They can be quite hazy, with complex transitional territories.

[2]Allman and Kaas (1971); and Zeki (1974). See their books (Zeki, 1993) and Allman (1999).

the large-scale architecture employed? After all, cortico-cortical fibers make up the bulk of the white matter beneath the cortex. Studying where they come from and where they go to should make it possible to determine whether every area is connected to every other, whether areas are randomly thrown together, or whether some sort of hierarchical order can be discerned.

Forward and Feedback Connections Give Rise to a Hierarchy

The neuroanatomists Kathleen Rockland and Deepak Pandya observed that connections among cortical areas fall into at least two groups. They had the insight to propose that these constitute forward and feedback pathways for information flow. Their classification revolved around the critical role of layer 4. Recall from Chapter 4 that layer 4 within the cortical sheet making up V1 is the site where the bulk of the retino-geniculate input terminates. In general, a well-developed layer 4 is the hallmark of any sensory area.

A connection between two cortical areas is considered to be *ascending*, or *forward* if the axons predominantly terminate in layer 4. This is particularly true if the cell bodies of the projection neurons that give rise to these axons are sited in superficial layers 2 and 3. A *descending* or *feedback* connection is one in which the axons avoid layer 4, targeting the upper layers instead (in particular, layer 1, the most superficial one) and, on occasion, layer 6 (the deepest layer). The cell bodies of the pyramidal neurons that supply the feedback axons are usually found in deep layers.

John Maunsell and his doctoral advisor, David Van Essen, at the time at the California Institute of Technology, inferred from these anatomical patterns an explicit hypothesis of hierarchical organization. Given the Rockland-Pandya laminar rules, it is possible to determine the relative position of any one area within a hierarchy. If area A_2 receives a forward input into its layer 4 from A_1 and projects, via its superficial layers, into layer 4 of area A_3, then A_1 must be placed below A_2 which, in turn, must be below A_3.

The termination zone of axons feeding back information from a higher to a lower level is wider than that of forward projectiong neurons, making excitatory synaptic contacts with a larger set of neurons.[3]

Besides ascending and descending links, there are *lateral* connections too, which couple cortical areas at the same level in the hierarchy. Lateral connections can originate in all layers that project out of a cortical area (that is, from all except layers 1 and 4) and can terminate throughout the width of the cortical column in the recipient area.

---

[3] For example, areas V1 and V2 receive widespread feedback connections from inferotemporal and parahippocampal regions (Rockland and Van Hoesen, 1994; and Rockland, 1997). Salin and Bullier (1995) and Johnson and Burkhalter (1997) discuss cortico-cortical connections in detail.

With these rules in place, what had before looked like a chaotic jumble of cortico-cortical connections now took on some semblance of order. Earlier versions of this hierarchical organization were extended by Daniel Felleman and Van Essen. The resultant organizational chart with a dozen levels (Figure 7.2) resembles a maze of steam pipes in an old industrial plant; highly intricate, with myriad bypasses, shortcuts, and seemingly random additions. Yet despite the complexity of the linkages, not every area talks to every other one. In fact, only about one-third of all possible connections among areas have been reported so far.[4]

Like a set of Russian dolls nesting inside each other, each one of the rectangular boxes in Figure 7.2 is an elaborate neuronal network in its own right, with plenty of substructure. Two of these steam pipe plants, the left and right hemispheres of your brain, are heavily cabled together by tens of millions of callosal fibers, and are packed into a single skull. Similar hierarchies operate in the somato-sensory and auditory modalities.

What Does this Hierarchy Reflect?

The hierarchy revealed by these laminar rules does not look perfect. In the words of Felleman and Van Essen, various irregularities

> raise the issue of whether the cortex is inherently only a 'quasi-hierarchical' structure that contains a significant number (perhaps 10%) of bona fide irregularities and exceptions to any set of criteria that can be devised. Alternatively, the visual cortex might contain an essentially perfect anatomical hierarchy that has been imperfectly studied using inherently 'noisy' methods of anatomical analysis.

The hierarchy may not be unique, in the sense that many organizational structures can be generated that satisfy the same anatomical connectivity constraints but are more refined, with additional levels.[5]

---

[4]The three key papers describing this series of advances are Rockland and Pandya (1979), Maunsell and Van Essen (1983), and Felleman and Van Essen (1991). Related or alternate hierarchical schemes have been proposed by Kennedy and Bullier (1985); Barbas (1986); Zeki and Shipp (1988); and Andersen et al. (1990). For a thorough review, see Salin and Bullier (1995). Young (2002) infers the organizational chart of all 72 areas hitherto described in the monkey's cerebral cortex. Figure 7.2 has been updated to reflect a better knowledge of the areas and connections between the inferior temporal and the medial temporal lobes (Lewis and Van Essen, 2000; and Saleem et al., 2000).

[5]The idea of a *unique* hierarchy has been criticized by Hilgetag, O'Neill, and Young (1996), who used an evolutionary optimization algorithm to find those hierarchies that had the fewest departures from perfection. They concluded that the visual system, with around 300 cortico-cortical connections among its more than 30 areas, is surprisingly strictly hierarchical without being exact and that the number of levels in the hierarchy ranges between 13 and 24 (Young, 2002).

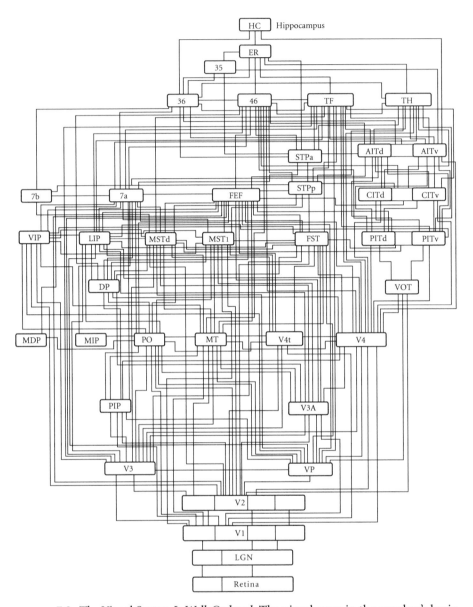

FIGURE 7.2 *The Visual System Is Well-Ordered* The visual areas in the monkey's brain have been assigned by Felleman and Van Essen to a highly stratified hierarchy, interconnected by a few hundred linkages, most of which are reciprocal. Rooted in the retina, this processing tree extends deep into frontal and motor structures. For more details, see footnote 4 on the previous page and the front endpages. Modified from Felleman and Van Essen (1991) and Saleem et al. (2000).

Despite some similarities between Figure 7.2 and the organizational chart of a university or a company, no president or chief executive officer oversees this entity. There is no single Olympian region that looks down upon the entire visual system. The areas at the top of the figure project either outside the cortex proper or onto regions in the frontal part of the brain, and from there onto (pre-)motor structures that execute the brain's commands. Indeed, as Zeki points out,[6] every cortical area—with no exception—sends its output axons somewhere. No region is a one-way nexus. If it were, it could not be a causal agent; it could not mediate any useful consciousness.

While evidence for an hierarchical organization is widely accepted for the sensory modalities at the back of the brain, it is unclear to what extent forward and feedback cortico-cortical projections can be identified in the front of the brain. This applies, in particular, to the connections between inferior temporal, posterior parietal, and prefrontal cortical regions.[7] In fact, shouldn't there be an inverted hierarchy—mirroring the one found in vision—reaching from the upper echelon of the prefrontal cortex down to the primary motor regions? More research on these questions is needed.

Brain scientists are puzzled as to why the hierarchy exists. One reason may be that such an architecture permits higher cortical regions to easily detect correlations among neurons in lower areas. At the next level, correlations between correlations can then be established, and so on. This will lead to an elaboration of receptive field properties (as described in the following chapter).

The hierarchy in the visual system is anatomical, not one that is necessarily reflected in the latencies of signals propagating up the rungs on the cortical ladder. In particular, all areas at any one level are *not* simultaneously excited by visual stimuli. As noted in Chapter 3, the magno- and parvocellular streams flow at unequal rates into V1. These temporal differences remain evident in further processing stages, such that the frontal eye fields in the front of the brain receive visual information prior to areas V2 and V4 at the back.[8]

Think of the nervous activity following an eye movement as a wave of spikes traveling up the optic nerve, through the lateral geniculate nucleus, and into the cortex. An analogy can be made with waves at a beach: The surf breaks up as it moves through the interstitial pools at the border between ocean and land; some of these water wavelets travel faster than others, depending on the depth of the pool and other factors. Likewise in the brain. Because cortical net-

---

[6] Zeki (1993).

[7] Indeed, Webster, Bachevalier, and Ungerleider (1994) concluded "... it may be that the rules that have been used for establishing hierarchical relationships within both the visual and somatosensory systems do not extend, in any simple way, to connections with frontal lobe areas." See also Rempel-Clower and Barbas (2000).

[8] Schmolesky et al. (1998) and Nowak and Bullier (1997) review signal timing across cortical areas.

works have both short and long-reach connections, this wave of activity may, in some cases, jump over intervening regions. The rapid increase in stimulus-triggered spiking propagates through the stations along the visual hierarchy without appreciably changing the steepness of the wave's leading edge. I call this a network wave or *net-wave*. Experiments have shown that the occurrence of net-waves is both reliable and precise. Even deep into the cortex, their signature can be detected with a jitter of 10 msec or less.[9] I argue in Section 13.5 that such a forward traveling net-wave can rapidly trigger quite complex, yet unconscious, behavior (see also Table 5.1), while consciousness depends on some sort of standing wave between the back and the front of the cortex.

The great majority of cortico-cortical pathways between areas are reciprocal. Thus, if area A projects to area B, then B usually projects back to A. Reciprocity holds as well for the multiple connections between thalamus and cortex, but is not universal. Major one-way projections include the optic nerve leaving the retina, the descending fibers from visual cortex to the superior colliculus, and the pathway from the frontal lobes to the basal ganglia.

7.3 | THALAMUS AND CORTEX: A TIGHT EMBRACE

The thalamus, a quail-egg shaped structure sitting on top of the midbrain, is the gateway to the neocortex. The thalamus and the cortex evolved in close relationship to each other. Except for the sense of smell, all sensory modalities are relayed through the thalamus on the way to the cortex.[10]

The thalamus is subdivided into discrete nuclei, each with their own, separate input and output channels and unique functional correlates.[11] Specific nuclei send somatosensory, auditory, visceral, and optical information onto the relevant cortical regions.

By far the best explored of these is the lateral geniculate nucleus (LGN), first discussed in Chapter 3. It is not the largest nucleus. That distinction goes to the *pulvinar*. Phylogenetically speaking, the pulvinar is the most recent addition to

---

[9]Marsálek, Koch, and Maunsell (1997); Bair and Koch (1996); and Bair (1999). The net-wave propagates through a cortical stage in 5–10 msec.

[10]The olfactory bulb, the recipient of the receptor output from the nose, projects directly into the olfactory cortex. A fiber bundle extends from the primary olfactory cortex, older and more primitive than the neocortex, down to the thalamus and back up to a secondary olfactory cortex. Other cortical afferents that bypass the thalamus are the widespread modulatory ascending brainstem and basal forebrain pathways (Section 5.1), connections from the amygdala, and projections from a small satellite of the neocortex called the claustrum.

[11]When I refer to the thalamus, I mean the *dorsal thalamus*. For the detailed anatomy of the thalamus, consult the monumental Jones (1985). Sherman and Guillery (2001) summarize its electrophysiological properties.

the thalamus. It appears as a relatively small but rather clearly outlined nucleus in carnivores, increasing progressively in size from monkeys to apes, until it reaches relatively enormous proportions in humans. The primate pulvinar has been partitioned into four divisions with at least three separate visual maps (and possibly many more).[12] Unlike the cortex, these representations are not interconnected. In fact, thalamic nuclei do not much talk directly to each other or to their counterparts in the other hemisphere.

Recall from Section 5.1 that the acute, bilateral loss of the intralaminar nuclei (ILN) of the thalamus interferes with arousal and awareness, sometimes profoundly. Clinical research, functional brain imaging, and electrophysiological recordings link these regions—as well as some of the pulvinar nuclei—to the infrastructure of vigilance, attention, and goal-directed visuo-motor behaviors, most noticeably in the form of eye movements. Staring intently at the foliage because you might have seen somebody hiding there or scanning the road ahead of you are both likely to engage the switching capacity of these thalamic regions.[13]

Neurons in these thalamic nuclei fall into two broad classes, excitatory projection cells that send their axons to the cortex, and local, inhibitory interneurons. Staining the thalamus for two common calcium-binding proteins has revealed another, hitherto hidden, aspect of its architecture. The projection neurons come in at least two flavors, core and matrix. *Core* cells aggregate in clusters and target precisely delineated recipient zones in the intermediate layers of cortical regions. The magnocellular and parvocellular relay cells of the LGN and their topographically organized termini in V1 are the classic examples of core cells. *Matrix* projection cells reach in a more diffuse manner into the superficial layers of several adjacent cortical areas. They are in an ideal position to disperse and help synchronize activity or to provide timing signals to large populations of cells. While the core conveys specific information to its cortical recipients, the matrix might help assemble the widespread neuronal coalitions that mediate the multi-faceted aspects of any conscious percept.[14]

---

[12] Some retinal ganglion cells send their axons directly into the inferior pulvinar nucleus. The rest of the pulvinar receives its visual input via the superior colliculus (see the front endpages). Three of the predominantly visual nuclei of the pulvinar are strongly and reciprocally interconnected with different visual cortical areas (including posterior parietal and inferior temporal cortices), while the fourth casts its net wider to include reciprocal connections to prefrontal and orbitofrontal areas (Grieve, Acuna, and Cudeiro, 2000).

[13] One well-controlled imaging study found that high vigilance, as compared to rest or random motor activity, is associated with focal midbrain and ILN activity (Kinomura et al., 1996). Robinson and Cowie (1997) review the involvement of the pulvinar in attentional shifts and eye movements.

[14] The emerging story of core and matrix thalamic cells is summarized in Jones (2002). The koniocellular neurons in the LGN (Section 3.5) are an example of matrix cells.

7.4 | DRIVING AND MODULATORY CONNECTIONS

A tacit assumption is that the connections between the areas in Figure 7.2 are all alike. This is most certainly not the case.[15] For instance, the geniculate axons that terminate in layer 4 can evoke a vigorous volley of spikes in V1 neurons of the appropriate stimulus proclivity. Without such input, these cells would not fire. Conversely, feedback from middle temporal cortex (MT) to V1 and other early visual areas mediates some of the observed nonclassical receptive field effects by modulating the primary, forward response.[16]

To a first approximation, Francis and I think of forward projections as *strong, driving* connections. They rapidly and reliably drive their target cells, as the projection from LGN to V1 or from V1 to MT do. Feedback projections, such as those from MT back into V1, usually terminate on the distal parts of the dendritic tree of pyramidal neurons whose cell bodies are located in deep layers. Such far-away input can regulate the firing behavior of these cells but is unlikely, by itself, to give rise to a vigorous spike discharge. Feedback *modulates* the response of recipient cells, setting the magnitude of the neuronal response (the cell's *gain*).

Strong, driving (forward) and weaker, modulatory (backward) connections can also be identified when considering the wiring from the cortex to the thalamus and back. The general rule here is that a cortico-thalamic axon originating in layer 6 is likely to modulate its thalamic target cells (as in the V1 to LGN pathway), while a layer 5 cortical projection to a thalamic nucleus is expected to be a strong one. For the reverse direction, the rule appears to be that a thalamic input into layer 4 or the lower part of layer 3 is usually a strong connection.[17]

When connections between brain areas are considered in this binary manner, two intriguing conclusions emerge. First, there appear to be *no strong loops* in the cortico-thalamic system—there are no thalamic or cortical areas that are, directly or indirectly, recurrently connected via strong projections. Put differently, there is no driving pathway from area A to area B (with possible intermediaries) that is paired by a driving pathway back from B to A. Although many parts of the brain are as yet uncharted, Francis and I nevertheless postulate that no such strong loops will be found. We surmise that strong reciprocal

---

[15] Barone et al. (2000) present a promising approach for quantifying the strength of forward and backward projections.

[16] Hupe et al. (1998) reversibly inactivate area MT while recording in V1, V2, and V3. The MT feedback acts in a push-pull fashion, amplifying the response to an optimal stimulus within the classical receptive field. At the same time, it reduces the response to low saliency, visual stimuli that are large enough to cover both the classical and the nonclassical receptive field regions.

[17] Ojima (1994); Rockland (1994 and 1996); and Bourassa and Deschenes (1995).

connections promote uncontrollable oscillations, as in epilepsy.[18] Second, the hierarchy of Figure 7.2 is, to a first approximation, a forward network that is modulated by feedback connections. This is also true if the appropriate thalamic nuclei are incorporated into this scheme. Seen in this light, information flows from the retina up the hierarchy until it reaches its apex in the medial temporal and prefrontal lobes; from there, the information descends to the motor stages. Shortcuts bypass some of this hierarchy and feedback pathways may be needed for many of its functions.

In the future, it will be critically important to distinguish types of connections according to their strength, time-course, and other characteristics. This should make it easier to comprehend the behavior of the system. The distinction is analogous to that between intramolecular and intermolecular forces in chemistry. Intramolecular forces are the strong covalent or ionic bonds that hold atoms or ions together in molecules or ionic crystals, respectively. Intermolecular forces, on the other hand, are the relatively weak dipolar interactions (such as hydrogen bonds and van der Waals forces) that exist between the atoms in neighboring molecules. It would be impossible to understand the structure of a protein molecule, for example, if all its intramolecular bonds and intermolecular forces were considered to be equally strong or equally stable.

Lavishly illustrated anatomy textbooks suggest that many (if not most) pathways in the human brain have been elucidated and catalogued. This is far from the truth. There is a tremendous need for a broad and sustained exploration of human neuroanatomy.[19] Without detailed knowledge of the wiring of the human brain, the quest for the NCC will be significantly slowed.

7.5 | VENTRAL AND DORSAL PATHWAYS AS A GUIDING PRINCIPLE

A watershed in thinking about the visual brain occurred in the early 1980s, when Leslie Ungerleider and Mort Mishkin at the National Institute of Mental Health outside Washington, D.C., proposed that vision in the neocortex proceeds along two separate cortical routes. Their argument was based on a synthesis of anatomical, neurophysiological, and clinical data.

Key were the results of experiments in which the visual abilities of monkeys with inferotemporal (IT) lesions were compared against those with destruction of their posterior parietal (PP) cortex (Figure 7.3). Monkeys with IT, but not

---

[18]The distinction between strong and modulatory projections and the no-strong-loops hypothesis were proposed in Crick and Koch (1998a). There may be interesting exceptions to this hypothesis at the level of individual neurons.

[19]Crick and Jones (1993) make an impassioned plea for such a program. One promising technique for tracing white matter tracts in living humans is diffusion tensor magnetic resonance imaging (Le Bihan et al., 2001).

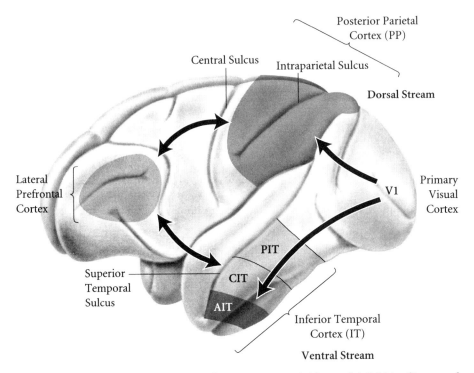

FIGURE 7.3 *Two Streams of Visual Information* Ungerleider and Mishkin discovered that the flow of visual information splits in V1 into two tributaries that reunite in the lateral prefrontal cortex. While the ventral or *vision-for-perception* stream handles form and object recognition, the dorsal or *vision-for-action* stream carries spatial information for locating targets and executing motor actions. Modified from N. Logothetis.

PP damage, had difficulties discriminating objects using sight. On the other hand, monkeys with PP, but not IT lesions, couldn't execute visuo-motor tasks, such as touching a visual target or reaching into a slot. Reinforced by data from neurological patients with focal brain damage, Ungerleider and Mishkin concluded that IT contains circuitry specialized for the discrimination and recognition of objects while PP is necessary for computing spatial relationships to guide the eyes or a limb to a target.[20] Subsequent functional imaging studies strengthened the Ungerleider–Mishkin distinction to the point where it is now a cornerstone of visual neuroscience.

---

[20]These two cortical streams are superimposed onto an evolutionarily older division of labor between cortical and subcortical visual centers (Ungerleider and Mishkin, 1982). Milner and Goodale's (1995) book provides an excellent historical perspective on the attempts of clinicians and neuroscientists to understand these distinctions. Psychologists had inferred separate cognitive and motor-oriented visual maps even earlier (e.g., Bridgeman et al, 1979).

Today, neuroscientists speak of two streams of information, the ventral and the dorsal. Diverting from V1, they converge again in the lateral prefrontal cortex. The ventral stream passes through V2 and V4 into IT, and projects from there into the ventrolateral prefrontal cortex. This pathway is responsible for the analysis of form, contour, color, and for detecting and discriminating objects. The inferior temporal cortex and associated regions have been implicated in conscious visual perception, a claim that is elaborated upon in Chapter 16. The dorsal pathway moves from V1 through MT and into the posterior parietal cortex. From there it sends a far-flung projection into the dorsolateral prefrontal cortex. PP neurons are concerned with space, motion, and depth. When an eye or limb needs to be moved to select one out of many targets, neurons in the posterior parietal cortex are involved. The dorsal stream processes visuo-spatial cues necessary for reaching and guiding the eye, hand, or arm (that is, for action). The ventral and dorsal streams are often called the *what* and *where* or the *vision-for-perception* and *vision-for-action* pathways, respectively.

The ventral and dorsal streams have plenty of direct cross linkages. Some areas, particularly in and around the superior temporal cortex, lie at the interface between the two pathways and defy any simple classification.[21]

7.6 | THE PREFRONTAL CORTEX: THE SEAT OF THE EXECUTIVE

While all of the neocortex behind the central sulcus, crudely put, deals with sensory input and perception, the concern of the frontal lobes, the large expanse of neocortex lying forward to the central sulcus, is action. Motor, premotor, prefrontal, and anterior cingulate cortices all belong to the frontal lobes (see the front endpages and Figure 7.3). Their function is to guide, control, and execute motor outputs, such as skeletal or eye movements, and the expression of emotions, speech, or internal mental states (as in unconscious thought processes; see Chapter 18). As organisms evolve, the complexity of their actions increases and their goals extend in space and time, coming to depend less on instinctual drive and more on prior experience, insight, and reasoning. This necessitates planning, decision making in uncertain environments and cognitive control, recall and the online storage of information, and the feeling of authorship. For these high-level, executive functions, the *prefrontal* cortex comes into its own.

---

[21] The areas on the left side of Figure 7.2 are part of the dorsal stream, while those on the right are part of the ventral pathway. Areas STPa, STPp, and FST, intermediate between these two, can't readily be assigned to either one (Saleem et al., 2000; and Karnath, 2001). Baizer, Ungerleider, and Desimone (1991) identify neuronal projections that link IT and PP.

The prefrontal cortex (PFC), the most forward located part of the cerebral cortex, is defined as the cortical recipient zones of axons from projection neurons in the mediodorsal thalamic nucleus. PFC increases significantly in size with phylogenetic development.[22] PFC is widely and reciprocally wired up to premotor, parietal, inferior temporal, and medial temporal cortices, the hippocampus, and amygdala. It is not directly connected, however, to either primary sensory or primary motor cortex. PFC is the only neocortical region that talks directly to the hypothalamus, responsible for the release of hormones. Prefrontal regions are therefore in an eminent position to integrate information from all sensory and motor modalities. Another of their roles is the short-term, online storage of information of relevance to the organism. I'll deal with this in Chapter 11.

The frontal lobes are intimately related to the *basal ganglia*, large subcortical structures that include the striatum and the globus pallidus. These ancient regions mediate purposive movements, sequences of motor actions or thoughts, and motor learning. In vertebrates with no or only poorly developed cortex, the basal ganglia are the most important forebrain centers.

Neurons in the deep layers of the cortex send their axons directly to the striatum. Via intermediate stations that include the thalamus, the basal ganglia project back to the cortex.[23] The basal ganglia are drastically affected in disorders such as Parkinson's or Huntington's disease, associated with severe motor deficits, up to a total loss of movement.[24]

---

[22]While accounting for only 3.5% of the volume of feline cortex, PFC occupies 7% of canine cortex (dog lovers, note), 10.5% of monkey cortex, and almost 30% of human cortex. The expansion of PFC relative to the rest of the brain does not hold true for the frontal lobes in general (Preuss, 2000). The exact hierarchical relationships among prefrontal areas, particularly the layers of origin and termination of specific neuronal subpopulations, remain murky (see, however, Carmichael and Price, 1994). Good references to the neuroscientific and clinical literature on PFC include Passingham (1993); Grafman, Holyoak, and Boller (1995); Fuster (1997); Goldberg (2001); and Miller and Cohen (2001).

[23]Projections between the frontal lobes and the basal ganglia are specific and reciprocal. Prefrontal area 9 projects to one part of the striatum which, by way of two intermediate stations, send fibers back to area 9, while premotor area 6 projects to a different part of the striatum that ultimately reciprocates this input.

[24]In a dramatic "natural" experiment, six young Californian drug addicts acquired all of the symptoms of severe, late-stage Parkinson's disease. Fully conscious (as they recalled later), they were unable to move or speak. They could open their eyes upon command, but it took a painful 30 seconds to do so. If the doctor held out the patient's arms in front and then released them, the arms would slowly relax and return—over three to four minutes—to the patient's side. A few days earlier, all six had taken a home-brewed concoction, a synthetic heroin. Unfortunately, the drug was tainted by a substance, MPTP, that selectively and permanently destroyed dopamine-producing neurons in their basal ganglia. These frozen addicts, described in a compelling book (Langston and Palfreman, 1995), made medical history and offered proof, once again—see Section 1.2—that consciousness does not depend on a functioning motor output.

7.7 | RECAPITULATION

This chapter introduced two further anatomical structures important to the quest for the NCC—the thalamus and the prefrontal cortex—as well as three broad organizational schemes to make sense of the myriad of thalamic nuclei and cortical areas.

A general principle of cortical architectonics is its hierarchical design. Based on cues about where the axons terminate and where the originating cell bodies lie, cortico-cortical projections in the back of the brain can be classified as forward, feedback, or lateral. Based on this determination, visual areas can be assigned to one of twelve or more levels within the Felleman–Van Essen hierarchy. Visual input triggers a rapidly propagating net-wave of spikes that passes through these stages until it reaches one or more effectors. The precise function of this hierarchical arrangement and how perfect it is remains controversial.

On the basis of the distinction between strong, forward, and modulatory feedback connections, Francis and I concluded that the cortex and thalamus have no strong loops that might drive the nervous tissue into uncontrollable oscillations. Lacking such loops, the visual system, including the LGN and the pulvinar nuclei, has the appearance of a largely forward network whose activities can be modulated by feedback pathways.

Visual information moves along two broad streams through the cortex, the ventral (vision-for-perception) and the dorsal (vision-for-action) pathways. Starting in V1, the two diverge and flow toward either the inferior temporal cortex (ventral) or the posterior parietal cortex (dorsal). From there, they project to different parts of the prefrontal cortex, where they reconverge. While the ventral system is responsible for conscious form and object vision, the dorsal pathway extracts information necessary for visual-driven motor actions.

Before returning to the central concern of the book, I must expand, in the next chapter, upon the remarkable properties of cortical tissue beyond V1 and how it analyzes and represents visual information.

CHAPTER EIGHT

Going Beyond the Primary Visual Cortex

Three Zen monks see a temple banner waving. The first monk states, "The banner is moving." The second monk says, "No, the wind is moving." Finally, the third monk remarks, "It is the mind that is moving."

From *The Dreams of Reason* by Heinz Pagels

The primary visual cortex represents the world in multiple low- and high-resolution maps. These emphasize canonical image features such as orientation, changes in the image, wavelength-specific information, and local depth. Yet it is but the first cortical area of many subserving vision. All in all, about one-quarter of the human cerebral cortex is involved with visual perception and visuo-motor behavior.

Any accessible part of the cortex can be "turned off" by cooling it with metal plates placed onto the surface. When V1 is shut down in this manner, visual responses throughout the ventral hierarchy are much reduced. Responses in some areas are so weak that a receptive field can't even be defined.

Cortical motion area MT (Section 8.3), however, is not so thoroughly suppressed by V1 inactivation. While the discharge of its neurons is substantially reduced upon cooling V1, they retain some degree of selectivity for movement. MT is fed, in the main, by two tributaries, both of which originate in the retina. One passes through V1 while the other reaches the cortex through a more circuitous pathway involving the superior colliculus. Consistent with this view is the observation that lesioning the corresponding regions in both V1 *and* the colliculus eliminates all responsiveness from MT cells. This subcortical bypass might be adequate to support the minimal, unconscious visuo-motor behaviors of patients whose V1 has been destroyed (these *blindsighted* individuals are examined in Section 13.2), yet insufficient to power the ventral pathway responsible for conscious object vision.[1]

---

[1] Bullier, Girard, and Salin (1994) review the role of V1 in mediating responses in extrastriate visual cortex. They suggest that V1 is *the* essential driver for the ventral, vision-for-perception stream, but not for the dorsal, vision-for-action one.

In the following section, I discuss the receptive field properties of neurons in some of these higher stages of the visual cortex. They are responsible for translating retinal information into conscious perception and action.

8.1 | MORE TOPOGRAPHIC AREAS: V2, V3, V3A, AND V4

The second visual area (V2) surrounds V1 and is about equal in size (Figure 8.1). Cells in the primary visual cortex project in a point-to-point manner onto counterparts in V2. As a result, V2 has the same skewed topographic representation found in V1 (Figure 4.2), with many more neurons dealing with central than peripheral vision.

The mapping between V1 and V2 extends in a continuous manner across the cortical sheet. This is also true for higher visual areas. There are no abrupt borders. Instead, the visual world is mapped, by and large, smoothly onto these areas. Modern cartographic methods employing *functional magnetic resonance*

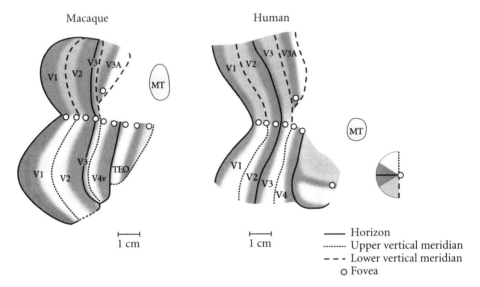

FIGURE 8.1 *Simian and Human Topographic Visual Areas* Functional magnetic resonance imaging has identified distinct maps in the human occipital lobe. Their exact shapes and extents are still being established. Homologous regions from the macaque monkey are also illustrated (only the central two-thirds of the eccentricity range is shown for humans). Retinotopy is indicated using the polar angle scheme on the extreme right. As in an impressionist collage, the outside world is represented multiple times by translation and mirror-reflection. The back of the brain (posterior) is on the left. Modified from Hadjikhani et al. (1998).

imaging (fMRI) confirm this (Figure 8.1);[2] the human occipital lobe contains multiple representations of the world, similar to those discovered in the monkey using microelectrodes.

Nothing like the remarkable receptive field transformation that occurs at the doorstep of the cortex—in the input layer to V1—is evident when moving from V1 to V2 or, for that matter, when transitioning into other cortical regions. V2 receptive fields are larger than those in V1, but that is to be expected because multiple V1 cells converge onto each V2 neuron. V2 cells are sensitive to depth, motion, color, and form. Many are *end-stopped*, responding best to short bars, lines, or edges. Their activity is reduced if the bar becomes too long.[3]

Illusory edges can delineate a shape, such as a triangle, that doesn't exist on the page (remember Figure 2.5?). No intensity change is present, yet you see contours. According to our activity principle, any such direct and immediate perception must be grounded in an explicit neuronal representation. Rüdiger von der Heydt and Ester Peterhans at the University of Zürich in Switzerland discovered neurons in monkey V2 that respond explicitly to both real and illu-

---

[2] These maps are described by Engel, Glover, and Wandell (1997) and by Tootell et al. (1998). Like its cousins, positron emission tomography and optical imaging of intrinsic signals, fMRI measures changes in the local blood supply in response to the increased metabolic demand of active synapses, neurons, and glia cells. Technological considerations currently limit the spatial resolution for human imaging to a bit more than one millimeter. The temporal dynamic is largely dictated by the speed with which local blood flow is regulated, typically a few seconds. It is generally assumed that hemodynamic activity is directly proportional to spiking activity. Thus, the larger the recorded fMRI signal, the higher the firing rate of the underlying neurons. This assumption has been corroborated in a few cases by indirect means (Heeger et al., 2000; Rees, Friston, and Koch, 2000), and, in a technically amazing tour-de-force, by simultaneously recording the local electrical signals *and* fMRI activity (Logothetis et al., 1999 and 2001). Unfortunately, the relationship between these two isn't always so simple. Vigorous hemodynamic activity can go hand-in-hand with a constant or even a decreasing neuronal firing rate (Mathiesen et al., 1998; Logothetis et al., 2001; and Harrison et al., 2002). Increases in the blood flow and oxygenation levels are most strongly coupled to synaptic activity, the release and uptake of neurotransmitter, and the restoration of metabolic gradients, but much more weakly to spiking activity. The metabolic demand of generating and propagating action potentials accounts for only a small fraction of the total energy demand of the brain. Thus, the fMRI signal may primarily reflect synaptic input to a region and local processing, rather than neuronal output—the trains of action potentials that are sent to more distant sites (Logothetis, 2002).

[3] The electrophysiological properties of V2 cells are catalogued by Livingstone and Hubel (1987); Levitt, Kiper, and Movshon (1994); Roe and Ts'o (1997); Peterhans (1997); von der Heydt, Zhou, and Friedman (2000); and Thomas, Cumming, and Parker (2002). V2 also has a distinct cytochrome oxidase architecture, related to the V1 blob system, as thoroughly described by Wong-Riley (1994). Unless otherwise mentioned, data in this chapter are obtained from the macaque monkey. Many of the details (but not the principles) will likely differ in the human cortex.

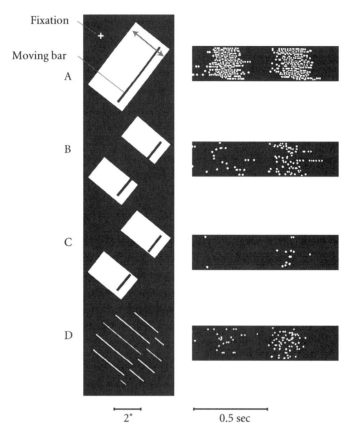

FIGURE 8.2 *V2 Cell Responding to Illusory Edges* This neuron recognizes oriented contours, real or imagined. While the monkey stares at the fixation mark, a dark bar moves back and forth over the bright background. A: The cell fires to an appropriately oriented bar. B: When the central portion of the bar is missing, the cell's response is reduced. C: Adding tiny terminators to the left and right bars abolishes both the illusory edge as well as the cell's firing. D: The neuron also responds to another anomalous contour, defined by the alignment of terminating lines. The spikes evoked by multiple sweeps of each stimulus are indicated on the right, with the two distinct halves corresponding to forward and backward motion. Modified from Peterhans and von der Heydt (1991).

sory edges (Figure 8.2). Such neurons are probably important for identifying partially occluded figures.[4]

Given these and other V2 cells that represent contours, defined by either contrast, motion, depth, or illusory edges, I conclude that a subset of V2

---

[4]Kanizsa (1979) and Gregory (1972) investigate the psychology of illusory contours. The electrophysiological results are described in von der Heydt, Peterhans, and Baumgartner (1984); and Peterhans and von der Heydt (1991).

neurons processes the information necessary to distinguish figures from their background and to identify the shape of objects. The physiological data that speak to the role of V2 in form vision are reinforced by behavioral evidence from monkeys whose V2 has been selectively destroyed.[5]

Directly adjacent to V2 is a third visual area (V3), with a split mirror-image representation of the visual world, one for the upper and one for the lower visual fields. In front of these are V3A and V4—two further regions that have their own retinotopic representation (Figure 8.1). V4 receives direct input from V1, as well as separate projections from V2 and V3. Its receptive fields are bigger than those of its inputs. Indeed, this is generally true as the visual processing hierarchy is ascended. The maps in the ventral pathway, however, retain a bias for stimuli at the fovea. This is, after all, the place at which you are usually looking.[6]

And on and on. Not much is known about the distinct functional roles this suite of cortical regions plays in vision. There are so many millions of neurons but only so few microelectrodes to listen to them!

8.2 | COLOR PERCEPTION AND THE FUSIFORM GYRUS

As emphasized by Arthur Schopenhauer, colors are a product of the mind and not of the external world.[7] Perceived hue depends on the relative activity in the different cone photoreceptor populations (Section 3.2) and is evaluated relative to the overall spectral distribution of the entire image. Psychologists talk about *color constancy*, the fact that large changes in the spectral composition of the light source causes only minor changes in the color appearance of objects. Hue perception is more or less independent of the vicissitudes of the illuminating light source. A ripe apple looks about the same under the whitish light of the full moon, the bluish light of the sky, or the yellow light of an incandescent light bulb. This is true even though the wavelength composition will differ significantly in all three cases.

In a series of influential papers, Zeki argued that V4 in the macaque monkey is involved in color perception. He based this hypothesis on his electrophysiological characterization of the wavelength-sensitivity of V4 cells in anesthetized monkeys. Many V4 neurons represent color, instead of raw wavelength. A

---

[5]Merigan, Nealey, and Maunsell (1993) ablated V2 and observed the monkey's deficits in behavior.

[6]The original monkey single cell experiments were reported in Burkhalter and Van Essen (1986); and Newsome, Maunsell, and Van Essen (1986). Tootell et al. (1997) identified homologous areas in the human brain on the basis of fMRI. Some dispute the need to divide V3 into separate areas (Lyon and Kaas, 2002; and Zeki, 2003).

[7]This has been demonstrated in many ways. See the primer on color by Bryne and Hilbert (1997).

double-opponent cell in V1 may fire whenever a set amount of, say, middle wavelength light impinges onto its receptive field, whereas a V4 cell responds to the middle wavelength region of the spectrum within its receptive field *relative to* the spectral distribution of stimuli in an extended region of the entire visual field.[8] Color selective cells are not limited to V4, but can be found in other regions.

In humans, lesions along the ventral surface of the occipital and temporal lobes, part of the fusiform gyrus (see the front endpages), can selectively disturb color vision. Patients with achromatopsia perceive the world in gray, not unlike having a color TV default to black-and-white. Hue perception is gone, even though form and other aspects of vision remain.[9] From this, Zeki infers the existence of an essential node for color in the human fusiform gyrus.

Functional brain imaging has established a number of regions in this part of the cortex that are selectively active during color perception and color judgments.[10] The extent to which highly discrete color regions can be found in a consistent manner across subjects remains uncertain.

Intriguingly, some color-tuned regions remain active when subjects experience color afterimages in the absence of any physical color. If you stare for a time at a saturated color, such as bright red, and then look at a uniform gray field, you will see its complementary color (in this case, green). This *negative afterimage* can be very compelling and fades within a minute. fMRI activity in a part of the fusiform gyrus follows the percept, increasing in response to the virtual color afterimage and decreasing back to baseline within a short time after the inducing color patch has been removed.[11]

In *colored-hearing*, certain words, sounds, or music consistently evoke particular colors. As in other forms of *synesthesia*, color-hearing is automatic, involuntary, and stable across many years. Celebrated famously in Aldous Huxley's *Doors of Perception*, it is a condition that some individuals are fortunate enough to enjoy throughout life without the use of any drugs. Hue percepts evoked by words trigger brain activity in the same part of the fusiform gyrus

---

[8]Zeki (1973 and 1983). These simian and the related human studies are summarized in a masterful monograph by Zeki (1993). The neighborhood-comparison computations that are key to color constancy occur at multiple stages, from the retina to V1 and V4 (Wachtler, Sejnowski, and Albright, 2003).

[9]Meadows (1974); Damasio et al. (1980); and Zeki (1990) discuss the relevant clinical literature. In one patient, the site of the lesion was so restricted that color perception was only lost in one visual field quadrant (Gallant, Shoup, and Mazer, 2000; see also, footnote 17 in Chapter 2). Remarkably, this patient—and others like him—do not notice that they see in grey in one part of their visual field and in color in another.

[10]Zeki et al. (1991); Cowey and Heywood (1997); Zeki et al. (1998); Hadjikhani et al. (1998); Tootell and Hadjikhani (2001); and Wade et al. (2002).

[11]Sakai et al. (1995); and Hadjikhani et al. (1998).

of synesthetes as colored stimuli. Noteworthy is the fact that V1 and V2 lacked any fMRI response during colored-hearing. These observations not only reinforce the specificity of the fusiform region for hue perception but also Francis's and my claim that the NCC for color does not have to rely on V1 activity.[12]

8.3 | CORTICAL AREA MT IS SPECIALIZED FOR MOTION PROCESSING

The middle temporal area (MT) is a small piece of cortical real estate, the size of a thumbnail (Figures 7.2, 8.1, and the front endpages). It is remarkably reactive to motion. All but a minority of its neurons prefer stimuli moving in one particular direction, with the average cell firing more than ten times stronger to motion in its preferred direction than to motion in the opposite direction. The neurons retain this selectivity over a considerable range of speeds, stimulus sizes, and positions.[13] In short, MT represents some forms of stimulus motion in an explicit manner.

MT Responds to Both Real and Illusory Motion

Until a few years ago, human MT could be identified only in corpses.[14] With the advent of MRI, however, MT is now routinely localized on the basis of its specific response to moving dots, gratings, or expanding circles in the living.[15]

What happens in MT when you think something is moving, but nothing actually does, as in the *waterfall illusion*? Will that also cause MT to be active? If you stare straight at a waterfall for a minute and then at the stationary ground next to it, you'll experience the eerie feeling of the trees and rocks moving skyward. Another way to induce a *motion aftereffect* is to gaze, for a minute or so, at the center of a rotating disk with spirals painted on top. If you then look at a friend's face, it will twist and contort in the opposite direction. You'll even see features on the face move, even though they don't change position! How can this be? Motion implies displacement, so this should be a physical impossibil-

---

[12]Nunn et al. (2002); and Paulesu et al. (1995). For background on synesthesia, see Cytowic (1993); Ramachandran and Hubbard (2001); and Grossenbacher and Lovelace (2001).

[13]This area was called MT by those who discovered it in the New World monkey (Allman and Kaas, 1971) and V5 by Zeki (1974) who first described it in the Old World monkey. Its human homologue is often referred to as MT/V5. I use the MT nomenclature. Albright (1993) and Andersen (1997) summarize the properties of MT and closely related motion-processing areas.

[14]This was done via myelin or antibody stains on post mortem material (Tootell and Taylor, 1995).

[15]Tootell et al. (1995); Goebel et al. (1998); Heeger et al. (1999); and Huk, Ress, and Heeger (2001) link fMRI activity in human area MT to various attributes of motion perception. Tootell and Taylor (1995) outline MT in the human brain using myelin, metabolic markers, and a monoclonal antibody.

ity. For a brain with distinct processes encoding position and motion, though, it is not that surprising.

What underlies the waterfall illusion? Cells that represent motion in the downward direction recalibrate after prolonged viewing of the falling water; their response for the same, persistent input becomes weaker. Because the neurons coding for upward motion do not respond to the water falling down, they do not adapt. Motion perception results from the competitive interaction between pools of neurons representing opposite directions of motion, those that code for motion in the downward direction and those for motion in the upward direction. The end product of extended viewing of one motion is that the balance is disturbed in favor of motion in the opposite direction. The neural substrate of illusory motion has been visualized using fMRI and illustrates the subtlety of the mind-body interface, as reflected in the epigraph at the beginning of this chapter.[16]

The Selective Loss of Motion Perception

What happens if MT is destroyed? In a monkey, small lesions cause modest and ephemeral deficits in its ability to judge the speed or direction of moving stimuli, while loss of the entire area leaves the animal with a permanently impaired motion perception. Likewise in people.

L.M., a neurological patient, strikingly demonstrates the highly particular nature of perceptual deficits that can be observed. She lost MT and other, nearby regions on both sides of her brain to a vascular disorder. This rare occurrence causes a devastating motion blindness or, to use Zeki's term, *akinetopsia*. According to the original report,

> She had difficulty, for example, in pouring tea or coffee into a cup because the fluid appeared to be frozen, like a glacier. In addition, she could not stop pouring at the right time since she was unable to perceive the movement in the cup (or a pot) when the fluid rose. Furthermore, the patient also complained of difficulties in following a dialogue because she could not see the movements of the face and, especially, the mouth of the speaker. In a room where more than two other people were walking she felt insecure and unwell, and usually left the room

---

[16]Based on this argument, a net reduction in the fMRI activity following an intense and constant motion stimulus *for the population of cells encoding that direction of motion* might be expected. This was confirmed in an elegant fMRI study by David Heeger and his colleagues (Huk, Ress, and Heeger, 2001). They reported direction-selective motion adaptation effects in most early visual areas, reaching a maximum in MT. In the monkey, cells that previously responded in the same way to upward and downward motion might have their balanced output disturbed following adaptation (Tolias et al., 2001). Today's researchers distinguish different motion aftereffects with distinct properties (e.g., for translating motion versus spiral motion). The monograph of Mather, Verstraten, and Anstis (1998) provides more details.

immediately, because "people were suddenly here and or there but I have not seen them moving." The patient experienced the same problem but to an even more marked extent in crowded streets or places, which she therefore avoided as much as possible. She could not cross the street because of her inability to judge the speed of a car, but she could identify the car itself without difficulty. "When I'm looking at the car first, it seems far away. But then, when I want to cross the road, suddenly the car is near." She gradually learned to "estimate" the distance of moving vehicles by means of the sound becoming louder.

L.M. could infer that objects moved by comparing their relative position in time, but she never saw motion. Nevertheless, she has normal color and form perception, spatial acuity, and can detect flickering lights. It was as if she lived in a world illuminated by a stroboscopic lamp, not unlike a disco in which the dancers are clearly visible, yet appear frozen, devoid of motion; or like watching a greatly slowed-down movie, in which the individual frames are visible, a key observation I shall return to in Chapter 15.[17]

Linking MT Neurons to Perceptual Decisions

Such observations motivated a classic study of how the firing of individual neurons relates to behavior. These experiments were conceived and carried out by neurobiologists William Newsome at Stanford University, Anthony Movshon at New York University, and others.[18]

Monkeys were trained to report the direction of moving dots—for example, translating either upward or downward (the 'signal')—embedded within a swirling cloud of dots that darted in all directions (the 'noise'). As the noise increased, diluting the motion signal, the task became more difficult and the animal made many more mistakes. In the limiting case of no signal, each dot could move in any direction, creating the visual appearance of a TV screen turned to a station that has gone off the air. The experimentalists recorded the

---

[17]The deficits of the late patient L.M. are detailed in Zihl, von Cramon, and Mai (1983), from which the quote is taken; Hess, Baker, and Zihl (1989); and Heywood and Zihl (1999). If an object moved slowly (< 10°/sec) in an unambiguous manner, L.M. could infer motion, most likely through a change in position. A German soldier whose occipital lobe was damaged by an exploding mine showed an absolute loss of motion (Goldstein and Gelb, 1918). He never experienced any visual movement, but could perceive tactile movement over the skin on his hand or arm. When asked to track the continuous motion of a hand on a watch, he would point to discrete locations, claiming that he only saw the hand 'here' and 'there' but 'never in between.' Zeki (1991) places such rare cases of akinetopsia in their historical context.

[18]The full details were reported by Britten et al. (1992). Shadlen et al. (1996) evaluated the implications for neural coding strategies. Schall's (2001) essay placed the experiments in the context of decision making. Cook and Maunsell (2002); Williams et al. (2003); and Ditterich, Mazurek, and Shadlen (2003) carried out ecologically more relevant reaction-time variants of these experiments.

firing rate of individual MT neurons while the animal performed this task. On the basis of a mathematical signal-detection analysis, the researchers derived a quantitative relationship between the animal's choices and the firing rate of MT neurons averaged over a 2-sec period. Overall, the cells did as well as the animal in extracting the weak motion signal from the noisy stimulus. That is, a mathematically astute observer with access to the number of spikes discharged by individual cells in response to the 2-sec long movie can infer, on average, the direction of motion of the signal about as well as the animal can.

Even when the motion signal was almost totally buried in noise, the animal could still detect the direction of motion with better than even odds (since the signal only moved up or down, a pure guessing strategy should yield the correct response—and the juicy reward—on half of all trials). For a given motion signal, the animal's response varied stochastically from trial to trial; the number of spikes fired by the MT cell fluctuated likewise. If MT neurons were causally involved in the animal's behavior—and, perhaps, in the underlying motion percept—the behavior should co-vary with the firing rate over repeated presentations. This was exactly what Newsome and colleagues found. Whenever a cell responded with a larger than average number of spikes, the monkey tended to choose *that cell's* preferred direction of motion *on that trial*. This was rather surprising, because it implied that behavior can be influenced by *individual* cortical neurons. Modeling studies bear this out; the monkey's decision could have been based on the weakly correlated activity of less than 100 MT cells.[19]

To further narrow the gap between correlation and causation, Newsome and his colleagues directly stimulated area MT while the animal was doing the motion task. That this *microstimulation* worked at all is a testimony to the columnar properties for motion (Figure 8.3). Suppose the neurons selective to different directions of motion were randomly scattered throughout MT; in this case, exciting neighboring cells would be unlikely to generate a net signal because the contributions of individual MT cells to the animal's decision would cancel out. If the electrode were to land inside a column coding for upward motion, however, stimulating these cells might bias the animal's decision in this direction.

The physiologists inserted an electrode into the cortical MT tissue capable of delivering electrical current pulses, activating neurons within a tenth of a millimeter or so from its tip. While viewing the moving dot display, the monkey was more likely to report upward motion when a cortical column coding for upward movement was stimulated. The consequence of microstimulation

---

[19]The computational metric involved is termed *choice probability* (Britten et al., 1996). It is a powerful computational technique that probes the physiology underlying perception in a rigorous manner (Parker and Newsome, 1998).

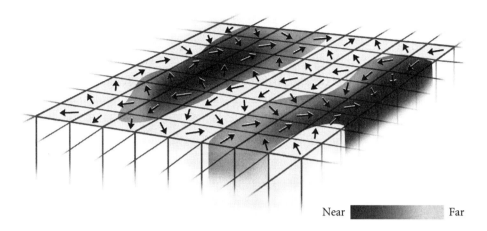

Near █████████████ Far

FIGURE 8.3 *Clustering for Motion and Depth* The world is mapped topographically onto area MT, with neurons expressing similar receptive field properties clustered across the thickness of the cortical sheet. That is, cells below a patch have similar direction-of-motion (symbolized by the arrows) and depth preferences (coded in gray-scale). This selectivity changes smoothly when moving *across* the cortical surface. For purposes of illustration, the discreteness of this clumping has been exaggerated. The area portrayed here is on the order of one square millimeter. Modified from DeAngelis and Newsome (1999).

was equivalent to increasing the motion signal in the upward direction by some fixed amount.[20]

What does the monkey see? By itself, microstimulation did not cause the animal to react. Thus, the electrical current was probably too weak to trigger a percept, such as a moving phosphene, but can influence its attributes.[21] Until this type of direct brain excitation is repeated in humans, possibly on epileptic patients during remedial surgery, we will not know.

---

[20]The effect of the electrical current delivered by the electrode was highly specific. The animal's decision was influenced only if the receptive field of the stimulated MT site overlapped with the location of the cloud of moving dots. On occasion, the stimulation electrode would bias motion in one direction; then, moving the electrode a mere 300 μm into a column for the opposite direction of motion (Figure 8.3), the same electrical stimulus would now influence this direction of motion (Salzman et al., 1992; and Salzman and Newsome, 1994).

[21]The effect may be implicit and unconscious, akin to the motion aftereffect obtained when staring at a blank screen. In such an empty field, the aftereffect can't attach itself to any contour, and no motion is seen.

Is Motion Sensation Generated within MT?

These findings implicate MT as an essential node for random-dot motion perception: If MT and nearby regions are removed, subjective feeling for motion,
as well as the associated behavior, is lost. Furthermore, area MT has a beautiful
columnar structure for direction-of-motion (Figure 8.3), suggesting that this
attribute is made explicit in the firing rate of these cells.

Just because area MT is an essential node for motion doesn't mean that it
would be conscious of motion if it were dissected out of the brain and placed in
a dish with its visual input attached. I think that MT has to enjoy *bidirectional*
interactions with other regions for motion awareness to occur.[22] MT projects
not only out of the cortex (via its layer 5 to the superior colliculus), but also to
the frontal eye fields and to several motion-sensitive areas in the posterior parietal cortex, including the lateral and ventral intraparietal areas and the medial
superior temporal (MST) area (see Figure 7.2 and the front endpages). Cells in
one part of MST respond selectively to different *optical flow fields* generated by
navigating through the environment (for instance, forward motion is associated with an expanding optical flow, while a turn of the head sets up a rotating
flow field). Neurons in a different part of MST help you track moving objects
with your eyes.

The advancing front of the net-wave triggered by motion onset and flowing
from the retina through V1 and into MT and beyond to other dorsal regions
is sufficient to mediate a rapid behavioral response.[23] Motion awareness, on
the other hand, probably requires feedback from the front of the cortex back
to MT and other motion-sensitive regions. This theme is picked up again in
Section 15.3.

---

[22] To help make better sense of the role of MT in motion perception, consider the following
analogy with biochemistry. Hemoglobin is a large protein consisting of two α subunits and two
β subunits. The iron at the heart of the heme group within each α and β chain can be thought
of as the essential node because that's where the oxygen binds. Interfere with oxygen binding
and bad things happen. Hemoglobin can also lose its activity, however, if some of its constituent
amino acids cannot properly fold around the bound iron-oxygen complex or if they somehow
prevent the four subunits of the molecule from coupling properly. On the other hand, the amino
acid sequence of hemoglobin shows considerable variability across species, implying that many
of the amino acids are not crucial to its function. Moreover, other molecules such as myoglobin
can also bind oxygen. And so it might be with the brain. MT is an essential node for motion but
not the only place where motion information is analyzed and expressed. Even cerebellar lesions,
quite removed from cortical MT, can interfere with aspects of motion perception (Thier et al.,
1999).

[23] The MT recordings of Cook and Maunsell (2002) provide some of the best evidence to date
that the leading edge of the net-wave ultimately determines how fast the animal can react to the
motion stimulus.

MT Also Encodes Depth Information

It is rare for any cortical area to subserve a single function. This is also true for MT. Neurons there encode not only motion but also depth. As you read in Section 6.5, the image of any object projects to slightly different parts of the left and right retinae. The relative separation of the image between the two eyes is the object's binocular disparity. Many MT cells care a great deal about disparity. Some will only fire if an object is close by, while others respond when the object is far away. Newsome and Gregory DeAngelis discovered that depth- or disparity-selective MT cells are found in islands positioned within a sea of neurons largely indifferent to disparity. At any one location, neurons within the column extending from deep to superficial layers showed the same disparity selectivity. This patchy organization is superimposed onto the columnar organization for direction of motion (Figure 8.3).[24]

Newsome's group repeated their microstimulation experiments with one modification—the animal now had to carry out a depth discrimination task. The external electrical current, delivered directly to MT, generated a bias signal that influenced the behavior and the depth perception of the animal, depending on the disparity tuning of the neurons near the electrode tip.[25]

8.4 | THE POSTERIOR PARIETAL CORTEX, ACTION, AND SPATIAL POSITION

Primates incessantly engage in myriad routine, 'mindless' sensory-motor acts, like picking fruit from a bush, reaching for a tool, stepping over an obstacle, or scanning a scene with their eyes. All of these tasks require visual guidance but probably not consciousness.

To extract the target location, its relative position on the retina needs to be converted into a form that the neuronal networks underlying reaching, grasping, and pointing can exploit to direct the eyes, head, arms, and fingers. Electrophysiological recordings in the monkey, clinical reports, and brain imaging in people implicate the *posterior parietal cortex* (PP) in combining and expressing position information and in relating it to action. PP is subdivided into half

---

[24]Maunsell and Van Essen (1983); DeAngelis, Cumming, and Newsome (1998); and Cumming and DeAngelis (2001) discuss the physiology of binocular depth perception in MT.

[25]An ingenious electrophysiological study by Bradley, Chang, and Andersen (1998) demonstrated that area MT combines depth and motion information. Grunewald, Bradley, and Andersen's (2002) related experiment strengthened the case against a direct involvement of V1 cells in perception (here for three-dimensional structure from motion cues), whereas MT cells do correlate with the animal's percept.

a dozen functionally distinct regions in the macaque, and more refined techniques keep uncovering additional ones (see Figure 7.3 and areas LIP, VIP, and 7a in the front endpages).

Common to these regions are neuronal responses that are neither purely sensory (visual as well as auditory and proprioceptive signal influence cells here) nor purely motor, but partake of both. Single-cell experiments indicate that PP is involved in such diverse functions as analyzing spatial relations among objects, controlling eye and hand movements, and determining where visual attention is to be allocated. Some cells encode the eye, hand, or arm movements that the monkey *intends* to execute within the next seconds. Others are strongly modulated by attention. A stimulus that is behaviorally important, perhaps because the animal has to look at it in order to get a sip of apple juice, will evoke an enhanced response relative to one that is irrelevant to the animal (I return to the theme of attention in Chapters 9 and 10).

PP is an important conduit for action-related information. Lesions in PP indelibly affect the monkey's ability to reach out and touch an object or to shape its hand and properly grasp it. The deficits can be so profound that earlier investigators believed that monkeys were blinded by such lesions, when in fact the animals could see but were, instead, unable to visually guide their limbs. The output pathways include direct projections from layer 5 of the posterior parietal cortex to the spinal cord and to brainstem motor structures, as well as massive, two-way cortico-cortical connections to pre-motor and prefrontal areas in the front.

In people, lesions in the posterior parietal cortex cause deficits in the perception of space and in visual behaviors. Of particular interest is *neglect*, characterized by severe disturbances of spatial awareness, and *optic ataxia*, a persistent inability to reach out or point to targets.[26]

The Encoding of Space via Gain Fields

How does the brain represent the location of objects? One elegant solution, popular in robotics and computer science, would be a global map of the environment in world coordinates. As in a common city map, such a representation informs the organism where things are with respect to external landmarks. As the subject explores the world, the map is updated using information from all sensors.

The brain pursues a different strategy. A number of maps encode object position using implicit representations (recall my explicit/implicit distinction

---

[26]Andersen (1995); Gross and Graziano (1995); Colby and Goldberg (1999); Snyder, Batista, and Andersen (2000); Batista and Andersen (2001); and Bisley and Goldberg (2003) discuss the posterior parietal cortex, attention, intention, and the encoding of space. Glickstein (2000) reviews connections between visual and motor areas. For more on neglect, see Section 10.3.

introduced in Section 2.2) that depend on the actuator concerned. Thus, the eye movement system contains a different representation of space than the brain region encoding visually guided reach movements. A case in point is the encoding of space in PP.

In most neurophysiology experiments, the monkey sits in a chair and is rewarded with a treat, like juice, if it keeps its eyes absolutely still in its head (which is often restrained to prevent turning or nodding). This allows the experimentalist to outline the neuron's receptive field in retinal coordinates. What happens if the animal shifts its eyes? Will the cell keep on responding as long as the stimulus keeps the same position with respect to the retina, as is the case for ganglion cells? Or is the stimulus encoded independently of the angle of gaze?

The empirically determined answer is neither. PP neurons systematically confound the two coordinate systems. Typically, the cell's firing response can be expressed as the product of a term that depends solely on the visual response relative to the retina—the cell's conventionally defined receptive field—and a term that varies with the position of the eye within its orbit. For instance, a neuron might respond maximally to some stimulus in its classic receptive field if the eye is positioned to the left, fire more modestly if the eye looks straight ahead, and be silent if the eye is shifted toward the right. Put differently, the output, or gain, of the receptive field is modulated by the position of the eye. This is known as a *gain field* strategy.[27]

Location, then, is encoded in an implicit manner. It can be recovered by combining signals from many such cells, a great example of population coding (Section 2.2). Other gain fields encode the position of the head relative to the shoulder. In this case, the response of the neuron can be described by the product of three terms, one of which depends on the visual stimulus relative to the retina, one on the location of the eye relative to the head, and one on the position of the head relative to the shoulder. I argued in Section 2.2 that an explicit representation is a necessary condition for the NCC. These findings can therefore be taken to imply that absolute spatial position is not accessible to consciousness. Instead, only relative position is—relative to eyes, hands, or body, or with respect to other objects in the field of view. This can be tested by assessing the coordinate system(s) underlying spatial awareness and contrasting them with those controlling visuo-motor behavior (see Section 12.2).

Some neurons in the brain do explicitly encode location. *Place cells* in the rodent hippocampus fire maximally when the animal is physically within a particular region in its environment (for instance, between the water-cooler

---

[27]This term was introduced in Zipser and Andersen (1988). Andersen et al. (1997); Pouget and Sejnowski (1997); and Salinas and Abbott (1995) review and discuss the computational consequences of this implicit representation of space.

and the door). Outside this restricted area, the cell is silent.[28] Can these cells be part of the NCC for perceived position? Perhaps. Right now, we don't know.

8.5 | THE INFERIOR TEMPORAL CORTEX AND OBJECT RECOGNITION

I conclude this chapter by moving from the dorsal to the ventral pathway. Originating in V1, the ventral stream passes in a series of stages through V2, V4, and the posterior inferotemporal cortex (PIT), until it arrives at the most forward, anterior part of the inferior temporal cortex (AIT; Figure 7.3 and the front endpages). One or two intermediate stages can be skipped, yet for the most part, the hierarchy is respected.

In the monkey, AIT is the last mainly visual processing region. Later stages are polysensory or are involved in action or memory. Besides sending highly processed visual information to the medial temporal lobe and to the striatum of the basal ganglia, AIT projects to the prefrontal cortex. The feedback from the medial temporal lobe probably serves to retrieve visual memories and load them into IT.[29]

The receptive fields of IT neurons, which almost always include the fovea, can be large, frequently encompassing information not only from the opposite field of view but from the same hemifield as well (mediated by axons routed through the corpus callosum). Little or no topographic organization is evident in AIT. This explains why IT does not show up in the fMRI mapping procedure used to generate parts of Figure 8.1.

One of the jobs of IT cells is to represent the form, shape, and surface features of perceived objects. If a monkey is looking at, or near, a target hidden in a crowded scene—think of Waldo in the popular children's book—but fails to detect it, AIT cells that otherwise fire to this target remain silent.[30] Chapter 16 summarizes the evidence that neurons in IT and beyond explicitly represent the current content of visual consciousness.

---

[28] Place cells, first described by O'Keefe and Nadel (1978), remain selective in the dark, as long as the animal has olfactory, tactile, or other cues to help orient itself. The spatial discrimination is sufficiently good that electrophysiologists can pinpoint the position of the animal to within a few millimeters by simultaneously recording the activity of a few dozen hippocampal place cells. Reconstructing the path of the rat as it moves through a maze based on the firing activity of 30-100 cells is described by Wilson and McNaughton (1993); Zhang et al. (1998); and Frank, Brown, and Wilson (2000). Rolls (1999) and Nadel and Eichenbaum (1999) describe place cells in monkeys and Ekstrom et al. (2003) in humans.

[29] Miyashita et al. (1996) and Naya, Yoshida, and Miyashita (2001) have amassed direct evidence for the essential role of this feedback pathway into IT in visual associative memory.

[30] (Sheinberg and Logothetis, 2001). Unlike neurons in the dorsal pathway, IT cells care little about eye movements.

It is in the inferior temporal gyrus and in the neighboring regions of the superior temporal sulcus (STS) that neurons with the greatest stimulus selectivity for objects are found. Examples include neurons that fire vigorously to paperclips twisted into particular shapes (Figure 2.1), trees, hands, or the sight of monkey and human faces viewed in perspective (Figure 2.4). This trend toward ever more sparse and explicit representations is characteristic of the ventral pathway. The story appears to be similar in humans, where some medial temporal lobe neurons are so exclusive in their selectivity that they only respond to very different views and pictures of specific, famous, or familiar individuals (Figure 2.2).[31] Such specificity is formed by experience.

Keiji Tanaka at Japan's RIKEN Brain Science Institute systematically explored the stimulus selectivity of AIT neurons in the monkey by developing a technique that allows him to home in on the visual stimulus that gives rise to the most vigorous firing response. The critical features that he finds are more complex than orientation, size, color, and simple textures, but—with the exception of human and monkey faces—they are not detailed enough to adequately and completely specify realistic objects.

Tanaka discovered a columnar structure for circles, corners, elongated and oriented blobs, common aspects of faces, and so on. This organization can be visualized by comparing metabolically active regions to inactive ones on the basis of the optical reflectance of the cortex (*optical imaging*). Any one moderately complex object gives rise to many hotspots of activity on the surface of IT, each about half a millimeter in diameter. The entire area could be parceled into more than a thousand such hotspots. The columnar representation is continuous: for example, as the viewing angle of a face changes, the positions of the blobs representing it shift systematically across the cortex. I interpret these data to mean there is an explicit representation for families of visual features, such as corners, geometric shapes and forms, facial identity, and angle of gaze.

Functional imaging of the human brain has revealed object-specific zones in the cortex. The ventral temporal cortex, including the fusiform gyrus and the lateral occipital region (see the front endpages), is selectively activated by the sight of objects. Most researchers agree that the sight of human faces preferentially activates the *fusiform face area* (FFA) in the fusiform gyrus.[32] Lesions

---

[31] Young and Yamane (1992); Tanaka (1996, 1997, 2003); Logothetis and Sheinberg (1996); DiCarlo and Maunsell (2000); Tamura and Tanaka (2001); Gross (2002); and Tsunoda et al. (2001) discuss visual response properties and columns in monkey IT cortex. The data from the human medial temporal lobe was alluded to in footnote 14 in Chapter 2.

[32] The FFA can be found in almost all subjects in the right mid-fusiform gyrus, with some having bilateral representation (Kanwisher, McDermott, and Chun, 1997; and Tong et al., 2000). Its activity is modulated by attention (Vuilleumier et al., 2001). The FFA is not the only brain region active for faces. Nor does all activity in the FFA relate uniquely to face perception (Haxby, Hoffman, and Gobbini, 2000). For other fMRI studies of visual object responses along the ventral pathway, see Epstein and Kanwisher (1998); Ishai et al. (2000); and Haxby et al. (2001).

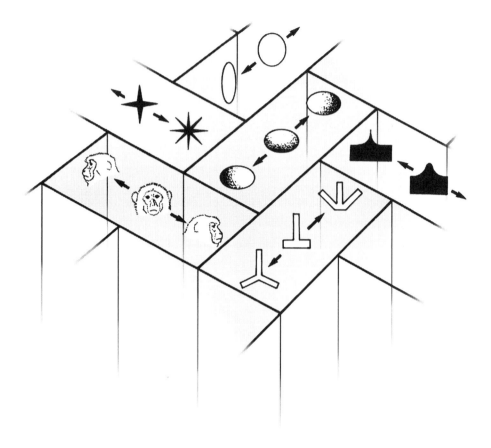

FIGURE 8.4 *Clustering for Complex Form Features* In the anterior part of monkey inferior temporal cortex, cells that encode similar high-level visual features, such as faces, corners, shaded blobs, and so on, are clumped together. A similar spatial organization most likely exists in humans and can be picked up by functional brain imaging. Modified from Tanaka (1997).

in this neighborhood are often associated with an inability to recognize faces, prosopagnosia.[33]

A debate currently rages between localists who assign one chunk of the ventral stream to the dedicated analysis of faces, another one to body parts, a third sector to houses and spatial scenes, and holists who argue that object recogni-

---

[33]Benton and Tranel (1993) survey the clinical literature. Wada and Yamamoto (2001) report on one patient with a highly circumscribed lesion who is unable to recognize faces.

tion is more widely distributed in patches of overlapping activity. As is often the case in science, both sides of this debate might be right.

8.6 | RECAPITULATION

This chapter took a bird's eye view of all of the visual cortex. Early areas V1, V2, V3, V3A, V4, and MT represent the environment in a series of distorted maps, with the center of gaze greatly emphasized. Neurons here analyze and encode form (including illusory contours), color, depth, and motion. Receptive fields become larger and their trigger features more specific when ascending this hierarchy. Simultaneously, retinotopy gradually erodes. While V1 and V2 exhibit a high degree of spatial order, this is lost in PP and IT. Everywhere, like-minded neurons cluster together, forming columns for different stimulus features.

Cells in V4 and neighboring regions in the human fusiform gyrus are tuned to color. Because destruction of these areas interferes with or even prevents hue perception, it can be inferred that this large cortical sector includes one or more essential nodes for color.

Area MT encodes the direction and speed of moving dots, gratings, or bars and their depth. Given the existence of a well-developed columnar organization for direction of motion and depth, these attributes are explicitly represented in MT. The decisions of a monkey in a motion discrimination task can be inferred from the strength of the firing activity of individual MT cells. Furthermore, the animal's behavior can be systematically biased by microstimulating small patches of this cortex. Functional brain imaging reveals that human MT is strongly active when subjects perceive either real or illusory motion. Finally, a patient with widespread bilateral destruction to MT and surrounding areas can't perceive rapid motion, although she can recognize the moving object. In Zeki's parlance, MT is an essential node for direction-of-motion and speed of simple moving percepts.

Other cortical areas besides MT respond to moving objects or to the optical flow fields induced by moving the eyes or the head. Each one is dedicated to different aspects of motion perception.

Neurons in the posterior parietal cortex combine visual, auditory, proprioceptive, and eye command information in an implicit manner. Part of the dorsal pathway, these cells encode the location of objects that guide the eye or hand toward them.

Neurons with highly refined visual response properties are found in and beyond the inferior temporal cortex. They provide the information necessary for recognizing objects. The existence of columns for complex features suggests that these attributes are made explicit here. It is in the inferior temporal cortex and medial temporal lobe—one of the output areas of IT—that cells that code for specific views of particular objects, or for different views of the same individual, can be found. I will argue in Chapter 16 that the activity in a coalition of neurons in these areas conveys the consciously seen attributes of objects, the NCC. The existence of large aggregates of neurons sensitive to the sight of faces, objects, houses, and places, has been confirmed by fMRI in the human ventral temporal cortex, including the fusiform gyrus.

This profusion of visual areas confronts brain scientists with a major puzzle: If no one brain region encodes all of the relevant information, how it is that we usually experience a single, integrated percept? This *binding problem* is addressed in the following chapter, in conjunction with the remarkable fact that the vast majority of sensory input is discarded by the conscious mind.

CHAPTER NINE

Attention and Consciousness

There is a further question about sensation, whether it is possible to
perceive two things in one and the same indivisible time or not, if we
assume that the stronger always overrides the weaker stimulus; which is
why we do not see things presented to our eyes, if we happen to be
engrossed in thought, or in a state of fear, or listening to a loud noise.

From *On Sense and Sensible Objects* by Aristotle

Seeing seems simple. You open your
eyes, look around, and quickly build up a stable representation of the world
in your head. You clearly see the books lined up on the shelves, the colorful,
abstract pattern woven into the Persian rug on the floor, and the motion of the
tree branches outside the window in the garden. From the user's point of view,
vision feels like an automatic process that maps external, physical reality in a
straightforward manner onto the inner, mental universe.[1]

A few minutes of self-observation reveal, however, that the relationship
between outer and inner worlds is far more complex. Experiences are not simply given, as some empiricists have asserted. Rather, your mind, implicitly or
explicitly, selects the few nuggets of information that are of current relevance
from the vast flood of data streaming in from the sensory periphery. As mentioned in Chapter 3, tens of millions of bits of information are flowing along
the optic nerve into the brain proper each second that the eyes are open. The
brain can't process all of this data; it deals with this informational overload by
selectively attending to a miniscule portion of it, neglecting most of the rest.[2]

---

[1]What you are conscious of is a refined view of the world in terms of fairly high-level objects,
such as letters on a keyboard, dogs running about, or mountains below a cobalt-blue sky. This
is one reason why rendering a realistic scene is so difficult. Untrained people draw the way they
see, using abstract objects, so the picture ends up looking childish, naive. It takes a lot of practice
to sketch using surface patches of differing intensity, edges, and subtle texture variations.

[2]Computational arguments for why the brain, with its massively parallel architecture, might
need focal attention are given by Ullman (1984) and Tsotsos (1990). An argument based on the
metabolic cost of spiking is provided by Lennie (2003).

By selectively *attending* to particular events or things out there, you choose one world to experience out of an uncountable number of universes.[3] I feel this most vividly when engaged by a demanding climb. Everything but the motion of my body over the rock and the howling wind is relegated to perceptual oblivion. Gone is the strain of the pack on my back, my aching muscles, the looming thunderstorm, and the siren song of the void beneath me. The mountaineer Jon Krakauer captured this well when he wrote:[4]

> By and by, your attention becomes so intensely focused that you no longer notice the raw knuckles, the cramping thighs, the strain of maintaining nonstop concentration. A trance-like state settles over your efforts, the climb becomes a clear-eyed dream. Hours slide by like minutes. The accrued guilt and clutter of day-to-day existence . . . all of it is temporarily forgotten, crowded from your thoughts by an overpowering clarity of purpose, and by the seriousness of the task at hand.

What you are conscious of is usually what you attend to. Indeed, a venerable tradition in psychology equates consciousness of an object or event with attending to it. However, it is important not to conflate these two notions. Attention and consciousness are distinct processes and their relationship may be more intricate than conventionally envisioned.

Let me begin by describing what selective attention is and how it operates. Attention is notoriously difficult to precisely pin down. Take this phenomenological definition from William James, the father of American psychology:[5]

> Every one knows what attention is. It is the taking possession by the mind, in clear and vivid form, of one out of what seem several simultaneously possible objects or trains of thought. . . . It implies withdrawal from some things in order to deal effectively with others. . .

At any point in time, only one or a few objects can be selected in this manner (how many will be taken up in Section 11.3). Two tasks, if carried out concurrently, interfere with each other if they both require attention.[6] Within

---

[3] Attention also has a more global connotation. A teacher admonishes her students to "pay attention" when she wants them to concentrate, to look at her, and to follow her instructions. This global form of attention, related to *alertness* and *vigilance*, implies a spatial orienting response—turning the eyes and the head—and dedicating mental resources to the task at hand. Lack of sleep or a hangover can interfere with alertness. Alertness depends on the locus coeruleus and other brainstem nuclei (Chapter 5).

[4] Krakauer (1990).

[5] From his monumental *The Principles of Psychology* (James, 1890).

[6] Modern surveys of selective attention include Treisman (1988); Nakayama and Mackeben (1989); Braun and Sagi (1990); Braun and Julesz (1998); Pashler (1998); Parasuraman (1998); and Braun, Koch, and Davis (2001).

the visual domain, a long-standing metaphor for selective attention is that of a *searchlight*. Items illuminated by the searchlight benefit from additional processing.

9.1 | CHANGE BLINDNESS, OR HOW A MAGICIAN FOOLS YOU

As pointed out in the chapter epigraph, which dates from the 4th century B.C., you often don't see what's in front of your eyes if your attention is engaged elsewhere. *Change blindness*, the failure to detect a large change between two otherwise identical images, is the most compelling demonstration of this troubling fact (Figure 9.1). The difference between the two pictures can be so pronounced that, once identified, it is impossible to ignore afterward. A jumbo jet repeatedly loses its engine, a bridge disappears and reappears from a scenic view, or the color of a shirt changes from red to blue and back.[7]

In a more natural setting, "Candid Camera"-like setups have been staged in which a psychologist engaged a random bystander in a conversation. Meanwhile, two "workmen," carrying a door, rudely walked between the experimentalist and the unwitting subject. Behind the cover of the door, one of the laborers swapped places with the experimentalist. Half the time the subject did not notice that he or she ended up talking to a different person![8]

If unexpected, subjects can even miss a single, well-isolated target flashed right in front of their eyes, an astounding phenomenon known as *inattentional blindness*.[9] Attentional lapses may be at the root of traffic or aviation

---

[7] Rensink, O'Regan, and Clark (1997) popularized change blindness using flashed, natural scenes separated by short, blank intervals (O'Regan, Rensink, and Clark, 1999). See also Blackmore et al. (1995); Grimes (1996); and Simons and Levin (1997). Change blindness can also occur in minimalist scenes (Wilken, 2001). The phenomenon itself goes back to experiments in the 19th century that measured the span of apprehension. You should experience some of these illusions yourself by surfing the relevant websites.

[8] Simons and Levin (1997 and 1998). Simons and Chabris (1999) reported how subjects that had to track two balls in a game could be blind to a student in a gorilla suit slowly walking across the court. Similarly, moviegoers usually fail to notice all but the most obvious *continuity errors* (Dmytryk, 1984). Actors, for example, may not be dressed the same from one cut to the next, the action in one scene may not be temporally locked to the next shot, or an actor's hair might be wet coming in from the rain but is suddenly dry inside the room. Are fans of Ridley Scott's *Blade Runner*, a dark science fiction film, aware of the more than two dozen mismatched shots, bits of flubbed dialogue, and other blunders throughout this cult classic (Sammon, 1996)?

[9] Inattentional blindness is described in the monograph by Mack and Rock (1998). Subjects had to fixate a cross and decide whether its horizontal arm was longer or shorter than its vertical arm. After three trials, an unexpected object, such as a small colored square or triangle, was added, without any warning, to the display. Immediately afterward, subjects were queried whether they noticed anything. After three more trials with just the cross, the same extra object was again added to the display. In the final, control trial, subjects were told to disregard the cross and to report the extraneous stimulus (while continuing to fixate the cross). Remarkably, a quarter of

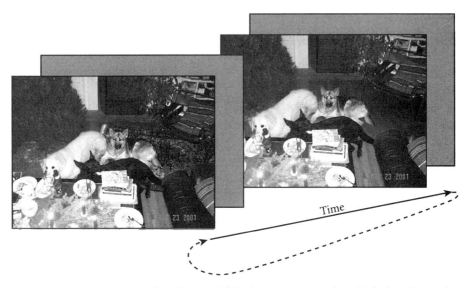

FIGURE 9.1 *Can You Spot the Change?* This short sequence, in which the picture in the first frame has been doctored and is shown in the third frame, is repeated in an endless loop until the thing that winks in and out of existence is seen. Remarkably, this can take a long time. The interposed blanks eliminate the strong, transient signal associated with the changed object that would otherwise give the game away.

accidents attributed to human error. Under conditions of high visibility, with no evidence of alcohol, drugs, mechanical failure, or foul play, drivers or pilots inexplicably crash into obvious obstacles. In one example, commercial airline pilots had to land a 727 in a flight simulator. On some approaches, the image of a small aircraft was unexpectedly superimposed onto the runway. Two out of eight pilots blithely continued with the landing maneuver, without taking any evasive action, a potentially disastrous failure of the perceptual apparatus.[10]

Stage conjurers have exploited inattentional and change blindness for millennia. Distracting the audience with a beautiful, bikini-clad assistant, objects vanish in plain sight. If you attend two consecutive shows and carefully track the hands of the magician, you'll see what I mean (it may spoil the fun of the illusion, though).

---

subjects did not see the stimulus when it was completely unexpected (on the 4th trial). The more observant ones could describe its orientation, color, motion, and location reasonably well. Nobody could distinguish its shape (e.g., triangle, cross, or rectangle). On the final trial, however, everybody unambiguously saw the extraneous object. In a variant of this paradigm, the cross was projected away from fixation so that it could only be seen out of the corner of the eyes. When the object was unexpectedly flashed right at the fovea while subjects had to complete the control task in the periphery, almost everybody failed to see it.

[10] When shown a video of these approaches, the pilots were dismayed at their lack of reaction (Haines, 1991). Gladwell (2001) argues that many traffic accidents are caused by a failure to attend.

Motion-induced blindness, encountered in Section 1.3, as well as flash suppression and binocular rivalry, introduced more fully in Chapter 16, are other examples of visual phenomena where the withdrawal of attention is likely to be critical in making these stimuli disappear.

The moral of these findings is that you can be oblivious to events taking place before your eyes, provided that focal attention is busy elsewhere. So much for the belief that you see everything around you. The truth is that you don't.

9.2 | ATTENDING TO A REGION, FEATURE, OR OBJECT

Allocating Attention to an Event Speeds Up Processing

In a classical *reaction time* experiment conducted by the neuropsychologist Michael Posner, at the time at the University of Oregon, subjects fixate a mark at the center of an otherwise empty monitor. At some point during the trial, a light is flashed at one of four locations on the screen. Subjects have to push a button as soon as they see the light, without moving their eyes. On many, but not all, trials the location of the upcoming flash of light is indicated by a *cue* (say an arrow) at the fixation mark. People take around 290 msec to respond to the light if they have no idea where it might appear, but require only 260 msec if cued. If prompted to attend to the left when the light actually appears on the right, reaction time increases to 320 msec. The simplest interpretation is that attention speeds up the detection of the flash of light by 30 to 50 msec. Focal attention also enhances the visibility of faint contrasts and subtle spatial features.[11] It is difficult to simultaneously attend to two separate locations.

These findings lend support to thinking of focal attention as a searchlight illuminating the world. However, while powerful and compelling, this is just a metaphor. To fully account for the data, the searchlight must conform to the shape of the illuminated object or region and its size must be adjustable based on prior expectations. Furthermore, whereas a searchlight sweeps continuously from one location to the next, attention does not. A more apt analogy would be a stage light that is extinguished at one location and turned on at another, illuminating different players as they take center stage.[12]

---

[11] Attention greatly reduces thresholds for spatial discrimination and detection tasks (Wen, Koch, and Braun, 1997; and Lee et al., 1999). The Posner experiment is described in Posner, Snyder, and Davidson (1980). The attentional benefit may be much larger than the 30–50 msec found in this experiment with an almost totally empty computer display.

[12] Cave and Bichot (1999) criticize the searchlight metaphor on the grounds that it provides erroneous insight into the action of attention. Sperling and Weichselgartner (1995) proposed the stage light analogy.

Visual Search, or How to Stand Out in a Crowd

A popular way to investigate attention is to ask subjects to look for something, such as a red 'D' hidden among other colored letters. Anne Treisman, now at Princeton University, and Bela Julesz, working at Bell Laboratories, pioneered these *visual search* studies. They focused on a deceptively simple question: How does the time taken to find the target increase as the number of distracting objects increases?[13]

For some combinations of target and distractors, the search is effortless. Subjectively, the target *pops out* of the display. Finding a red bar among 4, 8, 16, or 32 green bars scattered all over the place happens very fast, no matter how many green elements are present. If a bunch of 'L's are placed on the screen, the odd '+' sign stands out (Figure 9.2). In the parlance of computer science, the search proceeds in parallel (unless the individual elements begin to crowd into each other).

In general, pop-out occurs if the target is sufficiently different from the distractors in any one elemental attribute, such as color, size, form, or motion (as when you rapidly move your computer mouse back and forth to find the location of the pointer on the screen). Pop-out depends not only on the local stimulus configuration, but also on more global textural or figural effects emphasized by *Gestalt* psychologists.[14]

Integrating Features Using Selective Attention

For other target-distractor configurations, reaction time increases approximately linearly with the number of items in the display. This kind of *serial search* occurs when you look for a 'T' thrown in among the field of 'L's in Figure 9.2.[15] While targets defined by an unique feature, such as color or orientation, can be found in parallel, conjunctions of these features cannot; looking for a green and horizontal bar among green and vertical bars or red bars of any orientation takes more time if more potential targets are present.

To explain these findings, Treisman assumed that simple features were represented in topographic maps for orientation and color, found in V1, V2,

---

[13] On half of all trials, no target was present and subjects had to detect the target without moving their eyes (Treisman and Gelade, 1980; Julesz, 1981; Bergen and Julesz, 1983; Treisman, 1988, 1998; and Wolfe, 1992 and 1998a). The visual search paradigm has even migrated into children's books in which the reader looks for Waldo, in his red-and-white striped turtleneck and funny hat, among scenes populated by hundreds of zany people, animals, and other things.

[14] See the classic accounts of Koffka (1935) and Köhler (1969). Palmer's (1999) textbook offers a modern point of view.

[15] Note that small differences in the target can turn a parallel search into a serial one. In the case of Figure 9.2, the '+' pops out while the 'T' does not, even though both are constructed from the same two perpendicular lines, embedded among the distractors built from the same elements (Julesz, 1981).

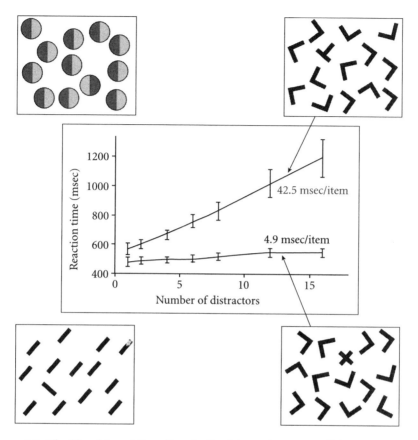

FIGURE 9.2 *The Visual Search Paradigm for Focal Attention* In *parallel search*, the target *pops out* (as in the two examples in bottom row). In practice, the time taken to detect the presence of the target increases mildly with the number of distractors in the search array. In *serial search*, detecting the target—a light-dark bisected disk among dark-light ones in the upper left panel and a 'T' among 'L's in the upper right panel—proceeds at a more ponderous pace as the number of distractors increases. The graph indicates the reaction times for eight subjects for the two tasks illustrated on the right. Modified from VanRullen and Koch (2003a).

and elsewhere. She then ingeniously proposed that determining which two elementary features, such as green and horizontal, make up any one object requires attentional resources. That is, making sure that both features are present requires attention. Because it takes time for the attentional searchlight to shift from one potential target to the next, reaction time increases as the number of objects that need to be inspected increases. Her theoretical framework, referred to as *feature integration theory*, is strengthened by the fact that the slope of the graph of the reaction time when no target is present versus the number of distracting items (Figure 9.2) virtually doubles compared to reaction times when a target is actually present in the display. If objects were randomly distributed across the field, the target would, statistically speaking, be detected after half of all items had been considered by the searchlight, while the absence of a target could be confirmed only after every item had been inspected, nicely accounting for the difference in slope.[16]

In Treisman's scheme, only the elementary features are explicitly represented, while their conjunctions are dynamically grouped, or *bound*, on an "as needed basis," according to the task demands.

The exegesis of these experiments launched an entire research program within psychology. Unfortunately, many of the original findings did not generalize well. Upon closer scrutiny, search slopes were found to vary in an almost continuous manner (from 10 to 150 msec per item or more) depending on the exact stimulus configuration. These data severely undermined the simple searchlight hypothesis. Furthermore, some conjunctive search tasks, such as those combining motion with depth or form, or those looking for an object defined by three features, are very easy and proceed in parallel. To reconcile these conflicts, interpretations radically different from a serial scanning of objects have been proposed. These hypotheses emphasized competition among groups of neurons that vie for dominance.

In all these experiments, abstract knowledge directs attention; a cue points to a location or you're told to look for a 'T.' This is called *top-down, task-dependent*, or *volitional-controlled attention*. Because you can pay attention to a circumscribed region in space, it is sometimes also referred to as *focal attention*.

Top-down attention can also be allocated to specific attributes, such as 'pink' or 'rightward motion.' *Feature-based* attention biases the search throughout the entire visual field in favor of the selected attribute. It pays to know, for example, that your daughter in that crowd of jostling kids is wearing a pink dress, or that the satellite you're trying to track in the night sky moves from east to west.

Selective attention can target an entire object or elongated contour. That is, when you attend to one feature of a stimulus, other features associated with it are selected for free. If you're gazing at two spatially interlocking objects, such as two letters printed on top of each other, you can selectively attend to one or the other. Remarkably, you will not be able to recognize the form of the unattended figure, even though it overlaps with the attended object.[17]

---

[16]This interpretation has been challenged by Chun and Wolfe (1996).

[17]The psychophysics of feature-based attention are nicely reviewed in Wolfe (1994). For the psychology of object-based attention, see Duncan (1984); Jolicoeur, Ullman, and MacKay (1986); Kanwisher and Driver (1997); and Driver and Baylis (1998). The classical experiment on attending to one of two overlapping figures is described in Rock and Gutman (1981).

In summary, attentional processing resources can be allocated to a region in the visual field, to one feature attribute everywhere, or to an extended object.

In most of the experiments cited, subjects are forced to look out of the corner of their eyes, that is, to attend to a location away from the fovea, the point of sharpest seeing. This is rather unnatural, given the almost irresistible urge to move the eyes to the target.[18] In real life, eye and attentional shifts are closely linked. The neural circuitry for the two overlap and an attentional shift is necessary to prepare for an impending eye movement.[19]

Salient Objects Attract Attention

Some things don't need focal attention to be noticed. They are conspicuous by virtue of intrinsic attributes relative to their surroundings. Examples include a red dinner jacket at a somber black-tie state affair, or a vertical line embedded among horizontal ones. These salient objects rapidly, transiently, and automatically attract attention (it takes willful effort to avoid glancing at the moving images on the TV placed above the bar in a saloon). The *saliency* of an object doesn't depend on any one task or behavior; it won't change from one mission to the next.[20] If a stimulus is sufficiently salient, it pops out because of this bottom-up form of attention operating throughout the visual field.

Computer modeling shows that a saliency-based selection strategy can explain many aspects of attentional shifts, eye movements, and object detection. Selection is controlled via an explicit *saliency map*. The neurons of this map do not encode particular stimulus attributes, such as color or orientation, but conspicuity—that is, how different the stimulus is from its immediate neighborhood. A winner-take-all mechanism selects the currently most salient location in the map and directs attention to it via a gating mechanism. After a short while, this location in the saliency map is inhibited and the searchlight automatically shifts to the next most salient location in the image.[21]

---

[18]In military boot camp, a drill sergeant frequently screams at some unlucky recruit for some minor offense, while the soldier must stand ram-rod at attention, staring straight ahead, thereby demonstrating the discipline needed to inhibit the superior colliculus by way of the cortex.

[19]The links between moving the eyes and shifting the "inner eye" are explored from the psychological point of view by Shepherd, Findlay, and Hockey (1986), and at the neurological level by Corbetta (1998) and Astafiev et al. (2003). According to the pre-motor theory, attentional shifts to a point in the visual field occur because the oculo-motor system is preparing to move the eyes to that location (Sheliga, Riggio, and Rizzolatti, 1994; Kustov and Robinson, 1996).

[20]Saliency can be manipulated without necessarily affecting the appearance of things (Blaser, Sperling, and Lu, 1999).

[21]Koch and Ullman (1985) originally proposed a retinotopic saliency map as an attentional selection strategy. Related ideas expressed within a psychological tradition can be found in Treisman and Gelade (1980) and Wolfe (1994). Itti, Koch, and Niebur (1998) and Itti and Koch (2000) implemented this scheme in a suite of vision algorithms applied to video or natural

TABLE 9.1 Two Forms of Attentional Selection

Property	Bottom-up	Top-down
Spatial specificity	Thoroughout field of view	Spatially proscribed (focal)
Feature specificity	Acts at all times and in all feature dimensions (saliency)	Can select specific attribute
Duration	Transient	Sustained (with effort)
Task dependency	No	Yes
Under volitional control	No	Yes

Combining this saliency-based, bottom-up form of attentional deployment with the focal, top-down selection discussed earlier gives rise to a two-component framework of attention (Table 9.1).[22] The former is automatic and transient, while the latter is voluntary and sustained (with effort). The willful engagement of attention is effective, but comes at a price. It takes time for the task information ("look for a plus sign") to affect the visual system. Focal attention then needs to dwell at the location of some potential target, disengage from it, and move on to the next location. Time estimates range from a few hundred milliseconds to half a second or longer for this entire process.

A binary theory accounts well for change blindness: You detect the object that appears and disappears if it is either highly salient or if you attend to it. Otherwise, it passes from view unseen.

---

scenes. Machine vision systems built around a saliency map do well in detecting, tracking, and identifying "interesting" objects (Walther et al., 2002). Neurophysiological and psychological evidence for saliency maps in the brain is reviewed by Itti and Koch (2001). Other models of attention (Hamker and Worcester, 2002; Rolls and Deco, 2002; and Hamker, 2004) avoid an explicit saliency map, relying instead on the dynamically recurrent interaction among cortical areas.

[22] This framework dates back to James (1890). These two sorts of attention are also called *exogenous* (bottom-up) and *endogenous attention* (top-down). See Nakayama and Mackeben (1989); Shimojo, Tanaka, and Watanabe (1996); Egeth and Yantis (1997); Braun and Julesz (1998); Duncan (1998); and VanRullen and Koch (2003a). I here use the term top-down attention as operationalized by dual-task and visual search paradigms.

9.3 │ DOES CONSCIOUSNESS REQUIRE ATTENTION?

As stated early on in this chapter, to most psychologists attention and consciousness are inexorably linked—you are only conscious of what you attend to. This doesn't quite jibe with the way the world looks, though. When I stare intently at a distant wall to determine its exact shape and decide whether it has enough holds to be climbed, the rest of the world doesn't turn an indistinct gray. The universe is not reduced to the area illuminated by the attentional spotlight.[23]

Doing Two Things at Once

One way to evaluate whether focal attention is necessary for awareness is to consider what you see when focal attention is tied down elsewhere. Jochen Braun, now in the United Kingdon at the University of Plymouth, is a master at exploiting this *dual-task paradigm*. He trains subjects in an attentionally demanding task at the fovea, where they fixate, while simultaneously having them perform a secondary task in the periphery, out of the corner of their eyes. In one such experiment, they had to identify a peripheral target embedded within an array of objects. If the target was sufficiently salient, if it stood out among the crowd of distractors, it was easily detected without interfering with the performance of the central task at the fovea.[24] Trained observers can even distinguish two bars in the periphery and name their color and orientation, all while successfully coping with the central task. That is, with top-down attention pinned down at fixation, subjects *see* one or two objects quite a distance away as long as they are salient enough. In Braun's words, "observers enjoy a significant degree of ambient visual awareness outside the focus of attention."

This paltry trickle of information about artificial stimuli outside the focus of attention turns into a gush once natural images are used. Dual-task experiments by FeiFei Li and Rufin VanRullen at the California Institute of Technology (Figure 9.3) demonstrate that focal attention is not needed to recognize the presence of one or more animals (or vehicles) in briefly flashed natural scenes (e.g., jungles, urban landscapes, savannahs, and so on). This result is

---

[23] Something like this does happen, however, in Balint's syndrome, a rare neurological condition discussed in Section 10.3.

[24] Sperling and Dosher (1986); Braun and Sagi (1990); Braun (1994); and Braun and Julesz (1998). Driving a car while using the cell phone is an everyday example of a dual task. Unfortunately, experiments show (Strayer and Johnston, 2001) that the attentional requirements of carrying out an engaging conversation significantly decrease the chances of detecting traffic signals and increases the driver's reaction time to them. Whether the phone was hand-held or hands-free made no difference. So, don't drive and call at the same time! See also de Fockert et al. (2001).

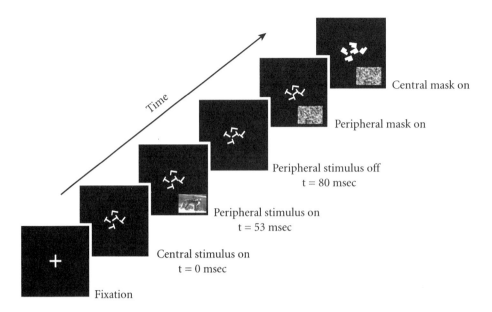

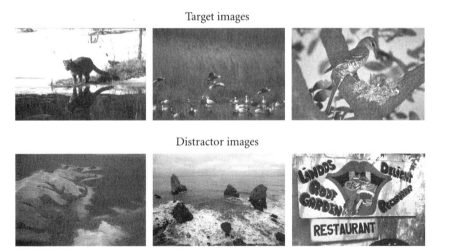

FIGURE 9.3 *Seeing Outside the Focus of Attention* In a *dual task,* subjects must carry out two jobs. At fixation, they have to decide whether the briefly visible letters are all the same or whether one is different. Simultaneously, they have to judge whether a colored photograph of a natural scene that is flashed somewhere in the periphery contains one or more animals (target) or none (distractor). Surprisingly, they can do this, even though they are stymied if the peripheral task is replaced by one in which subjects must decide whether either a red-green or a green-red bisected disk appeared somewhere in the periphery. Modified from Li et al. (2002).

quite surprising—detecting an arbitrary animal in a photo is fairly complicated from a computational point of view—and lacks an adequate explanation.
In stark contrast, a seemingly simpler task, distinguishing a bisected red-green
disk from a green-red one, requires focal attention.[25]

Gist Perception

One of the many pleasures of living in North America is driving in solitude
for hours on end across the high plateaus, deserts, and mountains of the West,
with its sweeping vistas. I can ponder life's mysteries or listen to the complete
Ring des Nibelungen without interruption. I drive as if on automatic pilot (an
example of an on-line or automatic system introduced in Chapter 12), while
I concentrate on the music but not on the scenery streaming past. Yet under
these spaced-out conditions, I am still conscious of the gently curving road
ahead, a slow moving truck in front of me, a billboard off to the right, the over-
pass coming up, and so on. Although little studied in the laboratory, humans
often wander through the world lost in thought.

What I see is the *gist*, a high-level, semantic representation of familiar scenes
that can literally be apprehended in a flash. It's a vignette, a succinct summary
of what is in front of me, devoid of details—a crowd at a football game, a
lone cyclist, a mountain. Gist might even include the fact that some animal is
present, without knowing its identity or location (as in the experiment that I
just discussed). I suspect that gist perception does not require focal attention.[26]

Neurons in the upper stages of the visual system may directly encode gist
explicitly. These semantic neurons might respond, for example, to any animal,
or to office scenes, or to a crowd of kids.[27] Gist perception probably occurs
before you are aware of the details of the scene.[28] Because gist neurons are
found in the upper stages of the hierarchy (while the details are represented in
earlier areas), they may very quickly establish a dominant coalition, sufficient
for conscious perception of the gist. I argue in Chapter 15 that the NCC require
some sort of feedback from the prefrontal cortex, affecting higher areas before
it influences lower ones. This explains why, if the image is only flashed for a
very brief time, you still have the distinct feeling of seeing everything in front

---

[25] Li et al. (2002); see also Rousselet, Fabre-Thorpe, and Thorpe (2002) and the extensive commentary by Braun (2003). Similar experiments demonstrate that focal attention is not needed
to distinguish men's faces from women's (Reddy, Wilken, and Koch, 2004).

[26] Gist is immune from inattentional blindness (Mack and Rock, 1998).

[27] For the psychophysics of visual gist, see Potter and Levi (1969); Biederman (1972); Wolfe and
Bennett (1997); and Wolfe (1998b). Individual neurons in the medial temporal lobe of humans
respond to fairly high level semantic categories, such as images of animals or famous people
(Kreiman, Koch, and Fried, 2000a). They may be part of the neuronal correlate of gist perception. Gist is, by its very nature, invariant to large changes in the content of the scene. Thus, the
gist stays the same during the image manipulation that occurs in change blindness (Figure 9.1).

[28] A similar argument is made in Hochstein and Ahissar (2002).

of you without being able to report any of the particulars. This is precisely what the gist is: seeing the forest but not the trees!

Focal Attention May Not Be Strictly Necessary for Perception

When you pay attention to something, you usually become conscious of it. I've added the qualifier "usually" since if processing time or resources are severely curtailed, attentional amplification of a weak stimulus may not be sufficient for it to reach consciousness.[29] What about the converse? Can you become conscious of something without necessarily focusing attention onto the event?[30]

Focal attention acts as a gatekeeper, but not the only one, to conscious perception. Its role is two-fold.[31] First, as postulated by Treisman's feature-integration theory, attention must dynamically generate neuronal selectivities that are not explicitly present at the level of individual neurons. It solves the binding problem for novel stimuli (this is explained in the next few pages). Second, attention helps resolve the competition that arises when two or more objects share overlapping neural representations. This occurs for natural scenes containing many things. In this case, attention biases the coalition coding for one object, thereby suppressing competing assemblies and reducing neuronal uncertainty. Focal attention is not needed to detect isolated features or object categories that are explicitly represented by the firing of groups of cells high up in the ventral pathway (if this explanation seems opaque, fear not; I expand on these ideas in the following chapter).

Here I enter the realm of speculation; bear with me. Confronted with the real world, populated by a dizzying variety of dynamic and partially occluded objects in cluttered and noisy environments, top-down attention selects one (or a few; Section 11.3) object and boosts its neuronal representation until the associated coalition dominates. If this coalition persists for long enough, the conscious percept of "seeing" the object comes about. The coalition's victory is ephemeral, however, because attention swiftly selects the next interesting thing and the game begins anew.

It follows from these postulated functions of focal attention that if dynamic binding is not required (because a preformed, explicit representation exists already) and in the absence of any real competition (because only one or a few, spatially dispersed, objects are out there in the world) focal attention is not

---

[29]Naccache, Blandin, and Dehaene (2002) demonstrated that unconscious word priming only occurred if subjects attended to the stimulus. Without attention, no priming took place. Paying attention to the masked stimulus was sufficient for priming but not for *seeing* the word. Attention without visual awareness has also been reported in blindsight (see Section 13.2 and Kentridge, Heywood, and Weiskrantz, 1999).

[30]See also Lamme (2003) and Hardcastle (2003).

[31]VanRullen and Koch (2003a); and VanRullen, Reddy, and Koch (2004).

needed for consciousness. In a world consisting solely of familiar, isolated, and clearly visible stimuli—such as a single patch of moving dots or a face—focal attention isn't necessary to recognize them.

Because the saliency-based form of attention is always active, it gives rise to neuronal activity that may trigger some transient degree of visual awareness (see Table 5.1). The psychologist Ronald Rensink calls such metastable neuronal coalitions *proto-objects*. Without further attentional bias, these structures quickly dissipate.[32] As a result, an awake person always has some visual experiences. These can only be turned off by closing the eyes.

Such experiences, coupled with gist perception, have limited informational capacity—as change blindness attests to—yet they are powerful enough to mediate the cherished sense of the real, the belief that you see everything around you.

As discussed in the context of change or inattentional blindness, people have difficulty seeing the unexpected. This highlights a different role or even a different kind of attention, tied to the subject's *expectation*. For example, subjects have to receive extensive training before they successfully cope with dual-task experiments. Only when they have strong expectations about what they are likely to see, can they perform well on both tasks. Furthermore, I know from my own experiences that when looking at a very briefly presented visual stimulus the first couple of times, it is hard to make out anything except a vague feeling of "seeing something." Eventually, after a dozen or more trials, I experience a fully-formed stable visual percept.

If expectation is considered as a variant of attention, it is plausible that some form of selective attention is necessary, but not sufficient, for a conscious percept to form. Frustratingly, though, it is difficult to rigorously prove this claim without an operationalized definition of attention. Care must be taken to not gratuitously reify attention. At the neuronal level, attention may be but a set of mechanisms to transiently assemble coalitions of neurons and to influence interstimulus competition. When these functions are not required, attention may not be needed either. Contemporary psychological methods by themselves are not powerful enough to resolve this question decisively.

9.4 | THE BINDING PROBLEM

Chapter 2 introduced the binding problem. It arises from the brain's architecture, in which the outside world is represented by nervous activity in a hundred or more distinct regions.

---

[32] By attending to them, they can be strengthened and made accessible to memory or the planning stages (Rensink, 2000a, b). A related idea is James's *fringe consciousness* (James, 1962; Galin, 1997).

Suppose I am looking at a smiling young man. His face triggers activity in the fusiform face area and in other parts of the cortex dedicated to facial recognition. The hue of his skin activates color neurons. As his head sways back and forth, neurons in a plethora of regions subserving motion generate spikes. His voice triggers a torrent of neural activity in the auditory cortex and speech related regions, and on and on. Nevertheless, all of this disparate activity is experienced as a single, integrated percept: my son talking to me. von der Malsburg was among the first to explore how integration can be achieved in the far-flung networks of the brain.[33]

Binding Comes in Different Flavors

Several types of binding must be distinguished. As Francis and I wrote in 1990,[34]

> Binding can be of several types. In a sense a neuron responding to an oriented line can be considered to be binding a set of points. The inputs to such a neuron are probably determined by genes and by developmental processes that have evolved due to the experience of our distant ancestors. Other forms of binding, such as that required for the recognition of familiar objects such as the letters of a well-known alphabet, may be acquired by frequently repeated experience; that is, by being overlearnt. This probably implies that many of the neurons involved have as a result become strongly connected together. (Recall that most cortical neurons have many thousands of connections and that initially many of these may be weak.) Both these types of binding are likely to have a large but limited capacity.

This second category of binding may underlie much of the sights and sounds of everyday life. Suppose you're looking at a well-known politician. His face stares out at you so often from TV screens, newspapers, and magazine covers that neurons in the upper parts of the visual hierarchy learn to respond to him in a sparse and explicit manner (Figure 2.2). Firing of these neurons will come to symbolize him. Cells do this by detecting common correlations in their inputs and altering their synapses and other properties so that they can more easily respond to them. Exactly how this happens remains controversial. The existence of such neurons implies that the feature they symbolize may be

---

[33]The roots of the binding problem reach back, in some form, to Immanuel Kant at the end of the 18th century. Binding via neural synchrony was proposed in Milner (1974) and von der Malsburg (1981). For more recent accounts, see von der Malsburg (1995, 1999), Treisman (1996), and Robertson (2003). Some recent experiments, discussed in Section 15.2, have raised doubts about the temporal precision with which multiple attributes are bound into a single percept. At the time-scale of 50 msec, unitary perception may well be fragmented.

[34]Taken from Crick and Koch (1990a).

detected without utilizing top-down attention. This conjecture can be tested using the dual-task method.

Because such specific neurons are in all likelihood rapidly recruited to partake in the storage and recognition of newly learned sights, it is possible that most of what you experience on a daily basis is encoded by overlearning. The faces of family, friends, and celebrities, your pet, your car, the font you use for personal documents, the Statue of Liberty, and so on, might be represented by dedicated neurons, solving the binding problem in hardware.[35]

Francis and I then went on to postulate a third binding mechanism.

> The binding we are especially concerned with is a third type, being neither epigenetically determined nor overlearnt. It applies particularly to objects whose exact combination of features may be quite novel to us. The neurons actively involved are unlikely all to be strongly connected together, at least in most cases. This binding must arise rapidly. By its very nature it is largely transitory and must have an almost unlimited potential capacity, although its capacity at any one time may be limited. If a particular stimulus is repeated frequently, this third type of transient binding may eventually build up the second, overlearned type of binding.

It is this form of binding that needs, so we argue, focal attention. It permits you to see unfamiliar objects or familiar things in combinations you've never experienced before.[36] This form may be implemented using synchronized oscillations, such that the neurons in the various areas that encode for the attended object fire in concert, in a synchronized manner (see footnote 33 on the previous page).

Binding for Multiple Objects and Illusory Conjunctions

Binding a single object seems complicated enough, yet the brain faces an even more daunting challenge when confronted with multiple objects. In early topographic areas, such as V1 and V2, edges, colors, and other primitives associated with objects located at different points in the scene are encoded in correspondingly different parts of the cortex. For the most part, there is no or only minimal overlap. But what about high-level ventral areas that have

---

[35] How rapid this learning mechanism operates depends on the level in the processing hierarchy at which the relevant neurons are situated. In early areas, such as V1, learning low-level features requires numerous exposures, while a single experience can be remembered by the medial temporal lobe.

[36] There are hints from a patient with damaged parietal cortex that transient binding can occur without giving rise to awareness (Wojciulik and Kanwisher, 1998). That is, binding is not sufficient, by itself, for conscious perception.

no (or little) apparent topographic order? Two spatially distinct objects will often have overlapping neuronal representations, creating the potential for confusion.

Suppose you are looking at two dogs, a black German Shepherd with a red scarf around her neck and a white Kuvasz with a blue scarf. In brain areas representing colors and objects, at least four groups of neurons will be active— one for the German Shepherd, one for the Kuvasz, one for the red scarf, and one for the blue. How will the brain know, though, that the activity of the "red scarf" group goes together with the "black dog" group? All else being equal, the next stage could interpret this activity pattern as a black dog wearing a blue scarf (an illusion, in other words). And, indeed, such illusions do occasionally happen. *Conjunction errors*—confusing the attributes of one object with those of another one—occur when processing time is severely curtailed.[37]

Nontopographic regions of the visual brain might deal with this by wiring up cells that represent a black guard dog with a red scarf, but this costs time and ties up a large number of neurons. Alternatively, as von der Malsburg suggested, the brain could exploit temporal synchronization of the spike discharge to label the appropriate neuronal coalitions in different ways.[38] This difficulty is avoided in V1 and related topographic areas, because the images of the two dogs occupy different locations and thereby excite different populations of cells without ambiguity.

9.5 | RECAPITULATION

Neuronal selection mechanisms prevent information overload by letting only a fraction of all sensory data pass into awareness. Change blindness, inattentional blindness, and magic shows are compelling demonstrations that you fail to notice things before your very eyes unless you attend to them or they, themselves, draw your attention.

A large body of psychophysical evidence, based on the visual search and dual-task paradigms, can be summarized by postulating two selection mechanisms, namely bottom-up, transient, saliency-based attention and top-down, sustained, focal attention. Saliency-based attention is driven by intrinsic image qualities, such as the presence of some feature relative to its neighborhood.

---

[37] Treisman and Schmidt (1982), and Treisman (1998). Tsal (1989) and Wolfe and Cave (1999) offer alternative accounts.

[38] Multiple attributes could be bound to multiple objects either by using different frequencies, different phase delays within one particular frequency, or by multiplexing two frequency bands, a low frequency carrier and a high frequency signal, as in FM radio (Lisman and Idiart, 1995). You may want to return to Section 2.3, to the analogy with the electric lights flickering on the Christmas tree.

It acts rapidly, automatically, operates throughout the entire visual field, and mediates pop-out. In the normal course of events, this form of attention can only be turned off by closing the eyes. Willful, top-down attention takes longer to deploy and can be directed to a proscribed region in space, to individual objects, or to specific attributes throughout the visual field.

Attention and consciousness are distinct processes. Some type of attentional selection is probably necessary, but may not be sufficient, for conscious perception. When attending to something, the rest of the world doesn't disappear. Even when lost in thought, you remain conscious of the gist of the scene in front of you. In combination with proto-objects—neural assemblies that don't have enough time to properly establish themselves—the neuronal representation for gist mediate the rich sense of seeing everything. One role of focal attention is to resolve competition when two or more objects are represented within the same neural network. In that case, attention biases the assembly coding for one object, thereby suppressing the other.

I discussed the binding problem: How can a percept be experienced as unitary, when its underlying neural representations are dispersed all over the brain? This problem becomes more severe when the attributes of two or more objects need to be represented; when there isn't enough processing time, errors in binding can occur, illusory conjunctions.

The brain possesses at least three distinct integration mechanisms to deal with the binding problem. One is the confluence of information laid down in the genes and early sensory experience, leading to neurons that explicitly respond to the combination of two or more features. A second mechanism involves rapid learning. If confronted with the same object numerous times, neurons rewire themselves to explicitly represent it. This strategy is efficient and does not require an inordinate amount of hardware. A third type of binding deals with novel, never-before-experienced objects or combinations thereof. It dynamically generates neuronal selectivities that are not explicitly present at the level of individual cells and depends on focal attention.

How are attentional selection mechanisms implemented? How does attention influence the firing of neurons? Understanding this will provide us with important lessons for the NCC. Read on.

CHAPTER TEN

The Neuronal Underpinnings of Attention

Everything should be made as simple as possible, but not simpler.

Attributed to Albert Einstein

You are oblivious to much of what goes on around you. As you just learned in the previous chapter, you selectively attend to places, objects, or happenings in the world, devoting additional processing resources to their analysis. In particular, you usually become conscious of them. Everything else is pretty much tuned out. Selective processing, therefore, comes at a price—a vast sea of never-perceived events. This strategy works only if the way that attention selects things is fast, fairly clever, and can learn to cope with new threats.

How do these selection mechanisms operate? Psychologists speak of processing limitations and the bottleneck of attention, yet the brain has a quintessential massively parallel architecture, with the environment mapped onto numerous cortical regions. How does the serial character of attention and awareness arise out of these enormously dispersed networks?

Before discussing the relevant data, recall the election metaphor introduced in Section 2.1. Democratic elections in a populous country, such as India or the United States, each with hundreds of millions of independently voting citizens, are truly massive parallel affairs. Ultimately, however, only a single person from a single party can be prime minister or president. This corresponds to the winning neuronal coalition that represents what you are conscious of. With some regularity (occasionally interrupted by resignations or assassinations), leaders are replaced, as the focus of attention shifts from one object to the next. Getting elected or passing legislation requires temporary alliances to be forged among competing interests. For example, big business may temporarily side with labor unions to defeat a candidate who promotes stringent environmental regulations, but once that goal is accomplished, they may fight over the liberalization of markets. The number of relationships among individuals—their connectivity—can be quite large. Most people, though, are not quite as gregarious as some pyramidal neurons that receive input from, and output to, thousands of other cells.[1]

With this analogy in mind, let me turn to how attention influences the neuronal networks of the brain. Given the tight, though not exclusive, relationship between attention and awareness, there are lessons with direct relevance to the NCC to be learned.

10.1 | MECHANISTIC ACCOUNTS OF ATTENTION

Recall from Section 9.3 that two functions of attention are to dynamically bind features for objects that do not have an explicit neuronal representation, and to resolve the competition that arises when multiple objects or events are represented within the same network.

Unfortunately, a direct test of the binding hypothesis is an uphill battle against a sort of neuronal Heisenberg uncertainty principle. That is, the more the brain is probed, the more it changes. Evaluating synchronization during focal attention requires teaching a monkey some sort of visual discrimination task. The necessary training is extensive. It takes a few hours a day, day in, day out, over many, many months. By the time the monkey can adequately carry out the task, it has seen the stimuli thousands of times, ensuring the formation of an explicit neuronal representation that comes to symbolize the various inputs. That is, binding may shift from being implemented dynamically across a large neuronal population to being solved at the single neuron level. Overlearning can be avoided by using objects that are unfamiliar to the animal, but unless precautions are taken, this will likely confuse it. Quite a bit has been learned, on the other hand, about how attention influences interneuronal competition.[2]

---

[1] The philosopher Olaf Stapledon suggested in *Star Maker* that galaxies could evolve toward some form of (self-)consciousness (Stapledon, 1937). This is unlikely, however. Even though a large galaxy contains more stars than there are neurons in the human brain, and even though stars are complex entities, these stellar denizens are coupled to each other via gravitational forces whose influence decays homogeneously in space. There is no known astrophysical mechanism at these vast cosmic scales that would allow for specific, adaptable interactions between pairs of stars relatively independent of distance. It is these interactions, however, that are key to information processing, storage, and recall.

[2] Electrophysiological investigations of attention in behaving monkeys were pioneered by Robert Wurtz and Michael Goldberg at the National Eye Institute outside Washington, D.C. (Wurtz, Goldberg, and Robinson, 1982), and by Vernon Mountcastle at Johns Hopkins University in Baltimore, Maryland (Mountcastle, Andersen, and Motter, 1981).

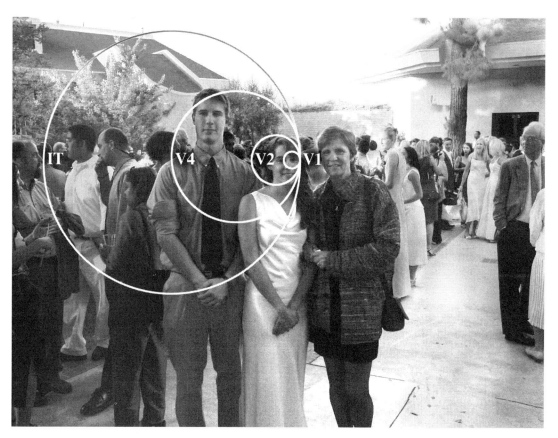

FIGURE 10.1 *The Need for Attention* Suppose you are looking at my family in this high school graduation photo. I've superimposed, in a schematic fashion, idealized receptive fields of exemplar neurons from four stages along the vision-for-perception pathway. Attention permits cells to effectively limit their input to a subregion within their receptive field, enhancing their selectivity and responsiveness.

Biased Competition or the Origin of the Attentional Bottleneck

Receptive fields in V1—particularly those covering the fovea—are small (less than 1°). At successive stages in the ventral stream, receptive field sizes steadily increase until, in the inferotemporal cortex (IT), receptive fields can encompass a large fraction of the entire visual field (while retaining a bias for foveal stimuli). Under natural conditions, that means that neurons at these higher stages receive a mixture of objects as input, in Figure 10.1 a combination of my son's and my daughter's face. This is confusing to the cell and it is likely to only respond weakly. Much could be gained if the visual input could shrink around a single object, the one at the focus of attention.

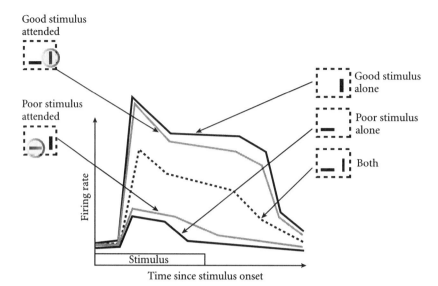

FIGURE 10.2 *Attention at the Neuronal Level* The competition among cortical neurons that sets in when more than one object is located within their receptive fields is resolved in favor of the attended item. Here a hypothetical V4 cell responds best to a lone vertical bar of light and poorly to a horizontal one within its receptive field (here schematized by a rectangle). When attention is directed away from both, the response amplitude to their joint appearance is intermediate between the responses to the individual bars. If the monkey concentrates on the vertical bar, the cell behaves as if the distracting horizontal bar was removed. If attention shifts to the horizontal bar, the neuron fires weakly, as if its trigger feature, the vertical bar, has been filtered out. Modified from Reynolds and Desimone (1999).

Let me discuss a simpler example of a scene containing but a vertical and a horizontal line (Figure 10.2). This input will activate tens of thousands (if not many more) of cells throughout the visual cortex. What is the effect of these dual stimuli on an individual neuron that responds preferentially to a single vertical bar, but barely to a horizontal bar, by itself?

As long as the monkey is attending elsewhere, the neuron's response to their joint appearance is less than the response to the vertical bar by itself. This reduction in firing is due to interneuronal tug-of-war and has profound consequences when looking at the real world, filled with adjacent or even overlapping objects. Without attention, cortical neurons would respond to all of this stuff, but without gusto; thus, it would be difficult for any one coalition to establish itself. As a consequence, the prefrontal cortex would hear only a cacophony of weak voices.

Things change, though, if the animal attends to the vertical bar. Now the cell's original vigorous response is almost restored. It is as if all cells whose preferred orientation is vertical receive a boost, enabling them to successfully fight off the inhibitory influence of the nonpreferred stimulus (Figure 10.2). The same logic also applies when the monkey attends to the cell's nonpreferred (horizontal) stimulus, but in an opposite way. Boosted by attentional bias, the horizontally-selective cells in a nearby orientation column will fire more strongly. They can therefore more effectively suppress the response of neighboring cells that encode for other orientations, such as the vertical cell.[3] The net result of attending to an object in the presence of competing stimuli (nearby objects) is to mimic the cell's response to the object shown in isolation. Extending across multiple levels, these effects are compounded such that the neuronal representations of objects within the searchlight are much stronger than those not benefiting from attention (unless they are, by themselves, highly salient).

The cellular manifestations of attention can be understood as helping one budding coalition establish dominance over other nascent coalitions. This principle was enunciated by the electrophysiologist Robert Desimone at the National Institute of Mental Health and the psychologist John Duncan at the MRC Cognition Unit in Cambridge, England.[4] Their *biased competition* framework assumes that attentional signals—top-down or bottom-up—influence the competition in favor of the attended stimulus.[5]

The action of attention depends on the distance between the stimuli and at what level in the hierarchy they are represented. Little interference is expected as long as the relevant neuronal networks don't overlap and, consequently, are not directly competing with each other. This principle explains much of the dual-task performance of Section 9.3.

Bottom-up, saliency-driven, and top-down, volitionally-controlled attention bias the competition until only the coalitions for one or a few items sur-

---

[3]Moran and Desimone (1985); Miller, Gochin, and Gross (1993); and Rolls and Tovee, (1995). Numerous experiments have manipulated what monkeys attend to while recording from cells in areas V2, V4, MT, MST, and IT (Chelazzi et al., 1993; Treue and Maunsell, 1996; Luck et al., 1997; Reynolds, Chelazzi, and Desimone, 1999; Reynolds and Desimone, 1999; and Rolls, Aggelopoulos, and Zheng, 2003). Competitive suppression has been observed in extrastriate human cortex on the basis of fMRI (Kastner et al., 1998).

[4]Desimone and Duncan (1995). In Crick and Koch (1990b), Francis and I had similarly postulated that spatial attention turns on, or greatly strengthens, competition among two stimuli within a cortical column. Computational modeling of increased competition among banks of tuned filters accounts quantitatively for a lot of psychophysical thresholds measured with and without focal attention (Lee et al., 1999).

[5]This attentional bias can often lessen the cell's response, as in the second curve from the bottom in Figure 10.2. Reynolds and Desimone (1999) observed that stimulus saliency modulated the competition between two stimuli within the cell's receptive field. Suppose, for example, that the horizontal bar in Figure 10.2 was low contrast. Increasing its contrast while the monkey attended to this stimulus would further decrease the cell's output, despite the continuing presence of the cell's preferred stimulus. This makes perfect sense within the competition framework.

vive in the anterior part of the inferior temporal cortex.[6] These items are the ones the subject becomes aware of. The suite of cortical regions that are fed by the output from IT, namely the memory systems of the medial temporal lobe and the planning and decision making networks in the prefrontal region, are dominated by information pertaining to these attended objects.

In terms of the election metaphor, the counterpart of focal attention is the money used to run an aggressive advertising campaign. It biases the competition in favor of the candidate with the deep pockets and organizational power.

10.2 | ATTENTIONAL INFLUENCES OCCUR THROUGHOUT THE VISUAL HIERARCHY

How do attentional influences manifest themselves? Electrophysiological experiments in monkeys and brain imaging in humans show that focal attention can modulate responses throughout the cortex—including V1, V2, V4, MT, parietal and inferior temporal areas of the dorsal and ventral pathways, and premotor and prefrontal structures—and the thalamus. Depending on the exact context, attention may act at practically all levels beyond the retina.

The effects of attention can be seen as early as the lateral geniculate nucleus and V1.[7] They are spatially circumscribed and depend on the difficulty of the task.[8] Other studies characterized the neuronal signatures of feature- and object-based attention in early regions (V1 and MT).[9]

---

[6] V4 and posterior IT (PIT) are key players in the attentional modulation of perceptual tasks. Without these regions, animals can still discriminate an isolated target but not when it is embedded within a dense visual display. The brain needs V4 and PIT to sort the wheat from the chaff (DeWeerd et al., 1999).

[7] Attentional modulations of V1 cells in the monkey are described by Motter (1993) and Ito and Gilbert (1999). Many groups report attentionally modulated hemodynamic responses in human LGN and visual cortex (Watanabe et al., 1998; Somers et al., 1999; Gandhi, Heeger, and Boynton, 1999; Brefczynski and DeYoe, 1999; Kastner and Ungerleider, 2000; and O'Connor et al., 2002). Leaving aside eye movements—a form of attention—only the retina is immune from such attentional modulations, because no—or only very few (Spinelli, Pribram, and Weingarten, 1965; Brooke, Downes, and Powell, 1965)—fibers project back to the eyes.

[8] In a display with 10 independently moving balls, the *attentional load* increased as subjects had to simultaneously track 2, 3, 4, or even 5 balls that randomly bounced around. The amplitude of the fMRI signals increased proportionally to the difficulty of the task in selected parietal areas (Culham et al., 1998, and Jovicich et al., 2001).

[9] In one experiment, the monkey had to concentrate on a downward moving cloud of dots in one half of the visual field. This enhanced the firing of MT cells in the opposite field of view as well, provided that their preferred direction was also downward (Treue and Martinez-Trujillo, 1999; see also McAdams and Maunsell, 2000). The most compelling fMRI study of feature-based attention in people is that of Saenz, Buracas, and Boynton (2002). In yet another laboratory, monkeys were trained to attend to one of two elongated curves. When the attended contour snaked across

Methods based on recording action potentials from individual V1 neurons find that attention increased firing activity, but only mildly. Conversely, techniques that measure hemodynamic signals in V1 observe large and robust attentional effects. This discrepancy might reflect feedback that generates synaptic activity and increases the local metabolism, seen with the magnetic scanner, without necessarily enhancing the firing rate of V1 cells.

In higher areas, both fMRI in humans and single cell recordings in monkeys report strong attentional modulation. John Maunsell at Baylor College of Medicine in Houston, Texas, and his student Carrie McAdams, quantified attentional enhancement as a function of the orientation of a Gabor patch—an undulating grating with a slant in one particular orientation. Recording from hundreds of V4 cells, they found that attention increased cellular responses, on average, by about one-third (Figure 10.3). The gain of the cell is turned up—like the volume on the radio—without affecting its tuning. Similar results have been reported when varying the direction in which an object moves.[10] Maunsell argues that attention amplifies the part of the cell's response that exceeds spontaneous activity, akin to increasing the contrast of the attended object. In this case, the searchlight metaphor is perfectly appropriate, because any object illuminated by attention stands out.

In general, the lower the contrast or saliency of the target, the higher the beneficial effects of attention. For high-contrast stimuli, often little effect is seen. In the election metaphor, running additional TV or radio advertisements for a candidate who is far ahead will not increase her lead by much more.

Attention not only affects the firing rate of cells, but also shifts the exact spike timing around. Two teams of monkey electrophysiologists found that top-down attention increased spike synchrony among cells whose receptive fields were covered by the attentional searchlight. Spikes from two cells responding to an attended object were much more likely to occur at the same time than if the object was not attended to. This will boost their postsynaptic punch compared to randomly-firing cells. As predicted ten years earlier by Ernst Niebur and myself, the stimulus saliency may be directly encoded by spike coherency.[11]

---

the receptive field of cells in V1, the neuronal response was enhanced by about one-quarter compared to the case where the animal didn't attend (Roelfsema, Lamme, and Spekreijse, 1998).

[10] McAdams and Maunsell (1999) and Treue and Martinez Trujillo (1999) observed a wide range of neural responses, possibly associated with discrete cell types. A sizable minority of V4 cells showed little appreciable orientation tuning without attention but became more discriminating with attention. Other cells were unaffected by attention. The timing of these attentional effects anticipates the timing of behaviorally relevant events (Ghose and Maunsell, 2002).

[11] Multi-electrode recordings in the visual (Fries et al., 2001b) and the somatosensory cortex (Steinmetz et al., 2000) of behaving monkeys revealed an increase in spiking synchrony among neurons that represented the attended feature. This effect was postulated, and modeled, by

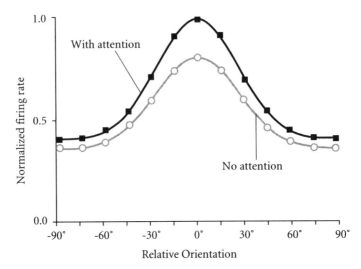

FIGURE 10.3 *Selective Attention Increases the Gain of Neurons* McAdams and Maunsell quantified one cellular manifestation of attentional selection by measuring the orientation tuning of V4 neurons with and without attention. Directing attention to a stimulus inside the receptive field increased the firing rate of the neuron by about one-third. Modified from McAdams and Maunsell (1999).

While attentional effects take around 100 msec or longer to develop in V1, they occur much sooner in higher areas. This might be due to the topography of feedback projection from the frontal lobe. It reaches strongly and quickly into higher visual areas but only weakly and belatedly into earlier ones.[12]

Where do the attentional signals that bias competition originate? The source of top-down, willful attention must be sought in prefrontal structures. As I shall discuss in Chapter 11, it is here that neurons retain information by elevating their firing rate over many seconds. These neurons might well be responsible for encoding the instructions needed to successfully carry out the visual search tasks described in the previous chapter (e.g., remembering that you're looking for a red, vertical bar).

Niebur and Koch in 1994 (see also, Niebur, Koch, and Rosin, 1993; and Niebur, Hsiao, and Johnson, 2002). van Swinderen and Greenspan (2003) observed something similar in the fruit-fly. Their discovery opens up attentional selection to the type of targeted, genetic interventions presently not practical in mammals.

[12]Noesselt et al. (2002).

Sources for bottom-up, saliency-mediated attention are numerous and include the pulvinar nuclei of the thalamus,[13] regions such as the lateral intraparietal area in the posterior parietal cortex,[14] and the frontal eye fields.[15]

10.3 | NEGLECT, OR PATIENTS WHO ARE NOT BLIND AND YET CAN'T SEE

It should not be surprising that damage to some of these structures can give rise to pathologies of attention. One such affliction is *spatial hemi-neglect* or, simply, *neglect*. It most commonly follows an infarct involving the right inferior parietal lobe.[16]

A patient with spatial neglect fails to notice objects on his left or to explore the left side of space.[17] Thus, he runs into the doorway on his left, doesn't eat food on the left side of his plate, doesn't notice if somebody approaches from the left, or walks into the ladies room because he missed the first two letters in "WOMEN." Usually, nothing is wrong with his eyes, primary visual cortex, or motor system. If the patient's attention is explicitly drawn to the neglected information, he may notice it, usually by directly looking at it.

Extinction is a variant of this syndrome, or possibly a milder form. The patient sees a single isolated stimulus in the left field. When a second stim-

---

[13] The dorsomedial region of the pulvinar plays an important role in saliency-driven attention (Robinson and Petersen, 1992; and Robinson and Cowie, 1997). The area contains a map of the opposite half-field and connects reciprocally to the posterior parietal cortex. Dorsomedial neurons respond either when the animal is about to make a saccade into their receptive fields or when it attends to a stimulus there (Desimone et al., 1990). Patients with gross thalamic damage have difficulties deploying attention to the opposite field of view (Rafal and Posner, 1987; and LaBerge and Buchsbaum, 1990). For a single, salient object, performance is unaffected by temporarily inactivating the pulvinar. This is not surprising when considered within the framework of "biased competition."

[14] Parietal representations are modulated by spatial attention (Section 8.4), in particular by stimulus-driven saliency (Gottlieb, Kusunoki, and Goldberg 1998; Colby and Goldberg, 1999; and Bisley and Goldberg, 2003).

[15] The frontal eye fields are heavily involved in controlling saccades and attentional shifts (Huerta, Krubitzer, and Kaas, 1986; and Schall, 1997).

[16] Robertson and Marshall (1993); Rafal (1997a); Swick and Knight (1998); Driver and Mattingley (1998); and Heilman, Watson, and Valenstein (2003). Why humans have a pronounced right dominance in spatial cognition remains a source of much theorizing (Husain and Rorden, 2003). The correct *façon de parler* would be to refer to the ipsi- and contra-lesional sides. This makes the writing cumbersome, however, so I assume that the damage is in the right cortical hemisphere, causing deficits in the left field of view. There is a lively debate about the exact area(s) affected in neglect. Karnath, Ferber, and Himmelbach (2001) finger the superior temporal cortex, rather than the more traditional inferior parietal lobe or the junction between the temporal, parietal, and occipital lobes, as key culprit and as critical for spatial awareness (Karnath, 2001).

[17] Recall that the left field of view is mapped to the right side of the brain and vice versa.

ulus is present in the right field, however, it grabs attention, leaving the left object perceptually invisible, unseen. The right stimulus extinguishes the left one.[18]

Neglect is not restricted to vision. It can occur in the auditory or somatosensory domains and can even extend to the patient's own body. In this case, the individual will insist that his left arm belongs to somebody else. Fortunately for the patient's well-being, true neglect often disappears within a few weeks of the trauma. Extinction, on the other hand, can linger indefinitely.

Subjectively, the neglect patient is not conscious of objects toward his left side. This region, similar to the space behind your head, is not gray or dark; it is simply not consciously represented. In this regard, spatial neglect is quite different from hemianopia, the total blindness in one field that occurs after the loss of V1 (Section 6.1). An hemianopic patient is aware of this loss and learns to cope by turning his eyes and head, quite unlike a neglect patient. Paradoxically, therefore, a hemianopic patient experiences a more absolute deficit, but fares better than a person with neglect. Such a patient might be able to deduce the loss indirectly, but this kind of rational conclusion has no lasting impact on behavior. A neurologist can help the patient discover that the hand hanging down from his shoulder is actually his and not somebody else's, but this insight is soon lost amid the overwhelming inaccessibility of sensory evidence that "this arm moving about is actually mine."

The neglected region of space is not coded in purely retinal terms (e.g., everything to the left of the center of gaze), but depends on the direction of the head and body or on the focus of attention. Thus, a neglect patient that copies a drawing may omit the left side of each object in the sketch. The Italian neurologist Eduardo Bisiach even showed that neglect occurs in imagery. Patients from Milan were told to imagine standing on the steps of the cathedral, overlooking the Piazza del Duomo. In this case, they couldn't visualize the left side of the market square. Subsequently, they were instructed to imagine being located at the other end of the Piazza, looking toward the cathedral. They still neglected the side of the square to the left of them, but this time it corresponded to a region they had visualized perfectly well from the other vantage point.[19] That is, the extent to which the information is available depends on the subject's perspective, whether real or imagined.

---

[18]To distinguish between neglect and extinction, have the patient steadily fixate your nose, then ask him whether he can see your hand moving in his left, impaired visual field. A neglect patient can't, but a patient with extinction can. If you simultaneously wave your other hand in the patient's right, normal hemifield, however, it will distract his attention and he will now fail to see your hand on his left.

[19]Bisiach and Luzzatti (1978); Driver and Mattingley (1998); and Mattingley et al. (1998).

Despite the lack of awareness in the neglected field, the patient does retain limited, unconscious processing capabilities there.[20] Suppose a picture of an animal or a vegetable is flashed into the functioning hemifield and the patient has to quickly decide which one it was. If an image from the same category (animal or vegetable) is simultaneously projected into the impaired field of view, the patient's response becomes faster. If the stimulus in the neglected part of space is from a different category, however, the patient responds slower. Thus, the affected hemifield can still carry out simple classifications. Other implicit measures of behavior indicate that color, form, or identity can be extracted from objects that remain invisible to the subject.[21]

A functional imaging study revealed the hemodynamic activity subserving this unconscious processing. A 68-year-old man with right inferior parietal damage and profound left-side extinction was shown pictures of faces and houses while lying in a magnetic scanner.[22] When the images were presented individually in either the left or the right fields, the patient correctly recognized them. When two pictures were presented simultaneously, one to the left and one to the right of fixation, however, he did not see the left image (extinction). Nevertheless, the magnetic resonance scanner registered brain activity in the primary visual cortex for the perceptually empty field. This activity was indistinguishable in time-course and amplitude from activity in response to a unilateral picture that he could see. The neurologists could even detect activity in the fusiform face area of the ventral pathway. Besides reinforcing my earlier conclusion that V1 activity does not correspond to the content of visual consciousness, these data also emphasize that the mere existence of a significant fMRI signal does not imply awareness for the features represented in that region. The right neurons may not be activated or might not fire vigorously enough.

If parietal regions were critical for visual experiences, the loss of both left and right lobes should give rise to profound neglect throughout the entire field of view, a total loss of vision. This is not the case, however. Patients with a rare condition known as *Balint's syndrome* have bilateral parietal lesions. The hallmark of this condition is a persistent fixation onto a single object. That's

---

[20]Neglect does not necessarily destroy the spatial representations associated with the lesioned hemifield. Consider the strange case of a patient described by Vuilleumier et al. (1996). After the first infarct to the right inferior parietal lobe, the patient displayed all the classical symptoms of left spatial neglect. In the clinic, he suffered a second stroke around his left frontal eye fields. While this caused a transient speech problem, his neglect symptoms disappeared, making this a rare case of a beneficial infarct. What this remarkable event suggests—supported by animal data (Sprague, 1966; Schiller, True, and Conway, 1979; and Payne et al., 1996)—is that neglect is caused by excessive competition, by unbalanced inhibition rather than by a total loss of spatial information.

[21]Berti and Rizzolatti (1992) and Driver and Mattingley (1998).

[22]Rees et al. (2000). See Vuilleumier et al. (2002) for a related case report.

all they see; everything else is neglected. They can identify and describe the object at their focus, but not where it is with regard to anything else. These patients are lost in a universe devoid of any discernible spatial structure, a space that contains only what is inside the spotlight of attention.[23] Clearly, neurons in the posterior parietal cortices encode spatial relationships among objects, imposing order onto the perceived world. Yet they are not needed to generate a particular visual percept.

10.4 | RECAPITULATION

The previous chapter dealt with selective attention and its two postulated functions—namely, to dynamically bind attributes of unfamiliar objects and to bias the competition among coalitions of neurons so that the representation for the attended object is enhanced, while nonattended stimuli are suppressed. This chapter focuses on the neuronal substrate of these effects. Almost nothing is known about the mechanisms underlying binding; on the other hand, plenty of physiological evidence has accumulated in favor of its second function. Interference between two stimuli occurs if their representations overlap (if they fall into the same receptive field). If they don't compete, attention isn't necessary to process them. This biased competition framework is general enough to accommodate both electrophysiological and imaging data.

When ascending the cortical hierarchy, receptive fields become larger, giving rise to more competitive interactions (because stimuli are more likely to excite the same neuron). After a few stages of this cascaded form of competition, only a few neuronal assemblies remain. These survivors get other groups of cells in the planning and memory centers in the front of the brain involved. Together, these neurons reinforce each other and establish themselves as the NCC, and the subject becomes conscious of their representational content. The attentional bottleneck arises out of hierarchical processing in a parallel architecture with overlapping representations.

The attentional bias strengthens the output of neurons whose receptive fields overlap with the searchlight of attention or that represent a particular attribute, such as downward motion. Almost none of the cortical regions inspected so far appear immune from attentional modulation. The potency and time-course of these effects depends on the exact task and the nature of the stimuli. Their origins are diverse. Regions in the posterior parietal cortex and the pulvinar provide bottom-up, saliency driven cues, while the prefrontal cortex provides top-down instructions.

If some of these regions are defective, as in unilateral neglect or extinction, competition breaks down. Patients lose awareness for stimuli in the affected

---

[23] Rafal (1997b); Robertson et al. (1997); and Robertson (2003).

field, even though some unconscious processing capabilities remain. Patients with Balint's syndrome, associated with bilateral parietal lesions, see nothing except what they are attending to. The posterior parietal cortices are needed to generate the attentional signals necessary to see an entire scene and represent spatial relationships among things in that scene, but they are not strictly necessary for conscious object perception. Thus, the quest for the NCC will have to be pursued elsewhere, primarily along the ventral stream and in the prefrontal cortex. (I will do so in Chapter 16). Next, I will dwell on the different types of memory systems and their relationship to consciousness.

Memories and Consciousness

Has it ever struck you, Connie, that life is all memory, except for the one present moment that goes by you so quick you hardly catch it going? It's really all memory, Connie, except for each passing moment.

From *The Milk Train Doesn't Stop Here Anymore* by Tennessee Williams

All creatures, great and small, live in the present. Only an abbreviated and heavily edited version of the past can be relived. I recall the time I got into a fight in seventh grade over an ethnic taunt or, decades later, when I fell while leading a short climb up a steep boulder. These memories may be so vivid that they seem real, but what I remember is only a paltry and pale imitation of the richer experience I had then. The voluntary ability to recall specific episodes from the past endows life with a sense of self, belonging, and purpose.

Understanding memory is a quest as old as civilization itself. Until the early 19th century, it was pretty much the exclusive domain of philosophers. Unfortunately, introspection and logical argumentation, the sole methods available prior to the systematic scientific exploration of the mind, are insufficient to unravel such a complex system. Truly decisive insights had to await the marriage of psychology with clinical studies in the 20th century. Augmented by animal models of memory and by functional brain imaging in humans, the brain sciences have made dramatic strides in revealing the organization of memory.

Primates use a multitude of distinct modules to retain information. These modules differ in what they store, how the material is acquired and for how long it can be accessed, their site of expression, and their biophysical mode of operation.[1] Yet almost none of these are needed to experience something. Less is known about the rapid forms of memory that are necessary for consciousness.

---

[1] Analogues to the plurality of biological memory systems are found in computers. There is high-capacity, slow access, long-term information storage on hard disks, tapes, and DVDs, faster but lower capacity RAM for short-term memory, and very fast, but very limited, cache memory on the CPU itself.

11.1 | A FUNDAMENTAL DISTINCTION

What is memory? In the most general sense, it is any change following an experience. This definition is far too broad to be helpful, however, because it includes injury, fatigue, and the changes that occur during childhood. A more useful, operational definition of memory, suggested by the Israeli neurobiologist Yadin Dudai, is *the retention of experience-dependent internal representations over time.*[2] At the neuronal level, a fundamental dichotomy exists between short-term, *activity-dependent memory*, and long-term, *structural memory*.

Activity-dependent memory is encoded by maintained spiking in cliques of neurons. Prefrontal neurons keep on firing, albeit at a reduced rate, if their trigger feature, say a picture of a red circle, has been removed from sight and the subject has to remember the stimulus. These cells are selective because they don't fire to the memory of a green triangle. Their elevated firing rate is a neural trace of this transient form of memory.

Structural memory arises from appropriate adjustments in the neuronal hardware itself, in particular, in changes in the strength of the synapses between neurons (*synaptic plasticity*). Synaptic receptors of the NMDA type (Section 5.3) in the hippocampus, in particular, have been implicated in consolidating long-term memories.[3] Learning and memory may result from nonsynaptic structural changes, too, such as adjustments in the ionic channel densities controlling the threshold and the gain of the cell's firing response or in its dendritic morphology. Long-lasting forms of plasticity require protein synthesis and the modification of gene expression in the cell's nucleus.[4]

By way of analogy, recall that computer memories also come in two kinds, namely RAM and ROM. Whereas the content of dynamic RAM lasts only as long as the chip is powered, ROM retains its information for years, without electrical power. Likewise in people. Knocking somebody out with a blow to

---

[2] Squire and Kandel (1999) and Eichenbaum (2002) are two superb introductory books to memory and its molecular and neuronal correlates. For additional insight, consult Dudai (1989), Baddeley (1990), LeDoux (1996), and Martinez and Kesner (1998).

[3] In one spectacular experiment, Joe Tsien at Princeton University and his colleagues genetically engineered mice to express the juvenile form of the NMDA receptor in adults in the hippocampus (Tang et al., 1999). Using a battery of tests, they showed that the transgenic animals had enhanced learning abilities and memory. The critical difference between the adult and the juvenile forms of the NMDA receptor lies in the decay time of the current flowing through the receptor. It is much longer in young animals, which might explain why children learn so much more easily than adults. Wittenberg and Tsien (2002) discuss more recent findings in this rapidly-moving field.

[4] The dichotomy between activity-dependent and structural memory is not as absolute as I have made out here. How, for example, should an elevation in the concentration of intracellular calcium ions at the soma, which causes a reduction in the firing rate, be considered?

their head, or an anesthetic, erases what was on their mind without, generally, interfering with their long-term memories.[5]

The distinction between activity-dependent and structural memories is important for consciousness, because the NCC depend on the former but not on the latter.

11.2 | A TAXONOMY OF LONG-TERM MEMORY

Long-term memory systems that store relevant information for hours, days, or years, come in many flavors. Their storage capacities are commodious and nearly limitless.

Nonassociative Forms of Memory

Simplest are nonassociative forms of learning, such as *adaptation, habituation,* and *sensitization.* The orientation-dependent aftereffects discussed in Section 6.2 are one example of adaptation. Habituation occurs when you're in the presence of some constant background noise. You might notice this hum early on but, given its constant, nonthreatening presence, it eventually fades from your perception. Were somebody to discharge a gun at this point, you would be surprised and, for some time after, any abrupt noise would startle you, because you would have become sensitized.

The molecular and cellular basis of these forms of learning have been dissected in considerable detail in the marine snail *Aplysia* by Eric Kandel and his colleagues at Columbia University in New York.[6]

Associative Conditioning

Classical conditioning was famously explored by Ivan Pavlov in Czarist St. Petersburg. This line of research resulted from the observation that dogs salivated at the sight of the approaching attendant who fed them. The animals learned to associate the sight of the person with food, triggering the digestive reflex. Slugs, flies, birds, mice, monkeys, and humans can all be conditioned.

---

[5] In *hypothermic circulatory arrest* during cardiovascular surgery, the beating of the patient's heart is slowly stopped. To minimize neurological damage, the blood is cooled to a mere 10° C. This reduces brain metabolism to about one-tenth of its baseline value and suppresses almost all EEG activity. Nevertheless patients retain their long-term memories (McCullough et al., 1999). Francis Crick underwent such a procedure a few years ago, in which his EEG remained flat for about a half an hour, to no ill effect.

[6] This work culminated in a share of the 2000 Nobel prize in Physiology or Medicine for Kandel (Kandel, 2001).

To do so, two disparate events are associated with each other. The *conditioned stimulus*, initially meaningless to the organism, must be followed by a reinforcing event, the *unconditioned stimulus*. It is called unconditioned, since this stimulus, by itself, will elicit a predictable reflex, such as salivation or a startle response.[7]

In *fear conditioning*, an electric shock, loud noise, or a scary picture is combined with a tone. After one or a handful of such pairings, the tone reliably induces a conditioned response. In humans, this can be a change in heart rate or an increase in the *galvanic skin conductance*. You become anxious and start to sweat when you hear the tone (the basis of the lie detector test). In mice, *freezing*, in which all body movements cease (except for breathing), is usually taken as a measure of fear.

In a variant called *context fear conditioning*, subjects avoid the context—the location, odors, sights, and sounds—in which bad things have happened to them in the past. For example, if a mouse is dropped into a cage in which it was previously shocked, it will freeze for many minutes before gingerly exploring its new surroundings.

An ongoing debate revolves around the question of whether successful conditioning requires awareness of the conditioned and the unconditioned stimuli and of the relationship between them (for example, the tone is usually followed by a shock, while the ssssh-like noise never is). In this context, the neuroscientist Larry Squire, a pioneering explorer of human memory, and Robert Clark, both from the University of California at San Diego, made a crucial discovery when studying two variants of *eye blink conditioning*. A tone is combined with a puff of air to the eye. After a hundred or more of these pairings, subjects blink when they hear the tone. Their brains have come to expect the puff of air following the tone and reflexively move to protect their eyes by blinking.

Clark and Squire had one group of volunteers learn this association when the tone and the eye irritation took place at the same time. For arcane reasons, this is called *delay conditioning* (like in Figure 11.1). In a second group of subjects, the tone was followed, a half or a second later, by the air puff. This is called *trace conditioning*. In all other ways, both forms of conditioning are the same. Most subjects learned that a particular sound predicts the puff of air and blinked.

Remarkably, this minute difference—having the puff of air follow the sound rather than overlap with it—makes conditioning much more difficult. It becomes so demanding, in fact, that subjects must attend to the two events and need to be aware of the relationships between them in order to be condi-

---

[7]The conditioning literature is immense. For reviews, see Mackintosh (1983); Gallistel (1990); Tully (1998); Squire and Kandel (1999); Fendt and Fanselow (1999); Eichenbaum (2002); and Medina et al. (2002).

tioned. To demonstrate this, Clark and Squire distracted subjects during the conditioning procedure. Similar to the dual-task attentional experiments of Section 9.3, subjects had to track rapidly appearing numbers, or watch a movie while being bombarded with tones and puffs of air. Distraction had little effect on delay conditioning; subjects still learned to associate the tone with the puff of air, even if they failed to consciously note that the sound and the annoying blast of air occurred together. This was not the case for trace conditioning. If subjects were sufficiently engaged by the secondary task competing for their attention, the trace interval interposed between the tone and the puff of air prevented conditioning.

With the aid of a post-experimental questionnaire, Clark and Squire found that only those subjects who were conditioned under the trace paradigm could describe the relationship between the events. Those who were not conditioned were confused about which stimuli preceded the puff of air and which did not. It seems as if attention and awareness are needed to bridge the gap between the unconditioned and the conditioned stimuli.[8]

A Test for Consciousness in Mice

These findings acted as clarion call for me. I figured that this procedure, applicable to mice, could be one of a battery of operational tests for the presence of attention and awareness. The development of a sort of Turing test for consciousness would be very exciting. Let me tell you why.

The bulk of the ongoing experiments looking for the NCC involve humans and other primates (e.g., Chapter 16). For ethical reasons, human brains are, by and large, off-limits to the types of rigorous, controlled procedures that are necessary to tease apart the circuitry underlying the NCC. With proper care and compassion, electrophysiological or pharmacological interventions can be done in nonhuman primates, such as monkeys. Yet immense practical problems (gestation time, size, costs) severely constrain their widespread use.

---

[8]Clark and Squire (1998) actually employed a somewhat more sophisticated version of conditioning than described here. In their experiments, one sound, say a pure 2 kHz tone, predicted the puff of air, while a second sound, say a hissing noise, was never followed by the unconditioned stimulus. Subjects who conditioned under the trace paradigm could describe the relationship between the two types of sounds and the reinforcing puff of air (e.g., "the tone was followed by an air puff a short time later while the noise was not"). Those who didn't condition, couldn't describe the relationship between the three events. Such explicit knowledge made no difference to delay conditioning (see also Clark and Squire, 1999). It has long been surmised that many forms of associative conditioning require awareness (Baer and Fuhrer, 1970, and Dawson and Furedy, 1976). For related experiments, see Öhman and Soares (1998); Carrillo, Gabrieli, and Disterhoft (2000); Knuttinen et al. (2001); Carter et al. (2002); and Lovibond and Shanks (2002). In light of the close relationship between attention and awareness (Section 9.3), future work must clarify the exact role that both play in conditioning.

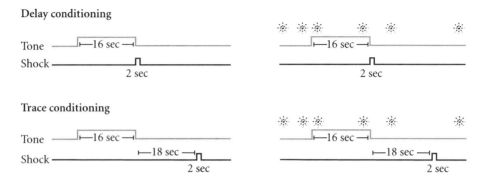

FIGURE 11.1 *An Assay for Attention and Awareness* Mice learn to associate a tone with an immediate (delay conditioning) or a retarded (trace conditioning) electrical shock. When bright lights are flashed at random in the gloomy cage during the tone-shock pairing phase, trace conditioning is much weaker, as if the flashes prevent the mice from attending to, and being aware of, the relationship between the tone and the shock. Distraction doesn't work when the shock immediately follows the tone. Modified from Han et al. (2003).

Molecular biology is coming to the rescue, however, by delivering technologies to cheaply and quickly manipulate genetically identifiable neuronal populations in another mammalian species, mice. It has not proven possible to routinely train mice to carry out visual discrimination or detection tasks popular with people or monkeys: Hence the importance of developing alternative operational means of routinely, rapidly, and conveniently evaluating consciousness in mice.

Two post-doctoral fellows, C.J. Han and Colm O'Tuathaigh, working in David Anderson's laboratory and mine at Caltech, in collaboration with Michael Fanselow and Jennifer Quinn at the University of California at Los Angeles (UCLA), have taken a huge step in this direction. First, Han had to design a protocol for robust trace and delay fear conditioning in mice. Six pairings of a beeping tone with an electrical shock proved to be sufficient to reliably induce freezing in the rodents upon hearing the tone (Figure 11.1). In a second step, O'Tuathaigh demonstrated that a visual distractor—flashing lights in an otherwise dimly lit cage—selectively interferes with the acquisition of trace conditioning but not with delay conditioning. It is as if the flashing lights distract the animals from attending to the relationship between tones and the shocks, leading to much more modest trace conditioning without interfering with learning in the delay context.[9]

---

[9]Contextual fear conditioning is also not reduced during the distracting procedure. These experiments are described in Han et al. (2003).

Based on the human data, one interpretation is that the flashing lights reduced murine awareness of the relationship between the tone and the shock when they didn't occur at the same time. If tone and shock directly follow each other—as in delay conditioning—no or only little awareness is needed. This would explain the selective interference.

This protocol offers an effective means to test, with the aid of pharmacological or genetic manipulations, which regions and which specific classes of neurons underlie a task that, in humans, involves awareness of the conditioned and unconditioned stimuli.[10] With this practical assay in place, large-scale screening of behavioral mutants becomes feasible. Indeed, it is quite possible that among the thousands of inbred strains of laboratory mice there are some that can't bridge the trace interval, either because they lack attentional selection mechanisms or some other aspect of the NCC. Such nonconscious mice would not survive for long in the wild, but might not show much of a deficit when reared in laboratories. It would be a pity to miss them for want of looking. Similar operational tests and screens might also usefully be applied to other species, including the genetic model animal *par excellence*, fruitflies.[11] Despite people's strong intuitions about the automata-like character of flies, these and other insects might harbor dim feelings, qualia for pain, odors, or sexual pleasure. How many neurons are really needed for a brain to express consciousness? 10,000, one million, or one billion nerve cells? Right now, we just do not know.

Another major form of associative learning is *operant conditioning*, made famous by Skinner and his eponymous Skinner box for training animals. Here the organism learns the consequence of its actions in order to seek a reward or to avoid a punishment. For instance, the rat will press a lever to obtain food pellets. Operant or instrumental learning is central to goal-directed behaviors.

Procedural Learning: Skills and Habits

Procedural learning is at the basis of the skills and habits that dictate the patterns of our life. Knotting a tie, driving a car, riding a bicycle, dancing, writing,

---

[10]We have shown, by injecting drugs that destroy the anterior cingulate cortex in mice, that this part of the frontal lobe is necessary for the acquisition of trace but not of delay or contextual fear conditioning (Han et al., 2003). In a parallel effort, we have demonstrated that trace fear conditioning in humans is susceptible to disruption by concurrent working memory or attentional tasks (Carter et al., 2003).

[11]This is not as outlandish as it sounds. Fruitflies are capable of complex behaviors, including choice and selective, saliency-based attention (Heisenberg and Wolf, 1984; Tang and Guo, 2001; and van Swinderen and Greenspan, 2003). Moreover, they can learn to associate odors with electric shocks under either the delay or the trace conditioning paradigms (Tully and Quinn, 1985). Could trace, but not delay, conditioning be disrupted by distracting flies with the yummy smell of rotting fruits? For a general discussion of animal consciousness, see Griffin and Speck, (2004).

keyboard typing, and so on, require extended practice. Once learned, these sensory-motor procedures last for a lifetime and are comparatively immune from the ravages that the passage of time visits upon explicit memories.

It is notoriously difficult to teach sensory-motor skills in the abstract—that is, by talking about them. Instead, they must be practiced and rehearsed, which is why some coaches speak about "muscle memory" (these skills are, of course, stored in the brain). Procedural learning gives birth to the zombie agents that labor on in submental obscurity, responsible for much of daily behavior. Zombie agents are the topic of Chapters 12 and 13.

The inability to directly and consciously recall skills is why procedural learning is thought of as *implicit* or *nondeclarative memory*. But attention and consciousness are, probably, still necessary to learn these skills.

The neuronal structures that acquire and maintain skills and habits include sensory-motor cortex, the striatum and related basal ganglia structures, and the cerebellum.

Declarative Memories: The Stuff Making up the Past

To most people, memory is the conscious evocation of facts or events from their past. Here, two categories must be distinguished: *episodic memory* and *semantic memory*.

Episodic, or autobiographical, memory endows you with the notion of who you are, where you come from, the experience of last week's movie, and what you had for breakfast this morning. Semantic memory, on the other hand, stores abstract facts, relationships, the meaning of words, and all the other things that constitute the fabric upon which culture, law, science, and technology are built.

Both forms of memory are *declarative*, because information is retrieved consciously and you know that you are accessing stored information. As a result, you don't confuse the memory of an event with the event itself. The storage of this information is not conscious. Before you read the words "Statue of Liberty," there was no active neuronal coalition in your brain that encoded the picture of this fair lady. That only existed as a distributed synaptic pattern.

A distinction between declarative and implicit memories had long been surmised but remained controversial until the storied patient, H.M., was brought to the notice of the neuroscience community. To control massive epileptic seizures, substantial chunks of his medial temporal lobes (MTL) were removed on both sides.[12] H.M. has no obvious perceptual deficiencies, but suffers from

---

[12]The original paper describing H.M.'s deficits, Scoville and Milner (1957), remains one of the most cited articles in behavioral brain research. Follow-up studies are described in Milner (1972); Corkin et al. (1997); and Milner, Squire, and Kandel (1998). Scoville, the neurosurgeon,

severe memory losses. He is severely *amnesic*[13] for events that occurred since a couple of years prior to his operation. He forgets events as soon as they are out of his sight and mind. He can, with effort, retain a three-digit number by continual rehearsal. When he is distracted, though, the number is gone. When a person leaves the room and reenters a few minutes later, H.M. can't recall having met them before. An hour after a meal, he is unable to remember what he had eaten or even whether he had eaten at all.[14]

Nevertheless, H.M. has no specific intellectual loss, has normal immediate memory, and can learn and retain new skills, such as mirror-drawing, although he is unable to remember how he had acquired these abilities. And he is most certainly conscious. He can describe and experience his environment, he correctly answers questions about immediate events, and so on.

The pattern of his deficits proves that declarative memories are acquired and stored at distinct sites from procedural memories. While the former system is impaired in H.M., the latter is not. Subsequent animal work confirmed the critical role of the hippocampal formation and the adjacent entorhinal and perirhinal cortices for declarative memory. Bilateral MTL lesions induce profound amnesia. The hippocampus, however, is not the ultimate storage site for explicit memories—the final repository is the neocortex, particularly the temporal and prefrontal lobes. The hippocampus combines the information coming from all sensory modalities for the to-be-remembered event and consolidates these in the relevant cortical areas over many weeks.

The continual presence of consciousness in the face of an almost complete loss of declarative memory is exemplified most dramatically by Clive Wearing. A gifted musician and scholar, he suffered a viral brain infection that almost killed him and destroyed parts of both temporal lobes. His case is extremely severe, both in the extent of his retrograde amnesia—he has only the haziest idea of who he is—as well as in his inability to learn anything new. His musical capacities have largely remained, however.[15] Clive consciously experiences only

---

excised the amygdala, perirhinal and entorhinal cortices, and the anterior hippocampus, on both sides. The parahippocampal cortices and the temporal neocortex were largely spared.

[13] *Amnesia* refers to a permanent inability to learn new facts or events (*anterograde amnesia*), a variable degree of loss of memory (*retrograde amnesia*), an intact short-term memory, and normal intellectual and cognitive abilities.

[14] In "The Lost Mariner," the neurologist Oliver Sacks recounts the story of another such patient who is permanently marooned in the past (Sacks, 1985).

[15] A few months following his illness, he started writing compulsively. His diary is filled, page after page, with entries such as "awake for the first time," "I just woke up for the first time," and "I am really awake and alive" (Wilson and Wearing, 1995). The case history of another man with a viral infection that wiped out anterior temporal regions and left him incapable of recalling or recognizing any episode from his entire life can be found in Damasio et al. (1985).

the present. He has no childhood, no past. Like an actor in a Greek tragedy, he moves through life, unaffected by events around him, impervious to the passage of time.[16]

Clive Wearing, H.M., and other profound amnesiacs are living proof that forming new declarative memories or remembering one's life is not necessary for consciousness. These losses leave them deeply impoverished, but conscious. Furthermore, as these patients can see, hear, and feel fine, it follows that the anterior hippocampus and other parts of the MTL are not strictly needed for consciousness.[17]

11.3 | SHORT-TERM MEMORY

Short-term or *immediate memory* is a catch-all term for the temporary storage of information over tens of seconds. Looking up a phone number and dialing it would be impossible without a temporary buffer to store the digits. Compared to long-term memory, immediate memory is more labile and has only a very limited capacity.

There is no single, dynamic, RAM-like buffer in the brain through which all information moves on its way to oblivion or more permanent storage. Instead, different sensory modalities have their own temporary memory capacities operating in parallel.

Psychologists have replaced the relatively vague concept of short-term memory with *working memory*, composed of a *central executive* and several slave modalities, such as the *visual buffer* or *scratchpad* for visual information and the *phonological loop* for language.[18]

---

[16]A compelling depiction of what it feels like to live forever in the present is the film noir *Memento*. Told from a subjective, reverse-chronological point of view, it is the story of Lenny, who sustained damage to his hippocampi during a botched burglary that left his wife dead. On a mission to avenge her murder, he improvises imaginative and terrifying ways to deal with his inability to remember events beyond his attention span. Besides being a haunting psycho-drama, *Memento* is also by far the most accurate portrayal of the different memory systems in the popular media. Directed by Christopher Nolan, the movie opened in 2001. Sternberg (2001) analyzes the film from a neuroscientific point of view.

[17]Given the strategic location of the MTL, in intimate contact with the upper stages of the visual processing hierarchy and prefrontal cortex, it is likely that the activity of some hippocampal neurons contributes directly to the current content of consciousness, but that their loss can be compensated.

[18]The idea of working memory owes much to the work of the psychologist Alan Baddeley (Baddeley, 1986, 1990, and 2000).

Working Memory Is Needed to Solve Immediate Problems

When you listen to somebody speak, short segments of what they said are stored in the phonological loop, serving as backup for off-line processing.[19] Adding numbers, following a recipe, planning to drive to the cinema, comparing the hue of two shirts, copying a line drawing, or filling out your tax return, are all activities that depend on working memory. Human intelligence, as measured by IQ tests, is intimately tied to the performance of working memory. Working memory is characterized by a small storage capacity, semantic representation, and short duration. Without active rehearsal, its content fades within a minute.

The central executive is the agency that controls access to the phonological loop, the visual buffer, and temporary storage for other modalities, via a sort of attentional selection process. Attention and working memory are closely intertwined, making it difficult to cleanly separate them. The more working memory is taxed, the less effective attention is at disregarding distractors. Anybody who has ever participated in a demanding psychophysical experiment (such as that in Figure 9.3) or the legions of people who chat away at great length on their cell phones while driving, know this well.[20]

One way to assess how much material can be stored in working memory is to present a random string of digits or letters at an even pace (say, ten numbers spaced out over twenty seconds) and have the subject repeat them in the correct order. The number of items that can be recalled is the subject's *memory span*. The span for spoken digits among undergraduates is between 8 and 10.[21]

How Many Things Can You See at a Glance?

The storage capacity of the visual buffer is probed by briefly presenting a scene. How much detail will you see? How much could you recall if you were prompted afterward?

Rufin VanRullen in my laboratory at Caltech flashed images, each containing discrete objects—a car, a bicycle, a dog—in their natural setting, for a quarter of a second on a monitor. To erase any lingering afterimage, a scrambled

---

[19]Have you ever had difficulty processing some utterance, queried the speaker about what she said, then suddenly understood it before she has had a chance to repeat the sentence? Presumably, this is the delayed effect of your language modality processing the speech segment stored in the phonological loop.

[20]See footnote 24 in Chapter 9 for the sobering story about cognitive interferences when driving while carrying on an engaging phone conversation.

[21]The original estimate of 7 ± 2, as much a rhetorical device as a summary of the data, was made in Miller (1956). Material with intrinsic significance that links one element to the next—birthdays, dates of historical events—is recalled better than a truly meaningless list (Cowan, 2001).

image followed each picture, thereby overwriting or *masking* (Section 15.3) the neural activity associated with the input. Immediately afterward, a list of twenty words appeared, ten of which described the ten objects in the scene and ten others which referred to things not in the photo. Subjects selected, on average, a tad more than two objects. They knew more were present, but couldn't identify them.

Subsequently, the observers had to choose additional objects from the list of 20 items until a total of 10 were selected. They were told to guess if they had no explicit recall of anything else. Correcting for chance hits, subjects detected nonconsciously a further two objects. That is, something about these objects must have left some trace in the brain. Psychologists refer to this phenomenon as *priming* (positive priming in this case).[22]

All in all, VanRullen concluded that his subjects registered a bit less than half of the 10 objects in some fashion. More than one item was seen—which one depended on its saliency, its familiarity, and other factors—but far short of all of them.[23] About five to seven things were registered by the brain, which is in line with the previous estimate for the capacity of verbal working memory.

Deficits in Working Memory

Consider patients with damaged working memory. Some can't even keep two numbers in mind, even though they have normal long-term memory.[24] Many speak haltingly, hesitantly, or agrammatically, and have difficulty finding appropriate words; but they are all conscious.

The British neuropsychologists Jane Riddoch and Glyn Humphreys tested three such patients.[25] All showed significantly reduced memory spans for spoken letters and words, for visually presented lists of words, and for nonlinguistic visual material. They had trouble correctly copying line drawings and in performing simple calculations requiring two or more mental operations (such as $132 - 47$ or 13×9). They committed many errors when judging whether two lines shared the same orientation or length, or whether two circles were

---

[22] Priming can last for a long time and is another instance of implicit memory.

[23] VanRullen and Koch (2003a). The number of objects consciously recalled increased by almost half if pictures of the objects were flashed, one at a time, a few minutes earlier. This is another compelling example of positive priming. That is, seeing an object once increases the probability of detecting it in a later image by almost 50%. In *subliminal priming*, the image doesn't even have to be consciously perceived for priming to occur (Bar and Biederman, 1998 and 1999). The strength and duration of subliminal perception is weak, though, and does not warrant the public debate and urban legends associated with it and the power of advertising (Merikle and Daneman, 1998).

[24] Shallice (1988) and Vallar and Shallice (1990).

[25] Riddoch and Humphreys (1995).

the same size. All three, however, could clearly see and name objects and had normal visual sensations.

This would suggest that working memory is *not* a prerequisite for consciousness. I don't think you need the phonological loop to perceive the deep blue sky stretching above you, but only for talking about it afterward. Testing this hypothesis would be difficult, however, because how could you properly tell somebody about your experiences if your entire working memory was knocked out? Allowances would have to be made for your inability to even briefly store data.

Furthermore, I question whether each item in working memory is simultaneously and consciously experienced. When you are actively maintaining seven to ten—as many of the students in my class can—digits in working memory, are you really conscious of them all? Doesn't it seem plausible that you are only conscious of one or two numbers while the others hover in the background, readily accessible, but outside the pale?[26]

While only a subset of the content of working memory is consciously represented at any given point in time, the presence of working memory in a normal, healthy brain appears to go hand-in-hand with consciousness. One may, therefore, take the presence of working memory capabilities in individuals who can't talk, such as newborn babies or animals, as one indicator for the presence of some sort of consciousness in these subjects.

Prefrontal Cortex and Working Memory

Where in the brain is working memory to be found? In early visual areas, the neuronal response quickly subsides if the image is removed from view. Not so in the prefrontal cortex of the macaque monkey (PFC). It was here that the neurophysiologist Joaquín Fuster at UCLA discovered neurons encoding an activity-dependent form of memory. Fuster characterized these cells with two related paradigms that remain popular today. In a *delayed response* trial, the animal was cued at one of two places. The cue disappeared and the monkey had to remember this location until he was allowed to point to it (Figure 11.2). In a *delayed matching-to-sample* procedure, the monkey briefly saw a target image. After staring at the empty screen for awhile, the target and a foil appeared and he had to quickly fixate the target image (and not the distracting one), no matter where it appeared on the screen. If he did, he was rewarded with a drop of tasty juice.

Fuster's experiments, as well as more recent ones by Patricia Goldman-Rakic and her colleagues at Yale University, identified neurons that fired

---

[26]Indeed, some retrieval experiments suggest serial access to stored working memory (Sternberg, 1966).

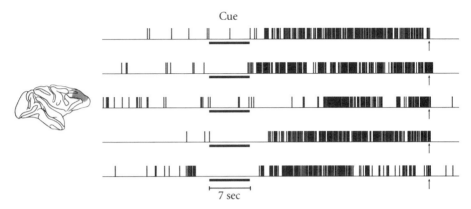

FIGURE 11.2 *Working Memory in the Prefrontal Cortex* The delayed response paradigm evaluates the monkey's ability to keep one of two locations in mind. The discharge of one class of responsive prefrontal cortex neurons (from the area indicated in gray in the inset) is silenced from their already low background levels during presentation of the cue but increases during the 32-second long retention period, when no stimulus is present. The cell stops responding when the monkey begins to reach out to the target (indicated by an arrow), when there is no more need to keep the location in mind. Modified from Fuster (1973).

during the delay period in the dorsal PFC, particularly in area 46 (top panel in Figure 7.1).[27] Furthermore, when the animal made an error, the delay activity faltered. During mock trials or when the cues were incomplete, the activity was often absent. It is therefore reasonable to argue that these cells are part of the infrastructure for working memory (although short-term changes in synaptic strength may have also played a role). Electrical recordings from a different neuronal storage site and computer models are compatible with the notion that such momentary storage of information can come about from the reverberatory interactions among a small and tightly coupled group of neurons.[28]

 Subsequent experiments probed the extent to which neurons store the identity of the remembered object, its location, or both. Earl Miller and his colleagues at MIT identified three classes of lateral PFC neurons, namely those that care only about the identity of the memorandum, those that encode its position, and those that encode both features and the position of the to-be-remembered object. The vision-for-perception and vision-for-action pathways converge in the lateral prefrontal cortex, representing both seen and remembered objects (Figure 7.3).

---

[27]Fuster (1995, 1997) and Goldman-Rakic, Scalaidhe, and Chafee (2000). Romo et al. (1999) carried out an elegant study of working memory for touch (haptic) information in the prefrontal cortex.
[28]Compte et al. (2000) and Aksay et al. (2001).

The prefrontal cortex does not act in isolation. Posterior parietal neurons fire to the location of objects and inferotemporal (IT) neurons respond to the identity of objects that have disappeared from sight. However, IT cells fail to maintain sample-selective information when the animal is attending to other stimuli. The delay activity of cells in the PFC is immune to intervening nonmatching images.[29] One interpretation is that the inferotemporal cortex retains a brief sensory trace (a snapshot) of the last attended—and therefore presumably conscious—stimulus.[30]

11.4 | FLEETING OR ICONIC MEMORY

An even briefer form of memory is probably essential to conscious experience. You can see the visual form in the reddish trail made by a glowing cigarette in the dark. If you are quick enough, you can draw a full circle in the air before the initial part of the trajectory fades. Such observations suggest decay times of a fraction of a second.

A more quantitative assessment was carried out in 1960 by the psychologist George Sperling. In these classical experiments, Sperling flashed six clearly visible letters, and had his subjects report as many letters at their relative location as they could. On average, they correctly recalled 4.3 letters. Lengthening display times to 0.5 sec made virtually no difference; people still only reported fewer than five characters, even though they could clearly "see" many more.

To get at this discrepancy, Sperling switched to displays consisting of three rows of four letters (Figure 11.3) and, ingeniously, combined this with a high, a medium, or a low-pitch tone *after* the image disappeared. The sound indicated whether the upper, middle, or lower line had to be read out. Now, subjects reported three of the four characters in the indicated row. Because they could not foretell which row they were supposed to report, subjects had to store an average of 3×3 letters, more than the 4.3 letters in the original design. Sperling also varied the time between the offset of the display and the cue. If the tone was delayed by one second, performance fell to the level observed in the noncued design.

This experiment suggested that the letters are read off from a high-capacity, rapidly decaying visual form of storage called *iconic memory*. It is quickly estab-

---

[29] That is, if the animal has to remember image 'A' and is then distracted with foils, a prefrontal cell continues to represent 'A'. Conversely, IT cells encode 'A' only as long as the monkey hasn't been distracted by the foils (Miller, Erickson, and Desimone, 1996). Miller's experiments on feature- and/or location-specific memory neurons in area 46 are described in Rao, Rainer, and Miller (1997) and in Miller (1999).

[30] Working memory tasks in humans activate frontal lobe areas, including the motor and premotor cortex, as well as some posterior cortical regions (Courtney et al., 1998; de Fockert et al., 2001; and Pochon et al., 2001).

```
P T F K
S X W Z
M B D O
```

FIGURE 11.3 *Testing for Fast Image Memory* A briefly flashed array of letters was followed, after a short delay, by a high-, medium-, or low-frequency tone. This indicated that the upper, middle, or lower row had to be read out. If the tone occurred within a few hundred milliseconds after image onset, most of the letters in that line were correctly recalled. This iconic or fleeting memory lasts for no more than a second. I believe it is critical to visual experience. Modified from Sperling (1960).

lished and persists for at least a few hundred milliseconds. Iconic memory has different components that can be separately studied by manipulating the display. Some of its content is *pre-categorical*, a large but undigested soup of blobs, shades, and edges. Some of it is *post-categorical*, classified as the letter A or as Albert Einstein's portrait.[31]

The duration of iconic memory depends not so much on the time of image *offset* as on its *onset*. That is, what matters is not the time after the display has been turned off, as in passive decay, but on how long the stimulus has been present (its total persistence). This suggests that one of its functions is to provide sufficient time to allow the brain to process brief signals. As a result, transient interruptions of the visual stream, as when the eyes blink, won't interfere with processing. Given my hunch that iconic memory is necessary for visual perception, this implies that a minimal processing period is needed for conscious perception (I refer the impatient reader to Chapter 15 for more).

Iconic memory is probably instantiated throughout the visual brain, starting as early as the retina and including the various cortical areas and their associated thalamic nuclei. As the net-wave triggered by the image races up the hierarchy, it activates, in turn, retinal ganglion and geniculate relay cells, neurons in V1, V2, IT, and so on. Think of iconic memory as the *neuronal afterglow* left in its wake, prolonged and amplified by reverberatory activities, both within local patches and by loops between the cortex and the various pulvinar nuclei.[32] In the retina, cells respond for another 60 msec after the stimulus has

---

[31]The classical experiment was done by Sperling (1960) as part of his Ph.D thesis. For more recent developments, check out Potter and Levy (1969); Loftus, Duncan, and Gehrig (1992); Potter (1993); Gegenfurtner and Sperling (1993); and the comprehensive edited volume by Coltheart (1999).
[32]Crick (1984) and Billock (1997) have proposed theories that emphasize reverberatory corticothalamic loops.

been removed, while the afterglow of neurons in IT and neighboring regions lasts up to 300 msec.[33] This is what you experience as fleeting memory.

I believe that iconic memory is essential for visual consciousness. I cannot conceive of how you could see something without the neural activity lasting some minimal amount of time. Given the distributed nature of the neural basis of iconic memory, this claim will not be easy to test.

Some Speculations Linking Iconic Memory to Visual Consciousness

The information in iconic storage is volatile, so it quickly fades away unless strengthened. Only some of its content, together with its gist, is made conscious. What data is transferred into consciousness's limelight depends on biases exerted by bottom-up saliency and top-down focal attention (Section 9.3). Because some letters are more noticeable than others, or because you've been told to pay attention to some object, attention reinforces the relevant neural coalitions. By prolonging their size and lifetime in the upper stages of the visual hierarchy, these coalitions activate neurons in the prefrontal cortex and elsewhere, which feed back to earlier areas, so that they can establish stable firing patterns that make up the NCC and that can be stored in working memory.

It is tempting to identify the post-categorical stages of iconic memory with areas in and around the IT and lateral PFC.[34] Here, information peculiar to object identity is made explicit and is maintained in the elevated spiking rate of neurons, even if the stimulus has disappeared. Activity in these regions can be thought of as a snapshot of the scene, with a handful of objects identified and labeled, and their spatial relationships encoded. As discussed in the previous chapter, interneuronal competition prevents all but a small number of objects from being represented in this manner.

I argue in Section 15.3 that this activity must last long enough and exceed some threshold in order to be sufficient for a conscious percept. This process involves reciprocal feedback loops between the IT, the PFC, the medial temporal lobes, and parts of the thalamus. As the winning neuronal assemblies coding for the handful of letters in the display become stable, they become sufficient for conscious sensation. Their vigorous, and possibly coherent, firing activity clears the way for this information to access working memory and the planning centers of the brain.

---

[33] Levick and Zacks (1970); Rolls and Tovee (1994); Keysers and Perrett (2002).

[34] Using computer-generated shapes that were morphed to look like cats or dogs or something in between, Freedman et al. (2001, 2002) demonstrated that while IT monkey cells care about images *per se*, PFC cells are more concerned about the category of the input, that is, whether it is a cat or a dog.

11.5 | RECAPITULATION

Memory, which feels monolithic, is a bestiary of many processes.

In associative conditioning, the organism connects two simultaneous or nearly simultaneous events to each other, such that one predicts the other. Some forms of Pavlovian conditioning require selective attention and awareness of the relationship between the conditioned and the unconditioned stimuli. Given the ease with which mice can learn, these forms of conditioning can be developed into an operational test for murine awareness.

Procedural memory contains instructions, such as how to ride a bike, tie shoelaces, or execute a sequence of climbing moves. Episodic memory encodes autobiographical events, while semantic memory deals with more abstract knowledge. Both are forms of declarative memory. In severe cases of amnesia, people are not only unable to form new declarative memories but also lose access to previously stored ones. These unfortunate individuals suffer from bilateral destruction of the hippocampus and associated medial temporal lobe structures, yet are certainly conscious. They conclusively demonstrate that consciousness does not depend on long-term episodic memories.

Shorter forms of storage rely on active neuronal circuits. Best characterized is working memory, which is quite limited in how much it can store. It does so in an abstract, categorical fashion. Unless continuously rehearsed, working memory decays within a minute. It is critical for all those daily tasks where data is briefly retained and manipulated.

In a well-functioning brain, working memory goes hand-in-hand with consciousness. Any organism with working memory capabilities is likely to be conscious, making the presence of working memory a litmus test for consciousness in animals, babies, or patients that can't talk about their experiences. The opposite, however, may not be true. I suspect that if a man were to be stripped of his working memory, he would remain conscious. He could still feel the world, even though he might not be able to talk about it afterward.

Iconic memory, on the other hand—a fleeting form of visual information storage that lasts for less than one second—is probably necessary for visual perception. Its neuronal substrate is the afterglow left by the waves of spikes sweeping up the visual hierarchy, amplified by local and more global feedback loops. The function of iconic memory may be to assure that even brief images last sufficiently long to trigger the NCC.

Retaining information over a few seconds, as in trace conditioning or working memory, is a common feature of many processes closely linked to consciousness. This idea is elaborated into a practical test for consciousness in Section 13.6. Before I come to that, however, let me tell you about the zombie within.

CHAPTER TWELVE

What You Can Do Without Being Conscious: The Zombie Within

> At this point, apart from a gnawing desire to be close to Belqassim all the time, it would have been hard for her to know what she did feel. It was so long since she had canalized her thoughts by speaking aloud, and she had grown accustomed to acting without the consciousness of being in the act. She did only the things she found herself already doing.
>
> From *The Sheltering Sky* by Paul Bowles

Zombies could be living among us. Or so claim some philosophers. These fictitious creatures are devoid of any subjective feelings, yet are endowed with behaviors identical to their normal, conscious counterparts. It does not feel like anything to be a zombie. They were invented by philosophers in their carefree way to illustrate the paradoxical nature of consciousness. Some argue that the logical possibility of their existence implies that consciousness does not follow from the natural laws of the universe, that it is an epiphenomenon. From this viewpoint, whether or not people feel makes no difference to themselves, to their offspring, and to the world at large.[1]

To Francis and me, this point of view seems sterile. We are interested in the real world, not in a logically possible never-never land where zombies roam. And, in the real world, evolution gave rise to organisms with subjective feelings. These convey significant survival advantages, because consciousness goes hand-in-hand with the ability to plan, to reflect upon many possible courses of action, and to choose one. I will expand upon this in Chapter 14.

What is of great interest is the observation that much of what goes on inside my head escapes me. As I grow older, reflecting upon a lifetime of experience,

---

[1] For the historical lineage of the philosopher's zombie see (Campbell, 1970; Kirk, 1974; and Chalmers, 1996).

it dawns upon me that large parts of my life lie beyond the pale of consciousness. I do things—complicated actions like driving, talking, going to the gym, cooking—automatically, without thinking about them.

Try to introspect the next time you talk. You will hear well-formed sentences come tumbling out of your mouth, but without any knowledge of what entity formed them with the appropriate syntax. Your brain takes care of that quite well without any conscious effort on your part. You might remind yourself to mention this anecdote or that observation, but the conscious "you" does not generate the words or put them in the right order.

None of this is new. The submental, the nonconscious—defined by exclusion as everything going on in the brain insufficient for conscious feelings, sensations, or memories—has been a scholarly topic since the latter part of the 19th century.[2] Friedrich Nietzsche was the first major Western thinker to explore the darker recesses of humanity's unconscious desires to dominate others and acquire power over them, often disguised as compassion. Within the medico-literary tradition, Freud spent a lifetime arguing for the existence of repressed desires and thoughts and their uncanny ability to influence behavior in hidden ways.[3]

Science has provided credible evidence for an entire menagerie of specialized sensory-motor processes, what I call *zombie agents*, that carry out routine missions in the absence of any direct conscious sensation or control. You can become conscious of the action of a zombie agent, but usually only after the fact, through internal or external feedback. Unlike the philosopher's or the voodoo zombie, though, zombie agents operate continuously in all of us.

These agents have one unfortunate practical consequence: The mere existence of some seemingly complex behavior does not necessarily imply that the subject is conscious. To the dismay of pet owners or new parents alike, the friendly dog wagging her tail or the baby smiling ever so cutely might be doing so automatically. Additional criteria must be devised to detect consciousness.

---

[2] Ellenberger (1970) provides a historical perspective on the non- and unconscious. The rigorous study of nonconscious sensory-motor behaviors is fraught with methodological difficulties. It is not easy to disentangle the rapid and automatic initiation of an action from a retarded but conscious signal triggered by the command to act or by the executed action itself. Another complication arises from the need for multiple trials, necessary to collect sufficient statistics. The repetition of the task can provide enough feedback that the subject—over time—can learn to become conscious of some aspect of the behavior. For reviews and relevant experiments, see Cheesman and Merikle (1986); Holender (1986); Merikle (1992); Kolb and Braun (1995); Berns, Cohen, and Mintun (1997); Merikle, Smilek, and Eastwood (2001); Destrebecqz and Cleeremans (2001); and Curran (2001).

[3] In general, I avoid using the term "unconscious" because of its Freudian overtones, preferring the more neutral "nonconscious" to refer to operations or computations not sufficient for phenomenal content.

12.1 | ZOMBIE AGENTS IN EVERYDAY LIFE

In some sense, zombie behaviors are like *reflexes*. Simple ones include *blinking* when something looms into your field of view, *coughing* when your breathing passages are obstructed, *sneezing* when dust tickles your nose, or being *startled* by an unexpected noise or abrupt movement. You may become aware of them only as they are happening. These reflexes are automatic, fast, and depend on circuits in the spinal cord or the brainstem. Zombie behaviors can be thought of as flexible and adaptive reflexes that involve higher centers. This chapter will describe their mode of operations in healthy people, while Chapter 13 will amass evidence from brain-damaged patients.

Eye Movements

Many nuclei and networks specialize in moving the eyes. By and large, they do so silently, without giving rise to awareness. The neuropsychologist Melvyn Goodale, from the University of Western Ontario in Canada, and two of his colleagues, demonstrated this quite vividly in the following way. A volunteer sat in the dark, fixating a single light-emitting diode. When the central light turned off and reappeared in the periphery, the subject shifted her gaze to the new location by a rapid eye movement—a saccade. Because the eyes usually undershoot, they compensate for this error by a second saccade that lands them right on target. That's their job.

On occasion, the researchers moved the light for a second time, while the subject's eyes were engaged in their saccade. Because vision is partially shut down during these rapid eye movements (recall saccadic suppression from Section 3.7), the subject didn't notice the jump in target position and had to guess the direction of the shift (Figure 12.1). Nevertheless, the subject's eyes didn't miss a beat and executed a correctly-sized saccade to the new position. Her eyes knew something that she didn't.[4]

The saccadic system is exquisitely sensitive to changes in the position of the goal. Given its high degree of specialization, there is little need to involve consciousness in its stereotyped actions. If you needed to be aware of each eye movement, to plan and execute it, you wouldn't be able to do much else besides. Why clog up experience with these details if they can be contracted out to specialists?

---

[4]If the motion of the target during the saccade became too large, subjects noticed the change and carried out a large, slower readjustment. The experiment summarized here is described in Goodale, Pélisson, and Prablanc (1986), based on earlier work by Bruce Bridgeman at the University of California in Santa Cruz. He specializes in uncovering dissociations between visual perception and eye or hand movements (Bridgeman et al., 1979; and Bridgeman, Kirch, and Sperling, 1981).

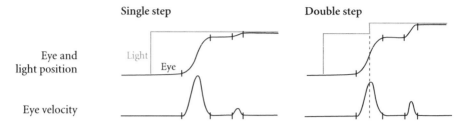

FIGURE 12.1 *Fooling Vision but not the Eye* Observers rapidly move their eyes when a light changes its location (left); a first, large saccade is followed by a smaller, corrective eye movement to place the target right onto the fovea. On some trials (right) the light is moved again while the eyes are in transition. Subjects don't see this jump in the position of the light; nevertheless, their eyes compensate for the perceptually invisible shift. Modified from Goodale, Pélisson, and Prablanc (1986).

Balancing the Body

Other nonconscious agents control head, limb, and body posture. As you weave your way through crowds of shoppers on the sidewalk, your trunk, legs, and arms continuously adjust themselves so that you remain upright, and avoid bumping into anybody. You don't give a thought to these actions that require split-second timing and a marvelous merging of muscle and nerve, something no machine has come close to achieving.

In one ingenious experiment, psychologists[5] had people stand inside a fake room, whose polystyrene walls were suspended from the ceiling within a larger room. As the foam walls gently rocked back and forth by a few millimeters, subjects adjusted their posture by swaying back and forth in tune. Most remained unaware of the motion of the room or of the compensatory adjustment of their body.

The networks mediating balance and body posture receive continuously updated information from many modalities, not just vision. The inner ears supply head rotation and linear acceleration, while myriad motion, position, and pressure sensors in the skin, muscles, and joints monitor the position of the body in space. All of this information is at the service of highly coordinated yet nonconscious zombie agents that prevent you from crashing into the approaching cyclist and that balance you when your friend unexpectedly slaps you on your back.[6]

---

[5] Lee and Lishman (1975).

[6] I recommend reading the inspiring case-history of a 19-year-old who suddenly lost all body sensation below the neck (Cole, 1995). In the absence of any proprioceptive feedback from his body, the patient gradually learned, with amazing tenacity, to consciously control his limbs by sight. The book brings home how utterly daily life depends on nonconscious processing.

Estimating the Steepness of Hills

When driving in the mountains, have you ever wondered about the "obvious" discrepancy between the slope indicated on the road sign and your feeling that the incline was much steeper? The psychologist Dennis Proffitt at the University of Virginia at Charlottesville confirmed this informal observation. It is but one striking example of a dissociation between perception and action.[7]

Proffitt and his assistants stood at the bases of hills and queried 300 passing students about the slope using verbal, visual, and manual measures. For the visual judgment, subjects had to set a disk mounted behind a concealed protractor to the angle that they thought best matched the inclination of the clearly visible hill. In the manual mode, volunteers adjusted a tilt board with a flat palm rest mounted on a tripod. To avoid "contamination" from vision, they were prevented from looking at their hand.

Subjects badly overestimated the slopes of these hills when judging verbally or visually, but were within the right ballpark when inferring the steepness using their hand (Figure 12.2).

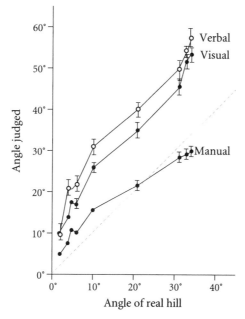

FIGURE 12.2 *Your Body Knows Better Than Your Eye* Subjects indicated the steepness of hills verbally, by a visual judgement, or by adjusting the tilt of their flat, outstretched hand. While comparatively accurate in the latter case, they consistently overestimated the slope using language or vision. Modified from Proffitt et al. (1995).

---

[7] Proffitt et al. (1995).

Remarkably, the mismatch between the perceived slope of a hill and visually guided actions, such as hand or foot placement, depends on the physiological state of the individual. Both verbal and visual overestimates of hill steepness increased by more than a third following an exhausting foot race, while the blind hand estimate was unaffected. If you're fatigued, therefore, hills do look steeper than if you're rested.[8] What you consciously see is not the same as what guides your actions.

Night Walking

I spent part of the summer of 1994 at the Santa Fe Institute for Complexity in New Mexico. Sandra Blakeslee, a science journalist living in the area, convinced me to join a nightly tour conducted by Nelson Zink and Stephen Parks, psychotherapists and writers operating out of Taos. I went along for a rather tantalizing experience that may be another example of an automatic visuo-motor behavior divorced from conscious perception.

We assembled on a floor of a canyon well outside town at night. The moonless sky was clear, with hundreds of stars shining down. Thus, visibility was low, but not zero. We wore baseball caps with a wire sticking straight ahead and a phosphorescent sphere attached to the end. Charged up by a flashlight, the sphere would faintly glow for minutes. The trick was to walk erect in the dark while looking at the sphere, suspended below the cap, and to keep fixating it despite the urge to inspect the ground ahead. At first, I gingerly moved forward on the sandy and rocky floor, exploring with my feet before committing the full weight of my body. After a surprising short time, however, I became more confident and walked at a comparatively brisk pace over the highly uneven ground, all the while staring at the sphere. Eventually, the sphere became superfluous and fixating the distant horizon or a star was sufficient to prevent central vision from aiding in the placement of the feet.

One explanation for this *night walking* is that information gleaned at some distance is stored implicitly and guides the placement of the feet once that location is reached. This would be a considerable feat in these canyons full of sandy hills, holes, and dried river beds.[9]

---

[8] A similar effect was found when subjects wore a heavy backpack, or were of low physical fitness, elderly, or in declining health (Bhalla and Proffitt, 1999). Proffitt argues that the variable relationship between actual and perceived steepness reflects the behavioral potential of the organism. The subjective slant percept corresponds to your ability to ascend hills. This is hard work and should not be undertaken lightly. It becomes even harder if you are tired, frail, or carrying a heavy load.

[9] I confirmed the need for peripheral vision since glasses that covered everything but the central part of the visual field made navigation impossible.

Alternatively, the extreme lower visual periphery may control the angle of placement of the feet, as well as the height to which they need to be lifted to avoid hitting the toes against rocks, without giving rise to any visual experience. The visual field representation in the superior colliculus extends to just about the feet, so the nervous system has access to this information.[10] There is little reason to classify objects at the rim of vision, explaining why conscious vision doesn't extend down there.

These ideas could be tested by determining the extent to which the lower peripheral field provides cues for navigating under low-light conditions. How well can night walkers describe the surface slant or the height of obstacles placed on the ground? How do these subjective judgments compare to the actual placement of their feet? Do the feet know something phenomenal vision doesn't?

12.2 | VISION-FOR-PERCEPTION IS DIFFERENT FROM VISION-FOR-ACTION

The neuropsychologist David Milner, at the University of Durham in England, and Melvyn Goodale argue for a multitude of visuo-motor systems, each controlling one specific behavior, such as eye movements, posture adjustment, hand gripping or pointing, foot placement, and so on, yet none giving rise to conscious sensation.[11] Think of each as carrying out a highly specialized computation in real time. Milner and Goodale call them *on-line systems*. These visuo-motor behaviors care about the here and now. They have no need to access working or declarative memory. That's not their function. Psychophysical experiments show quite conclusively that enforcing a delay of 2–4 seconds between a brief visual input and a required hand or eye movement taps into a different spatial map of the world, close to that used by visual perception, and quite distinct from the one used to execute a near-instantaneous motor response.[12]

These visuo-motor systems are like an army of zombie agents. Operating in parallel are the networks that mediate object classification, recognition, and identification—that is, the networks responsible for conscious perception (Table 12.1).

---

[10]Receptive fields in the ventral, vision-for-perception pathway are centered on or around the fovea.

[11]I recommend their comprehensive monograph, Milner and Goodale (1995). For a related view, see Rossetti (1998).

[12]Wong and Mack (1981); Abrams and Landgraf (1990); and, in particular, the study by Bridgeman, Peery, and Anand (1997).

TABLE 12.1 Milner and Goodale's Two Visual Systems Hypothesis

	Zombie Agents	Seeing System
Visual input	Simple	Can be complex
Motor output	Stereotyped responses	Many possible responses
Minimum processing time	Short	Longer
Effects of a few seconds delay	Does not work	Can still work
Coordinates used	Egocentric	Object-centered
Conscious	No	Yes

Because on-line agents help the organism to safely navigate the world, they need access to the true position of a target relative to the body. Perception, on the other hand, must recognize things and label them as "spoiled banana," "blushing face," and so on. These objects can be far away or close by, and must be recognized in the full light of the midday sun or at dusk, so that object perception must be invariant to distance, ambient light, exact location on the retina, and so on. As a result, the *spatial* location of what you see consciously is not as precise as the information accessible to your nonconscious agent planning the next move.

This strategy makes perfect sense from a computational point of view. The neuronal algorithms needed to reach out and grab a tool (vision-for-action) operate within a frame of reference and have invariances different from the operations that identify the object as a hammer (vision-for-perception).

In the normal course of daily events, zombie agents are tightly enmeshed with the networks mediating perception. What you perceive, learn, or remember is an interweaving of nonconscious and conscious processes and separating their contributions is no easy matter.[13] By investigating the seams, where vision-for-perception and vision-for-action come apart, Milner and Goodale probe the two in relative isolation.

Perception must recognize objects for *what* they are, no matter *where* they are. Conversely, the motor system must know about the exact spatial relationship of some to-be-manipulated object relative to the organism. In keeping with this view, Milner and Goodale argue that *size constancy illusion*—the fact that an object looks to have the same size no matter whether it is far away or close by—only applies to vision-for-perception, not to vision-for-action, whose job is to look at, point to, or pick up objects. This requires precise information about the object's size, location, weight, and shape. These seduc-

---

[13]The problem of separating conscious from nonconscious behaviors is known as the *process purity problem* (Reingold and Merikle, 1990; and Jacoby, 1991).

tive ideas have begun to be tested, but so far no firm conclusions have been reached.[14] Some dissociations between vision-for-action and perception have been uncovered—witness the previous section on slope estimation—but have failed to materialize elsewhere.[15]

The hypothesis of a collection of specialized visuo-motor zombie agents, complemented by a more general purpose, multi-faceted conscious vision module, is an attractive one. It nicely dovetails with our proposal, laid out in Chapter 14, that the function of consciousness is to deal with all those situations that require a novel, nonstereotyped response.

12.3 | YOUR ZOMBIE ACTS FASTER THAN YOU SEE

One of the cardinal advantages of zombie agents is that their specialized nature allows them to respond more rapidly than the general purpose perceptual system. You grab for the pencil before you actually see it roll off the table or you move your hand away from the hot burner before you feel its heat.

This last point is important, for it belies the notion that you jerk your hand away because you consciously feel pain. The withdrawal of a limb following an irritating or noxious stimulus is a spinal reflex; it does not require the brain. Indeed, decapitated animals as well as paraplegics whose lower spinal cord is disconnected from the brain, have such withdrawal reflexes. Consciousness does not have to be involved (keep this point in mind when I discuss the function of consciousness in Chapter 14).[16]

Marc Jeannerod from the Institut des Sciences Cognitives in Bron, France, is one of the world's leading experts in the neuropsychology of action. In one noteworthy experiment,[17] Jeannerod and his colleagues estimated the delay

---

[14]Geometry dictates that linear size is inversely proportional to distance. Yet somebody five meters away doesn't look twice the size they were 10 meters away. Aglioto, DeSouza, and Goodale (1995) provide evidence for size constancy operating in the perceptual but not in the visuo-motor domain, while Franz et al. (2000) found no such dissociation (see also Yamagishi, Anderson, and Ashida, 2001; Carey, 2001; and Milner and Dyde, 2003).

[15]In an experiment on spatial navigation, people judged the distance (between one and five meters) to a clearly visible target. This estimate was compared to dead reckoning, when subjects walked with their eyes closed to the (presumed) location of the target. Both measures consistently overestimated the distance to nearby points and underestimated it for more distant locations (Philbeck and Loomis, 1997). Since both deviated to the same extent from the true physical distance, both measures make use of the same information, unlike the slope estimate discussed in the previous section.

[16]For example, if a noxious stimulus is applied to the back of a headless frog, the appropriate limb tries to scratch at it. The remarkable sensory-motor abilities of decapitated or decerebrated animals were at the core of a debate in the second half of the 19th century over the extent to which consciousness was associated with the spinal cord (Fearing, 1970).

[17]Castiello, Paulignan, and Jeannerod (1991). Jeannerod (1997) provides a textbook treatment on the neuroscience of action.

between a rapid manual response and subjective awareness. Three dowels were placed in front of an observer with her hand resting on the table. Suddenly, the central dowel was lit from below and she had to reach out and grasp it as rapidly as she could. On occasion, the light was shifted to either the left or right dowel immediately as the hand started to move, and this one became the new target. As soon as the subject saw the new target light up, she had to shout.

On average, 315 msec would go by between the onset of the motor response and the vocalization. Indeed, in some cases, the subject had already lifted the second dowel before she realized that it was the new target—that is, action preceded awareness. Even when a generous 50 msec was accorded to the lag between the onset of muscle contraction of the speech articulators and the beginning of the shout, this still left a quarter of a second between the grasping behavior and the conscious percept that led to the shout. This delay is the price that must be paid for consciousness.

To put this into perspective, consider a track athlete. Assuming, with a grain of salt, that the 250-msec delay also applies to the auditory system, then the sprinter is already out of the starting block by the time he consciously hears the starting gun go off! Similarly, a baseball player facing a pitched ball approaching at 90 mph must begin to swing his bat before he is conscious of his decision to try to hit the ball or let it pass.

12.4 | CAN ZOMBIES SMELL?

Zombie agents are not limited to the visual domain. They are found in all modalities. One profitable sense to explore is smell. Although contemporary culture strongly frowns upon body odors—a sentiment that has given birth to endless hygienic products that seek to camouflage them—we do live in a redolent world, whether we are aware of it or not. Indeed, it has long been surmised that many sexual, appetitive, reproductive, and social behaviors are triggered by subliminal olfactory cues. This theory has been difficult to establish rigorously.

Examples where smell-based decisions have been studied extend from the banal, such as choosing a seat in a cinema, to the essential, such as choosing a sexual partner. The best-publicized example is the synchronization of menstrual cycles among women that live or work closely together (as in college dormitories or military barracks).[18] In one well-designed study, Martha

---

[18]McClintock (1998), Weller et al. (1999), and Schank (2001) lay out the evidence for and against menstrual synchronization. Gangestad, Thornhill, and Garver (2002) report how women's sexual interests, and the response of their male partners, waxes and wanes with ovulation.

McClintock at the University of Chicago applied odorless compounds from the armpits of women to the upper lips of other females. The menstrual cycle of the recipient was shortened or lengthened, depending on the phase of the donor.[19]

Such effects could be mediated by *pheromones*, volatile compounds secreted by one individual that alter the physiology or behavior of another individual. Some animals can respond to single molecules of pheromones.[20] In the case of humans, armpit secretions of men contains a testosterone derivative, while women exude a compound that resembles estrogen. Both airborne substances induce gender-specific physiological changes in deep neural structures.[21]

How might such nonconscious airborne signals be mediated? One culprit may be the *vomeronasal* organ. It is not widely appreciated that mammals possess not one but two senses of smell. The primary olfactory organ originates in the main epithelium of the nose and projects to the olfactory bulb and from there to the olfactory cortex. This organ is a broadly tuned, all-purpose system. A second module starts off in the vomeronasal organ at the base of the nasal cavity. From there, axons go to the accessory olfactory bulb and onward to the amygdala. The vomeronasal organ transduces *pheromones* and has been linked to gender-specific communication.[22]

Enough is known about mouse olfactory receptor molecules that their expression can be blocked in one but not the other organ, making it possible to study the molecular and neuronal correlates of genetically preprogrammed sexual or reproductive behaviors.[23]

In most people, the vomeronasal system, sometimes referred to as *Jacobson's organ*, may be vestigial—nonfunctional. Its job may have been taken over by the primary olfactory pathway. Another distinct possibility is that only a subset of adults express the relevant receptors. A vigorous research program could identify the individuals susceptible to 'odorless' smells for further genetic and physiological screening, to contrast the neural substrate of nonconscious and conscious olfactory processing.

---

[19] Stern and McClintock (1998).

[20] Pantages and Dulac (2000).

[21] The testosterone-derived pheromone triggers a response in the hypothalamus of women but not of men, while the estrogen-related substance excites the hypothalamus of men but not of women (Savic et al., 2001, and Savic, 2002). Even when the odor could not be detected by the subject, some brain activity persisted (Sobel et al., 1999).

[22] Johnston (1998) and Keverne (1999) review the scholarly literature, while Watson (2001) provides a popular account. Holy, Dulac, and Meister (2000) discovered that single vomeronasal neurons in the mouse are capable of distinguishing female from male urine.

[23] Researchers can now breed mice whose vomeronasal organ is knocked out. These transgenic animals lack male-male aggression. Instead they initiate courtship behaviors toward both males and females (Stowers et al., 2002).

12.5 | RECAPITULATION

This chapter reviewed the ample evidence for zombie agents—highly specialized, sensory-motor agents that work quite well without giving rise to phenomenal sensations. The hallmarks of a zombie agent are (1) rapid, reflex-like processing, (2) a narrow but specific input domain, (3) a specific behavior, and (4) the lack of access to working memory.

In the visual domain, Milner and Goodale argue for two distinct processing strategies, vision-for-action and vision-for-perception, implemented by networks within the dorsal and the ventral pathways, respectively. Because the job of visuo-motor agents is to grasp or point at things, they need to encode the actual distance between the body and these objects, their size, and other metric measures. The vision-for-perception mode mediates conscious vision. It must recognize things, no matter their size, orientation, or location. This explains why zombie agents access more veridical information about spatial relationships in the world than perception can. That is, while you may not see what is really out there, your motor system does. Prominent examples of such dissociations include tracking targets with the eyes, adjusting body posture, estimating the steepness of hills, and night walking.

Zombie agents control your eyes, hands, feet, and posture, and rapidly transduce sensory input into stereotypical motor output. They might even trigger aggressive or sexual behaviors when getting a whiff of the right stuff. All, however, bypass consciousness. This is the zombie you.

So far, I have said nothing about the differences between zombie and conscious processing modes at the neuronal level. The forward propagating net-wave triggered by a brief sensory input may be too transient to be sufficient for the NCC, but can mediate zombie behaviors. What is needed for conscious perception is enough time for feedback activity from frontal areas to build up stable coalitions. I will expand on this theme in Section 15.3.

Dissociations between conscious and nonconscious behaviors can be more prominent in sickness. This is the topic of the next chapter.

CHAPTER THIRTEEN

Agnosia, Blindsight, Epilepsy, and Sleep Walking: Clinical Evidence for Zombies

And as for sickness: are we not almost tempted to ask whether we could
get along without it?

From *The Gay Science* by Friedrich Nietzsche

Morbidity often accentuates or brings out traits that are barely apparent in good health. Historically, the clinic has been one of the most fecund sources of insight about the brain. The vagaries of nature give rise to anoxia, strokes, tumors, or other pathological aberrations that, if limited in their scope and correctly interpreted, can illuminate and guide my quest.

In the intact brain, zombie behaviors are so tightly interwoven with conscious ones that it is difficult to isolate them. For, even if the response was generated automatically, awareness may follow within the blink of an eye. Let me now turn to four clinical syndromes that better reveal the actions of zombie agents.

13.1 | VISUAL AGNOSIA

Pure *agnosia*, a relatively rare condition, is defined as a failure of recognition that cannot be attributed to elementary sensory defects (e.g., retinal deficits), mental or linguistic deterioration, or attentional disturbances. It is often limited to one sensory modality. Typically, a visual agnosia patient can't recognize a set of keys on a chain dangling in front of her. If she grasps them or if they are jingled, she immediately knows what they are.

Poetically termed *Seelenblindheit* (literally, blindness of the soul), it was rechristened agnosia by Freud and this term has remained. All sorts of quirky subcategories exist, including the inability to perceive color (*achromatopsia*; Section 8.2), the loss of motion perception (*akinetopsia*; Section 8.3), the inability to identify faces (*prosopagnosia*; Section 8.5), and *Capgras syndrome*, in which the patient insists that a loved one, say his wife, has been taken over by an imposter who looks, talks, and feels exactly the way she used to do before the alien replaced her.[1]

The often quite localized brain damage associated with agnosia implies that the NCC for specific perceptual attributes, such as color, motion, faces, or the feeling of familiarity, is restricted to a part of the cerebral cortex; that is, a particular brain region is an essential node for the perceptual trait in question. Armed with single-cell data from the monkey, Francis and I have hypothesized that the NCC in these essential nodes is based on an explicit, columnar representation (Section 2.2).

Take D.F., a patient who suffers from profound object agnosia, caused by a near-fatal carbon monoxide poisoning at age 34. The oxygen deprivation led to widespread and irreversible damage throughout her brain.[2]

D.F. does not recognize most objects by sight, but does well when she can touch them. She can't tell whether a pencil held in front of her is horizontal or vertical, whether she is looking at a square or a triangle, and she is unable to copy simple drawings (Figure 13.1). Yet she is not blind. She can see colors, she can identify some objects by their distinct texture or color (e.g., a yellow banana), and she can sketch things from memory. D.F. walks around on her own, steps over blocks placed in her way, and catches a ball or a wooden stick thrown to her. D.F. grasps objects placed in front of her with considerable accuracy and confidence, even though she cannot see them in any meaningful manner. She doesn't see the orientation of an elongated slot, she can't talk about it, nor can she rotate her hand to match its slant. When she has to place a card into the slot from arm's length away, however, she easily complies, rotating her hand to the correct orientation as soon as it starts to move toward the slot (Figure 13.2). She can even do this when the light goes off as soon as she initiates this action. In other words, the patient couldn't have used visual feedback to guide her hand.

D.F. scales her grip to the size of the objects she has to pick up, even though she can't tell a smaller from a larger one. The larger the object, the bigger the opening between thumb and fingers. When D.F. reaches for an object two sec-

---

[1] Farah (1990); Damasio, Tranel, and Rizzo (2000); Bauer and Demery (2003); and the exhaustive Grüsser and Landis (1991) review the clinical literature on agnosia.

[2] The original case report is Milner et al. (1991). See the two monographs by Milner and Goodale (1995) and by Goodale and Milner (2004) for details. Brain imaging confirms that the damage impacted D.F.'s ventral pathway much more than it did her dorsal one.

Original   Copy   Memory

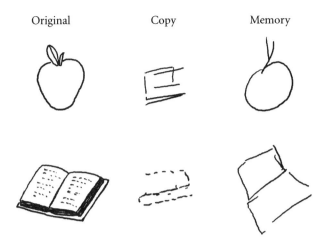

FIGURE 13.1 *Seeing and Drawing Objects in Visual Agnosia* The patient, D.F., couldn't recognize the two sketches on the left and performed miserably when trying to copy them (middle). She could, however, sketch an apple and an open book from memory (right). Modified from Milner and Goodale (1995).

onds after the article has been removed, however, her hand doesn't widen to accommodate its size. A normal person has no trouble pantomiming such a movement, including correctly scaling his or her grip, seconds after being shown the stimulus. This is an important observation, amplifying a point I

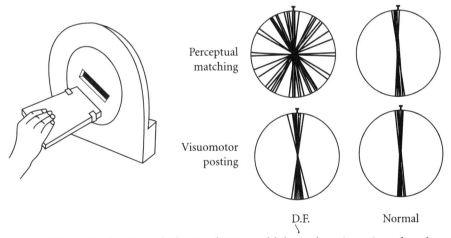

FIGURE 13.2 *A Zombie Controls the Hand* D.F. couldn't see the orientation of an elongated slot or match it to the orientation of a hand-held card (top row; compared to an age-matched healthy subject). She had no trouble, however, posting the card. She rapidly rotated her hand to the appropriate orientation and inserted the card (bottom row). Modified from Goodale (2000).

first brought up in Section 12.2. It implies that the networks responsible for D.F.'s reaching movements do not access working memory. Indeed, why should they? Because they are concerned with the here and now, they operate purely on-line.[3]

What this particular agnosia patient vividly exemplifies is that visual form and object information may be lost to consciousness yet continues to shape behavior. Milner and Goodale formulated their innovative two-visual-streams framework in light of D.F.'s pattern of lost and retained faculties: one for conscious vision and one for translating retinal input into motor actions without evoking any sensations. This is an elaboration of the Ungerleider-Mishkin "where" versus "what" distinction (Section 7.5); Milner and Goodale argue that the neuronal substrate for nonconscious, visuo-motor actions is located along the dorsal, vision-for-action pathway, while object detection and other tasks involving visual consciousness rely on the ventral, vision-for-perception pathway that has been severely compromised by anoxia in D.F. (Figure 7.3).

13.2 | BLINDSIGHT

Blindsight is an unusual condition in which the patient points at a target or correctly guesses its color or orientation, while strenuously denying any visual sensation. Different from visual agnosia, the patient doesn't see anything in the affected field of view. It is a strange syndrome that elicited disbelief and howls of derision when first reported in the literature. Due to the concerted and decades-long research efforts of the neuropsychologists Larry Weiskrantz and Alan Cowey at Oxford University and Petra Stoerig at the University of Düsseldorf in Germany, the initial criticisms have been adequately addressed. The syndrome proves the existence, in a handful of individuals, of some limited visuo-motor behaviors without seeing. Hence the oxymoronic name blind-sight.[4]

Blindsight results from damage to the primary visual cortex. Consequently, the patient fails to see anything in the hemifield opposite the impaired V1. He is blind there. Nevertheless, he can still point roughly in the direction of a bright

---

[3]These delay manipulations and their effect on reaching in D.F. and in normals are described in Goodale, Jakobson, and Keillor (1994) (see also Bridgeman, Peery, and Anand, 1997). Hu and Goodale (2000) further characterized the different computations underlying direct and pantomimed grasping in healthy subjects.

[4]The original report was based on patients with visual field defects who could detect stimuli in their blind field by pointing at them while denying seeing them (Pöppel, Held, and Frost, 1973). The most up-to-date reference is the extensive monograph by Weiskrantz (1997), while Cowey and Stoerig (1991) and Weiskrantz (1996) offer concise summaries. Kentridge, Heywood, and Weiskrantz (1997); Wessinger, Fendrich, and Gazzaniga (1997); and Zeki (1995) provide a taste of the ongoing controversy surrounding blindsight patients.

light: "I have no idea where the target is, but it could be over there." One such patient, G.Y., can nearly always surmise in which direction a spot of light is moving. If either the movement is too slow or the contrast of the target is too low, performance falls to chance levels—that is, the patient is truly guessing. Conversely, if the motion is salient enough, an ill-defined conscious percept may be reported, akin to "waving your hand in front of your eyes when they are closed," in the words of one patient. Other blindsight patients can distinguish a cross from a circle, a horizontal line from a vertical line, or can correctly guess which one of two colors is present.

Some blindsighted individuals can grasp at objects, even though they can't see their form. Their performance improves as the lag between stimulus and response decreases.[5] That is, the faster the patient points at an unseen target, the better her performance (recall that imposing a two-second delay eliminated D.F.'s grip-scaling abilities). The subliminal stimulus representations in blindsight are fragile. Without feedback from the perceptual system, the performance can't tolerate significant delays.

It is important to emphasize that blindsight patients don't have normal visual abilities *without* consciousness. There is no evidence that they can track one of several independently moving targets, can process information pertaining to multiple objects, or can recognize complex pictures. Most importantly, because they don't see, they can't use visual information to plan. If forced to, a blindsight patient might be able to correctly guess whether or not a water bottle was present in the blind field, but he wouldn't use this information to plan how to cross a desert. Information in the blind field is not used in any spontaneous, intentional manner. Blindsighted individuals, therefore, are a far cry from the philosopher's zombie.

In blindsight, the dominant retinal output—the geniculo-cortical channel—has lost its terminus in V1. So, how does visual information reach the motor regions? The most likely route involves the ganglion cell axons that connect the retina to the superior colliculus (Figure 3.6). From there, the information moves through the pulvinar of the thalamus into extrastriate visual cortices, bypassing the damaged V1.[6]

I expressed in the opening page of Chapter 8 my belief that this subcortical bypass into the visual hierarchy is too weak (either in amplitude or in duration) to corral neurons along the ventral stream for long enough into the necessary coalition to be sufficient for a percept. This pathway may be sufficient, though, to trigger some behavior under impoverished conditions (e.g., only a single target is presented, as in almost all blindsight studies). I suspect that when confronted with a more complex scene, the representations of the

---

[5]Perenin and Rossetti (1996), Rossetti (1998), and A. Cowey (personal communication).
[6]Minor projections from the LGN into V2 or higher cortical areas are another possibility.

objects interfere and, without focal attention, insufficient information can be extracted to trigger the right response.

What happens when neuroscientists try to create a blindsighted monkey by destroying V1 on both sides? The short answer is remarkably little. A few months after the operation, it is hard to find anything amiss in these animals. They clearly orient themselves using visual cues, they can find and pick up peanuts and avoid obstacles. This raises the interesting question, "Do these animals have any visual experience in their blind field?" To many, this query seems fundamentally unanswerable. How can something be inferred about the phenomenal aspects of seeing from a creature who can't speak or write about them?

Cowey and Stoerig proved these critics wrong.[7] After surgically removing V1 in one hemisphere in three macaque monkeys, the animals were trained to touch the location of a briefly flashed light on a computer screen (*forced-choice localization*). As expected, they could do this task well, whether the light appeared in their normal or in their blind hemifield.

Cowey and Stoerig then switched to a different test (*signal detection task*). As before, when a light was presented, the monkeys had to touch its location on the screen. What was new was that on occasion, a blank trial was inserted with no light. On these no-target trials, the monkeys were trained to press a special button, indicating an empty screen. Under this training regime, the animals pressed the "empty field" button if a bright patch of light was projected into the damaged hemifield, but not when the light was in the sighted field.

In other words, when the monkeys were forced to point at the target in their blind hemifield, they could do so without any problem, as could their human counterparts. However, when given a chance to respond "I don't see a target,"—for that, in effect, was what the special button signified—they did so. Phenomenologically, their blindsighted hemifield looked empty.

The Cowey-Stoerig experiments prove that we can find out what animals are conscious of!

13.3 | COMPLEX, FOCAL EPILEPTIC SEIZURES

In an epileptic fit, normal brain activity is disrupted in some way. There are many ways in which this can happen. Best known, because of their dramatic

---

[7] Cowey and Stoerig (1995). Stoerig, Zontanou, and Cowey (2002) followed up their seminal animal experiment by comparing one of these monkeys with four patients with unilateral field defects. This validated their approach, in the sense that the monkey and the people responded in similar ways, serving as a potent reminder that the neuroanatomy and psychology of vision is similar in both species.

manifestations, are generalized seizures (*grand mal*) that engulf the entire brain, with associated convulsions—the rhythmic tightening and relaxing of the muscles—and total loss of consciousness.[8]

Of more interest to students of consciousness are focal or partial seizures that begin in or involve one part of the brain. In a simple partial seizure, consciousness is not impaired. The characteristic rhythmic twitching might be limited to a limb and the patient can experience strange tastes, smells, or feelings. These symptoms, referred to as an *aura*, can be harbingers of worse things to come, when the simple seizure turns into a complex one.

Complex partial seizures are characterized by a marring or loss of awareness, accompanied by *automatisms*, such as chewing, smacking the lips, coordinated hand and arm movements—as if directing an imaginary orchestra—laughing, or acting scared, fiddling with clothes, verbal utterings, and so on. If not restrained, the person may wander about and "wake up" far from home or the hospital. Usually, the patient has no memory of any events during the seizure. Once the attack is over, some patients lapse into an exhausted sleep or a period of confusion while others are almost instantly fully responsive, as if a switch had been thrown.[9] Complex focal seizures often occur in the temporal lobe and last for a few minutes.

A patient experiencing one of these seizures may seem conscious, given her behavior and apparent display of emotions. On a subsequent attack, however, the same, though not identical, motor manifestations return. The patient once again smiles and tries to leave her bed. She behaves like an actor during an audition who goes through the same scene again and again, each time laughing on cue. After observing a few of these individuals, automatisms can readily be distinguished from conscious behaviors by their unnatural, forced, and obsessive quality.

---

[8] A seizure can be defined as an episode of hyper-synchronous, self-maintained neuronal discharge. Affected neurons fire in an elevated and highly synchronized manner, instead of in their usual disjoint and sparse fashion.

[9] I recommend Fried (1997) or Elger (2000) for an introduction to complex, partial seizures, Penfield and Jasper (1954) as the classic treatise on the subject, and Oxbury, Polkey, and Duchowny (2000) for its exhaustive coverage. For two thoughtful essays on the loss of consciousness during seizures, see Gloor, Olivier, and Ives (1980) and Gloor (1986). I am struck by the extreme heterogeneity of seizures (simple and complex seizures, absences, myoclonic seizures, and generalized tonic-clonic ones). Their origin, and their subsequent spread to other brain areas, varies tremendously, too, as do their duration, semiology, and associated auras. I am here mainly referring to focal seizures in the temporal lobes of adults. Another fascinating topic is *absence seizures* or *petit mal*. These are brief periods of wakeful unconsciousness. Most common in children, an absence seizure suddenly interrupts ongoing mental and physical activity for a few seconds, during which the child will stare motionless into space, before returning abruptly to the land of the living. Absence seizures involve the generation of abnormal oscillatory discharges in thalamocortical circuitry (Crunelli and Leresche, 2002). They can occur frequently, do not go hand-in-hand with muscle activity, and could be studied profitably using event-related fMRI.

Some patients can interact, at least in a limited manner, with their environment during these brief episodes. One patient can answer some routine questions. Another reported an attack while riding his bicycle to work. After setting out in the morning, he would occasionally find himself riding back home along his usual route, all while having a seizure. Others engage in nocturnal wanderings.[10] All of this raises the question whether these automatisms are remnants of zombie agents that animate the otherwise unconscious patient.

The extent to which consciousness is actually lost during the seizure is difficult to verify in a clinical setting. One way to assess whether anything but zombie behaviors are present is to evaluate working memory during a fit.[11] As mentioned in Chapters 11 and 12, the ability to store and make use of information over many seconds is a hallmark of conscious processes, and one not enjoyed by zombies.

It seems plausible that automatisms occur whenever the aberrant electrical discharges destroy the coalitions making up the NCC, while the neural activity underlying zombie behaviors is more resistant to such interference. Clinical evidence suggests a hemispheric bias. Partial seizures with left or bilateral temporal lobe involvement are more likely to interfere with consciousness than right temporal lobe seizures.[12]

To study automatisms in any rigorous manner is not easy. They occur unpredictably, and the patient may be unable to carry out the previously rehearsed motor program because his brain won't cooperate. What is clear is that some fairly elaborate sensory-motor behaviors are retained without much, if any, conscious sensation.

13.4 | SLEEPWALKING

What about people who walk in their sleep? Are zombie agents at work during *somnambulistic* activities, which range from the prosaic—sitting up in bed and

---

[10] Pedley and Guilleminault (1977).

[11] Suppose, for instance, that the patient hears either a low- or a high-pitch tone during the attack. A few seconds later, the same or a different tone is presented again and the patient has to point with his hand, arm, or head to the ground if the two tones are the same and point skyward if the tones are different. To perform this experiment, the patient must remember the task instructions during the seizure, have at least some limited degree of control over his limbs, and be able to hear the tones (M. Kurthen, T. Grunwald, and C. Koch, personal communication).

[12] Ebner et al. (1995), Inoue and Mihara (1998), and Lux et al. (2002). The left hemisphere is usually dominant for language (Chapter 17), prompting speculation about a relationship between loss of consciousness as measured at the bedside and aphasia. In at least one case (C. Elger, personal communication), loss of responsiveness occurred following a focal seizure in the left temporal lobe of a patient whose right hemisphere was dominant for language (as assessed by the Wada test). Thus, the link between no behavior and no consciousness and the left temporal lobe transcends language. The minimal brain structures that must be engulfed by the epileptic discharges for consciousness to be lost remain unknown (Reeves, 1985).

mumbling incomprehensibly—to the more unusual—dressing and undress-
ing, going to the bathroom, and moving furniture—to the bizarre—climbing
out of the window or driving a car? Sleepwalkers sure seem unconscious while
they stumble around their bedrooms, don't respond when spoken to, and don't
recall anything out of the ordinary the next morning.

Sleepwalking episodes last from a fraction of a minute to half an hour. They
are more frequent in children than in adults, occur during the nonrapid eye
movement phase of sleep, and leave no explicit, conscious recollection upon
awaking.[13]

Sleepwalkers display zombie traits instantly recognizable by any horror
movie fan—absence of sensations and feelings, glazed eyes,[14] the extraordinary strength, and the clumsy movements. To wit,

> They appeared, although in a state of frenzy and intense autonomic arousal, as
> automatons unaware of what they were doing and unresponsive to stimuli from
> their environment.[15]

Occasionally, sleepwalkers turn violent and become a danger to themselves,
their sleeping partners, and others. Rarely, this has ended in death. When these
cases come to trial, some sort of *noninsane automatism* defense is invoked,
based on the argument that the defendant wasn't himself when the homicide
occurred. By today's medico-legal standards concerned with *conscious intention*, a sleepwalker *is* like a zombie, a person with limited behavioral repertoire
and no conscious sensation.[16]

Little is known about the spectrum of behaviors expressed during som-
nambulism. Within the visual modality, is saliency-based attention operating?
Probably. Can the sleepwalker pay (top-down) attention to events or objects?
Probably not. Is working memory functioning? Unlikely. Are the sensory-
motor agents that control eye movements, posture, reaching, and gait, active?
Probably, to some extent.

What are the underlying pathological mechanisms? Because sleepwalking
occurs in deep sleep, the low level of arousal signals from the brainstem may be

---

[13] Sleepwalkers are characteristically deep sleepers, are hard to awaken, and have low dream
recall. For reviews on sleepwalking, see Kavey et al. (1990); Masand, Popli, and Weilburg (1995);
and Vgontzas and Kales (1999). The possible relationship to consciousness is discussed in
Revonsuo et al. (2000).

[14] Something Shakespeare recognized long ago. In Act V, Scene I of *Macbeth*, the doctor notes
that Lady Macbeth is wandering around. He says, "You see, her eyes are open," to which the
Lady-in-Waiting comments, "Ay, but their sense is shut." See also Jacobson et al. (1965).

[15] Page 738 in Moldofsky et al. (1995).

[16] For a thoughtful discussion of one sleepwalking case that resulted in mayhem and death, and
the attendant legal implications, see Broughton et al. (1994). Other examples are discussed by
Moldofsky et al. (1995) and Schenck and Mahowald (1998).

insufficient to support the sustained feedback activity needed for a dominant coalition to establish itself as NCC (that is, the NCC_e's of Chapter 5 are not fully present), but adequate to mediate the more transient, feedforward activity sufficient to power zombie agents. Answering these questions in any decisive manner will be difficult unless a method to reliably induce sleepwalking in human volunteers, monkeys, or mice is discovered.

13.5 | ZOMBIE AGENTS AND THE NCC

Now that you've learned there's an army of nonconscious zombie agents in your head, how does this aid the quest to understand the NCC?

First, it puts to rest the idea that the computational complexity of a sensory-motor task can separate nonconscious from conscious actions in any straight-forward manner. Zombie agents mediate nontrivial motor programs, and not mere reflexes. Imagine, for example, the web of processes necessary to evaluate the optical flow patterns impinging upon the eyes, combining this with information from the vestibular sense, and adjusting the skeletal-muscular system accordingly to retain an upright posture. As long as these procedures occur over and over, however, they can be learned (Section 11.2) by the cortex in collusion with the basal ganglia. Any distinction between nonconscious and conscious processes has to take this learning aspect into account, something I will develop more fully in the next chapter.

Second, what about the pathways underlying zombie actions? One possibility is that they might be physically distinct and separate from the networks that generate the NCC. That is, neural activity in some regions of the brain mediates behavior without consciousness while activity elsewhere is sufficient for sensations. Milner and Goodale argue forcefully that vision-for-action is carried out by the dorsal pathway while vision-for-perception is consigned to the ventral pathway. Another possibility is that the same network operates in two distinct *modes*. One is based on a transient net-wave that originates in the sensory periphery (e.g., in the retina) and quickly moves through the various cortical processing stages until it triggers a stereotyped nonconscious response. This traveling net-wave is too ephemeral to leave elevated firing in its wake. This would be the zombie mode of action in which the brain operates in what is essentially a feedforward manner, without significant active feedback (Table 5.1).

If the input is more sustained and is boosted by top-down attention, on the other hand, a sort of standing wave or resonance might be created in the network, with vital contributions from the feedback pathways. Both local and more global feedback could cause neurons to synchronize their spiking activity above and beyond the degree of synchronization that results from the sensory input by itself. This increases their postsynaptic punch compared to when they fire independently. A powerful coalition of neurons could be assembled in this manner, able to project its influence to the far reaches of the cortex and below. This would be the slow mode that underlies conscious perception.

Although these ideas are still inchoate, they can guide more detailed investigations. Given the highly variable nature and time course of the neurological deficits discussed here and the ethical limits on human experimentation, such investigations need to focus on appropriate animal models. Studying patients is essential to fully characterizing the phenomenology of deficits as they relate to consciousness. But untangling the underlying neuronal circuits demands interventions that selectively target discrete cellular components in the vast fields of the brain, and this can't be done in humans.

13.6 | A TURING TEST FOR CONSCIOUSNESS?

In 1950, the mathematician Alan Turing published a paper in which he considered the question of "Can machines think?" within the framework of an *imitation game*. Known today as a *Turing Test*, it involves carrying on an extended conversation with an entity, via typed natural language, on a variety of arbitrary topics, from the mundane to the esoteric. If, after a while, the observer is unable to decide whether this entity she has been interacting with is a machine or a human, it must be deemed intelligent.[17] The Turing test offers a practical means to gage progress in designing intelligent machines. A similar operational means to distinguish automatic zombie behaviors from those that require consciousness would be desirable.

Of tremendous significance is the evidence from normals, D.F., and blindsight patients that a delay of more than a few seconds virtually eliminates many of their zombie behaviors. In Chapter 11, I surmised that sophisticated actions that require the retention of information over seconds, such as trace conditioning or working memory, might be further litmus tests. Jointly, such a battery of operations might distinguish automatic from conscious behaviors.

Take your favorite sensory-motor routine in some species and enforce a waiting period of a few seconds between the sensory input and the execution of an action. If the subject can't perform the task with the delay, it was probably mediated by a zombie agent. If the organism's performance is only marginally affected by the delay, then the input must have been stored in some sort of intermediate, short-term buffer, implying some measure of consciousness. If the subject can be successfully distracted during this interval by a suit-

---

[17]The original paper bears reading for its simplicity and elegance (Turing, 1950). Millican and Clark (1999) provide a historical perspective and the current status of the Turing test.

salient stimulus (e.g., flashing lights), it would reinforce the conclusion that attention was involved in actively maintaining information during the delay period.

Dogs, probably like all mammals, easily pass this test. Think of hiding a bone well out of sight and teaching the dog to sit still until you tell her to "go fetch the bone."

This is not meant to be an infallible test, but good enough to be practical and useful at the bedside or in the laboratory. Of course, such tests are irrelevant for investigating questions of machine consciousness, since computers, robots, and other man-made artifacts are constrained by radically different forces than biological organisms.

13.7 | RECAPITULATION

In this chapter I examined pathologies that offer tantalizing glimpses of what humans can do without consciousness.

In visual agnosia, patients lose one or more specific aspects of visual perception (color, motion, faces, form). Patient D.F. is a case in point. She can't identify objects or recognize their shape or form. Yet she retains remarkable visual reactivity: she can slide her hand into a slit of variable orientation, she can grasp things appropriately, and she can walk around without bumping into objects placed in her way. Blindsight patients are blind in part of their visual field, but they can, if forced to, point to a bright light, move their eyes toward it, guess at the color of an invisible stimulus, and so on.

Some of these behaviors break down if a delay of several seconds is interposed between stimulus presentation and action, suggesting that these patients lack the necessary facilities to store information for more than a few seconds. The delay test proposed here constitutes a practical means to experimentally differentiate zombie agents from conscious systems in animals, babies, or severely disabled patients.

Some patients with complex, focal seizures or people who sleepwalk exhibit fairly elaborate learned motor patterns; they wander around, move furniture, or drive a car. They typically don't respond to verbal commands nor do they recall events that occurred during their episodes. These automatisms follow an internal program that can be influenced—to a limited extent—by the environment.

What underlies the distinction between automatic behaviors and those that rely on consciousness? Conceptually simplest is the possibility that distinct networks mediate zombie and conscious actions. Zombie agents might live outside the cortex proper as well as in the dorsal stream, while conscious visual perception is mediated by the ventral pathway. Like a long-time married couple, they each have their own vices and virtues, but manage to harmoniously work together.

Alternatively, the same network may operate in two modes. A transient net-wave is propelled from the sensory periphery through the cortical hierarchy to the output stages. This happens so quickly that each neuron contributes only a few spikes, leaving no long-lasting activity in the wake of the net-wave. This is sufficient to initiate stereotypical actions without any associated sensation. If the input is more sustained or is boosted by a top-down attentional bias, on the other hand, it sets up long-lasting reverberatory activity that is powerful enough to generate the coalitions sufficient for conscious perception.

If zombies are so wonderful, what is the function of consciousness? Why bother with consciousness at all? In tackling these questions next, I'll have to grapple with the two concepts central to the mind-body problem—qualia and meaning.

CHAPTER FOURTEEN

Some Speculations on the Functions of Consciousness

Introduction to Psychology: The theory of human behavior. . . . Is there a
split between mind and body, and, if so, which is better to have? . . .
Special consideration is given to a study of consciousness as opposed to
unconsciousness, with many helpful hints on how to remain conscious.

From *Getting Even* by Woody Allen

Why bother with consciousness at all?
The last two chapters dealt with sensory-motor agents in healthy and brain-damaged people. I emphasized the rapid and flawless manner in which they execute learned, stereotyped behaviors. The existence of these agents raises troubling questions. If so much processing can go on in the dark, without any feelings, why is a conscious mental life needed at all? What evolutionary advantage favored conscious brains over brains that are nothing but large bundles of zombie agents?

Consciousness is a property of particular types of highly evolved biological organs.[1] So phenomenal experience very likely serves a purpose. In a fiercely competitive world, consciousness must give the organism an edge over non-conscious zombies.

Within the last two decades, novelists, philosophers, scientists, and engineers have written extensively on the function of consciousness. Most of these speculations adopt a computational stance, identifying one or several information processing tasks as critical to and for consciousness.

---

[1] Not all complex and highly evolved organs are sentient, of course. The liver isn't, nor is the immune system. The *enteric nervous system*—100 million or more neurons that line the intestinal walls in your bowel—appears to operate nonconsciously (if the gut has a mind of its own, it is not telling the brain). And this is a good thing too, for the sparse signals it does provide are responsible for the feeling of a bloated stomach or of nausea (Gershon, 1998).

The list of putative functions is substantial, including

promoting access to short-term memory,
perceptual categorization,
decision making,
planning and control of action,
motivation,
setting long-term goals,
learning complex tasks,
detecting inconsistencies and anomalies in the world and the body,
labeling the present moment,
implementing top-down attentional selection,
creativity,
forming analogies,
self-monitoring,
making recursive models,
working with noncomputable functions,
inferring the state of other animals or people,
and the use of language.

Because some of the most advanced computers are based on parallel computer architectures, the artificial intelligence pioneer Marvin Minsky thinks consciousness emerges out of the complex interactions of a large number of autonomous and fairly simple-minded agents. The cognitive scientist Johnson-Laird sees consciousness as an operating system that controls a hierarchical but parallel computer made up of many individual modules. It calls on some routines and inactivates others, but is also powerful enough to generate a model of itself, giving rise to self-consciousness. All in all, this is quite a motley collection of proposed functions, though some may be more relevant than others in explaining the functions of evolved consciousness.[2]

A word of warning: Up to this point the book has, by and large, remained close to the facts, focusing on the relevant work in psychology and the brain sciences. This chapter is different in that I will share with the reader Francis's and my speculations about the functions of consciousness and of qualia. What is perhaps different from many of the proposals outlined in the previous

---

[2]For a more thorough discussion, see Johnson-Laird (1983), Minsky (1985), Velmans (1991), Mandler (2002), and Chapter 10 in Baars (1988). Thinking of the brain/mind as a parallel computer is just the latest in a long line of technological metaphors that extends back from parallel and von Neumann computers, telephone switchboards, steam engines, clocks, and waterworks, all the way back to wax tablets in ancient Greece.

paragraph is that our perspective leads to some specific and empirically verifiable predictions. If you don't like such speculations, then jump directly to Section 14.7.

14.1 | CONSCIOUSNESS AS AN EXECUTIVE SUMMARY

In our earliest published work on consciousness, Francis and I felt it was premature to speculate as to its purpose without a better understanding of how and where it acted in the brain. We reconsidered this position a few years later and stated our hunch as to its function as follows:

> Our ... assumption is based on the broad idea of the biological usefulness of visual awareness (or, strictly, of its neural correlate). This is to produce the best current interpretation of the visual scene, in the light of past experience either of ourselves or of our ancestors (embodied in our genes), and to make it available, for a sufficient time, to the parts of the brain that contemplate, plan and execute voluntary motor outputs (of one sort or another).[3]

The central nervous system, like so many people in today's hyperconnected world, suffers from information overload. So much data about the constantly changing environment is streaming in along the sensory pathways that the brain is unable to process all of it in real time. Recall from Chapter 3 that millions of bits of information are transmitted along the optic nerve every second. Your body moves continuously and adjusts its position, sending spikes into the brain that encode the joint angles, the extension of muscles, and so on. You are embedded in clouds of odor molecules that float about and interact with the mucus in your nose. A symphony of sounds constantly impinges on your ears. Out of this melee of sensory events only a few privileged events make it into phenomenal feelings, while the rest are discarded into an experiential limbo.

Natural selection pursued a strategy that amounts to summarizing most of the pertinent facts about the outside world compactly and sending this description to the planning stages to consider the organism's optimal course of action. Such a summary inevitably means that information is lost. In a dynamic environment populated with predators, however, it is usually better to come to some conclusion rapidly and act, rather than to take too long to find the best solution. In a world ruled by the survival of the fittest, the best can be the enemy of the good.

These few items, labeled with qualia, are then sent off to the planning stages of the brain to help decide a future course of action. For example, you may see a dog in front of you, baring its teeth and growling, and an open door to your right. At that moment, everything else is irrelevant.

---

[3]Crick and Koch (1995a).

This function of consciousness is related to the strategy that many leaders of large organizations adopt, namely, "I need a concise summary of all the relevant facts and I need it *now*." Former U.S. President Ronald Reagan was famous for demanding that his aides reduce any topic that he had to consider, from tax reform to strategic missile defense, to a single page. This *executive summary* was then used to make final policy recommendations. Vastly more background information on each topic can be supplied by assistants or by accessing databases, but frequently time pressures force a decision to be made based on this sparse collection of opinions and facts and the experience of the chief executive.

We argue that a similar situation applies to the brain. A single, compact representation of what is out there is presented, for a sufficient time, to the parts of the brain that can choose among different plans of action. This is what conscious perception is about. Since only a few items are represented in this manner, the information can be dealt with quickly.

The purpose or purposes for which consciousness originally arose in the course of evolution might be complemented or even supplanted by other functions in the meantime. There is no question that consciousness is important for language, for artistic, mathematical, and scientific reasoning,[4] and for communicating information about ourselves to others. Furthermore, once information is consciously accessible, it can be used to veto and suppress zombie behaviors, actions, or memories inappropriate to the situation at hand.[5] However, as the birth of conscious creatures probably predated the arrival of modern humans by millions of years,[6] these higher aspects of consciousness—limited to hominids—couldn't have been the decisive factor favoring the evolution of conscious phenotypes over zombies.

All animals with thousands or more visual, tactile, auditory, and olfactory receptors are faced by the same onslaught of sensory information and would benefit from an executive summary that enables them to plan what to do next.

---

[4]Though, much reasoning can occur without consciousness (Chapter 18).

[5]Waiting impatiently at a red traffic light, your instinct is to gun your car forward as soon as it turns green; but this impulse must be checked if a pedestrian is still crossing the street. Evidence of the suppression of memories and behaviors is offered in Anderson and Green (2001) and Mitchell, Macrae, and Gilchrist (2002).

[6]In *The Origin of Consciousness in the Breakdown of the Bicameral Mind*, psychologist Julian Jaynes (1976) sees consciousness as a learned process that originated somewhere in the second millennium B.C. when humans finally realized that the voices inside their heads were not the gods speaking to them but their own internalized speech. The book is highly readable, full of interesting archeological, literary, and psychological observations, yet devoid of any brain science or testable hypotheses. Its central thesis is certainly totally wrong. The philosopher W. V. Quine asked Jaynes what it was like for people to have experiences before they "discovered consciousness" and he is reputed to have replied that in those days, people had no more experience than a table! (Ned Block, personal communication).

I am not implying that planning or decision-making are necessarily, themselves, conscious mental activities. Indeed, copious evidence suggests otherwise. What I *am* proposing is that awareness occurs at the interface between sensory processing and planning.

Take all of these musings about the function of consciousness with a large grain of salt. What is important is the extent to which these speculations reveal something about the NCC. I'll return to this theme in Section 14.7.

14.2 │ CONSCIOUSNESS AND THE TRAINING OF SENSORY-MOTOR AGENTS

Our hypothesis is quite compatible with the existence of a multitude of stereotyped sensory-motor behaviors that bypass consciousness. A pool of specialists, however, can't deal easily with novel or surprising situations. This is where awareness comes in. Because the NCC correspond to some sort of sustained activity that projects selectively but widely throughout the forebrain, lots of computational and memory resources become available once an event is consciously registered. Moreover, motor systems stand by to execute the desired action. Thus, consciousness can deal with the many real-world tasks encountered in daily life with their often conflicting demands (such as quickly orienting yourself in an unfamiliar neighborhood).

But the price to be paid for this is that it takes several hundred milliseconds for a sensory event to give rise to consciousness—a fraction of a second that may spell the difference between life and death in the fight for survival.

Fortunately, given the amazing ability of brains to learn, a zombie agent can be trained to take over the activities that used to require consciousness. That is, a sequence of sensory-motor actions can be stitched together into elaborate motor programs by means of constant repetition. This occurs when you learn how to ride a bicycle, sail a boat, dance to rock-and-roll, climb a steep wall, or play a musical instrument. During the learning phase, you are exquisitely attentive to the way you position and move your hands, fingers, and feet, you closely follow the teacher's instructions, take account of the environment, and so on. With enough practice, however, these skills become effortless, the motion of your body fluid and fast, with no wasted effort. You carry out the action beyond ego, beyond awareness, without giving any thought as to what has to be done next. It just comes naturally.[7]

---

[7] This is not to say that all learning requires consciousness. A substantial body of research investigates *implicit learning*, in particular the nonconscious learning of motor sequences (Cleeremans et al., 1998; and Destrebecqz and Cleeremans, 2001).

At this stage, paradoxically, consciousness often interferes with the smooth and rapid execution of the task. If you compliment your tennis opponent on her impressive backhand, her subsequent attention to her return may cause her performance to diminish over the next few ball exchanges. A similar thing happens when performing a highly practiced piece of music that you haven't played in a while. It's best to let the "fingers do the playing," because thinking about the individual motifs and sequences of notes can lead you astray.

A baseball player might spend hour after hour in fielding practice, improving his eye-hand coordination, until catching the ball and throwing it to first base becomes "mindless." He is actively wiring up a zombie agent. Circuits in the posterior parietal and medial prefrontal cortex are initially involved, in conjunction with the basal ganglia and the cerebellum. Once training is complete, the prefrontal cortex loses its importance, because the striatum and other basal ganglia structures have taken over the routine, goal-directed behavior. These coordinate the interplay of muscles, optimizing performance and avoiding the delays inherent in depending on the output of the conscious, planning stage. That's why athletes, warriors, and performance artists rehearse over and over for situations where a fraction of a second spells the difference between victory and defeat.

Pick up a training manual for any sport and you'll read words to this effect. A wonderful example is to be found in one of the gems of contemplative literature, Eugen Herrigel's *Zen in the Art of Archery*. Toward the end of this slim volume, Herrigel explains how mastery in the art of swordsmanship is achieved:

> The pupil must develop a new sense or, more accurately, a new alertness of all of his senses, which will enable him to avoid dangerous thrusts as though he could feel them coming. Once he has mastered the art of evasion, he no longer needs to watch with undivided attention the movements of his opponent, or even of several opponents at once. Rather, he sees and feels what is going to happen, and at that same moment he has already avoided its effect without there being "a hair's breadth" between perceiving and avoiding. This, then, is what counts: a lighting reaction which has no further need of conscious observation. In this respect at least the pupil makes himself independent of all conscious purpose. And that is a great gain.

Humans revel in and glorify these kinds of achievements. Keep in mind, however, that this level of proficiency is only useful within a narrow context (except for those fortunate few at the top of their profession who make a living exploiting such situations). That's why a more general-purpose mechanism for dealing with novel or infrequently encountered situations is needed. It provides access to planning, intelligent reasoning, and decision-making. Their action is more flexible but, unfortunately, also slower.

14.3 | WHY THE BRAIN IS NOT JUST A BUNDLE OF ZOMBIE AGENTS

If these sensory-motor, on-line agents are so fast and efficient, why not dispense with consciousness altogether? Perhaps the organism would come out ahead in the long run if the slower, conscious planning stage were replaced by a bundle of nonconscious agents. The disadvantage would be the lack of any subjective, mental life. No feelings whatsoever!

Given the many senses—eyes, ears, nose, tongue, skin—that flood the brain with information about the environment, and given the diverse effectors controlled by the brain—eyes, head, arms and fingers, legs and feet, the trunk— breeding zombie agents for all possible input-output combinations is probably inefficient. Too many would be required as well as something that coordinates their actions, in particular when they pursue conflicting aims. Such a nervous system would, in all likelihood, be bigger and less flexible than a brain that follows a hybrid strategy of combining zombie agents with a more flexible, conscious module.

I am not claiming that such an *Über*-zombie could not exist or could not be built by artificial means. I don't know about that. What I am claiming is that natural selection favored brains that make use of a dual strategy.[8]

A helpful analogy can be found in embedded digital processors. These small, fast, and low-powered microprocessors are dedicated to one particular task and are ubiquitous in mobile phones, video game machines, washing machines, personal digital assistants, and automobiles. Contrast these with the bigger, more expensive and power-hungry, but also more powerful, processors for personal computers. A truly adaptive robot or other artifact will make use of both. And so it may be with our brains.

14.4 | DO FEELINGS MATTER?

None of the preceding ideas makes the central aspect of the mind-body problem any more comprehensible. Why should planning, indeed, why should *any* function go hand-in-hand with feelings?

Most thinkers through the ages have accepted the existence of sentience and qualia as given facts of life. But many are still stumped when it comes to assigning a function to consciousness. They therefore conclude that consciousness must be an *epiphenomenon*, with no causal powers, like the noise

---

[8]If evolution on this planet had not brought forth conscious creatures, you and I could not be wondering about consciousness. In this sense, the situation may be analogous to the *anthropic principle* in cosmology, the postulate that the physical laws in the universe appear to strongly favor the emergence of life (Barrow and Tipler, 1986).

the heart makes as it beats. The sound is useful to a cardiologist when diagnosing a patient, but is of no consequence to the body. Thomas Henry Huxley, the British naturalist and defender of Darwin, expressed this belief memorably as follows:

> The consciousness of brutes would appear to be related to the mechanism of their body simply as a collateral product of its working, and to be completely without any power of modifying that working as the steam-whistle which accompanies the work of a locomotive engine is without influence upon its machinery.[9]

The belief that phenomenal consciousness is real but impotent to influence events in the physical world continues to be remarkably widespread among modern philosophers. While this belief cannot, at this point, be shown to be false, it can be undermined since it is based on a trick, a sleight-of-hand.

All functional aspects of consciousness are lumped into one category, called *access consciousness* by the American philosopher Ned Block. The ability of consciousness to attend to and flag special events, to plan and then decide, to remember situations and so on, are all examples of access consciousness. Because these processes have a function, it is—in principle—straightforward to imagine how nervous systems carry out these functions (although practical, instrumental, and conceptual limitations will extend the process of discovery over decades). This is why Chalmers considers them to be part of the *Easy Problem* of consciousness. If you think of a new function, fine, just move it into access consciousness.

What remains are feelings—*phenomenal consciousness*. This is the raw experience of the haunting, sad vibes of Miles Davis's *Kind of Blue* or the ecstatic, near-delirious feeling of dancing all night. These qualia exist, but they serve no function. The fact that yesterday's root canal treatment makes you want to crawl under the covers of your bed belongs to the access realm of consciousness, while the ineffable, bad quality of pain—the subjective part—is phenomenal. Chalmers famously refers to the problem of how the physical world at large generates qualia as the *Hard Problem*, arguing that since qualia have no function, there will never be a reductionist explanation of the Hard Problem in terms of the Easy Problem.[10]

---

[9]This quote comes from a remarkable speech that Huxley delivered in 1884 to the British Association for the Advancement of Science. He took issue with Descartes's belief that animals were mere machines or automata, devoid not only of reason but of any kind of consciousness. Instead, Huxley assumed that for reasons of biological continuity, some animal species did share certain aspects of consciousness with humans. He was at a loss, though, when it came to the function of consciousness.

[10]Block (1995) introduced the distinction between access and phenomenal consciousness (see also Block, 1996). The volume edited by Block, Flanagan, and Güzeldere (1997) expands on this

I find this reasoning unpersuasive. Just because somebody can't *imagine* qualia having a function, doesn't imply that they *don't have* any. All it might mean is that the person's conceptual framework is inadequate. Let me present an alternative view.

14.5 | MEANING AND NEURONS

To do so, I need to tackle the related problem of meaning. The neuron illustrated in Figure 2.1 responds to a twisted paperclip seen by the monkey from one vantage point. The neuroscientist knows this by looking at the experimental setup, the paperclip in front of the animal, the cell's response, and so on; but how do the neurons in the monkey's brain that receives input from this cell know this? This is the problem of *meaning* (what philosophers also refer to as the problem of *intentionality*).

Meaning has traditionally been addressed within the context of linguistic *semantics*. Given the rise of symbolic logic and theories of computation in the past hundred years, meaning has usually been analyzed in terms of linguistic representations. Questions such as "How can the word 'lion' actually mean the real lion out there?" have been endlessly debated, analyzed, and re-analyzed. Yet the representations for language must have evolved out of spatial, visual, and auditory representations that are shared by humans and animals alike. From the standpoint of understanding how brain states can be about something, or can refer to something, the nearly exclusive concern with logic and language has been a comparatively barren enterprise. Fortunately, it is now slowly giving way to *neurosemantics*, which focuses on how meaning arises out of brains shaped by evolution.[11]

Two key problems stand out. First, where in the world does meaning arise? Second, how is meaning instantiated by squishy neurons?

---

topic. As I stated in Chapter 1, I don't distinguish between access and phenomenal consciousness. See Chalmers (1996) for the sophisticated, eristic arguments concerning the *Easy Problem* and the *Hard Problem*. This dichotomy has generated a large secondary literature (Shear, 1997). There is no doubt that today, in the early part of the 21st century, the phenomenal aspects of consciousness are very, very puzzling: a truly *hard* problem. Whether it will remain a hard one with a capital H remains to be seen. Other philosophers recoil from the very idea of qualia having any sort of real existence (e.g., Dennett, 1991). To them, the mind-body conundrum would disappear once we understood access consciousness and its material manifestations in the brain.

[11]The literature on intentionality, meaning, and mind stretches back more than two thousand years to the Stoa in classical Athens. By and large, how meaning emerges out of the brain is something that has occupied scholars only within the last decades (Dennett, 1969; Eliasmith, 2000; and Churchland, 2002).

On the Sources of Meaning

There are many sources of meaning in the world. One set is genetically prede-termined dispositions. Infants are not born as blank slates, with empty minds. They seek pleasure, such as sucking milk from their mother's breasts, and avoid pain. Getting the basic hedonistic drives right by specifying them in an innate fashion is clearly useful for survival.

A second, richer source of meaning is the myriad sensory-motor interac-tions you have constantly engaged in since the day you were born. These give rise to tacit expectations that inform everything you think, do, or say. If your head moves, your visual brain expects the image on the retina to shift accord-ingly. When you reach for something that looks like a hammer, you expect it to be reasonably heavy and adjust your muscles accordingly. You know that when you pick up a glass filled to its rim with water, you must be careful lest you spill its contents. Your nervous system learned these expectations in the past with the aid of experience-dependent learning rules and projects them, implicitly, into the future. A purely sessile organism, or somebody who was born com-pletely paralyzed, couldn't experience this aspect of meaning.

A third source of meaning comes from the fusion of sensory data within and across modalities. A rose is red, with a particular fragrance, and the thorns on its stem can prick you. When you look at somebody talking, you expect the movement of their lips and jaw to be synchronized to their voice. When this doesn't happen, as in a movie that has been dubbed in another language, it's disconcerting. Fancier brains, with more sensory input and motor output modalities, thus have richer meanings than simpler nervous systems.

In humans, meaning also derives from abstract facts about the world and from your autobiography. On stage, for example, Brutus betrays his trusting friend Julius Caesar; in geometry, π is the ratio of the circumference of a circle to its diameter; in your childhood, your grandfather held you in his arms. Such unspoken facts and memories weave the tapestry, the cognitive background, on which your life plays out.

How Can Neurons Mean?

How is meaning instantiated at the neuronal level? Francis and I believe that this takes place in the postsynaptic connections made by the winning coalition, the NCC, onto other neurons outside this assembly.

Consider the "Clinton" neuron of Figure 2.2, which is a member of the coali-tion responsible for the percept of seeing former President Bill Clinton. If its axon terminals were poisoned, preventing the release of synaptic vesicles, it would continue to generate action potentials but it wouldn't contribute anything to awareness because it couldn't affect any of its targets.[12] If the output of the entire coalition in your head were blocked in this manner, you would have difficulty quickly identifying President Clinton or imagining him and you might have trouble thinking of related concepts. A neurologist might diagnose you as suffering from a specific and limited form of what could be called *a-cognita*.

The meaning associated with any one conscious attribute is part of the post-NCC activity emanating from the winning coalition. Coalition members are highly networked with each other but also establish outside contacts with non-members. For instance, the Clinton neuron and others like it will excite cells that represent the concept of the "presidency" or the "White House," that are linked to neurons that recall the unmistakable voice of President Clinton and so on. These associated neurons make up the *penumbra* of the NCC.[13]

This implies that a brain with more explicit representations for sensory stimuli or concepts has the potential for a richer web of associations and more meaningful qualia than a brain with fewer explicit representations. Or, expressed at the level of cortical regions, the more essential nodes, the richer the meaning (Section 2.2). The extent any one attribute is represented in an explicit manner can be assessed by probing individual neurons within a cortical column. Such an operational means would permit, in principle, the meaningfulness of any one conscious experience to be measured and compared within different sensory modalities, across time in the same individual, or across species.

The penumbra expresses the various associations of the NCC that provide the perceived attribute with meaning, including past associations, the expected consequences of the NCC, the cognitive background, and movements (or at least possible plans for movement) associated with NCC neurons. A coalition representing a rope, for example, influences plans for climbing. The penumbra is outside of the NCC proper, although some of its elements may participate in succeeding NCC (for instance, when your train of thought moves from President Clinton to the current President of the United States).

I do not know whether mere synaptic activation of the penumbra is sufficient to generate meaning or whether the NCC need to trigger action potentials within the cells making up the penumbra. The answer probably depends on the extent to which projections from the penumbra back to the NCC support or maintain the NCC.

---

[12] It is not impossible that the immediate loss of one such cell might lead to subtle behavioral differences that could be picked up with a sufficiently sensitive test.

[13] This term, suggested to us by Graeme Mitchison, was used in this context already by William James (1890).

The penumbra is not, by itself, sufficient for consciousness, though part of it may become part of the NCC as the NCC shift.[14] Neurons within the penumbra that project back to the NCC may help to sustain the underlying coalition. The penumbra provides the brain with the meaning of the relevant essential nodes—its aboutness.

14.6 | QUALIA ARE SYMBOLS

The preceding discussion emphasized that any percept, such as my son's face, is associated with an enormous amount of information—its meaning. For the most part, these associations are not made explicit in the brain *at that point in time*, but are there implicitly, in the penumbra. How he looks, when I last saw him, what I know about his personality, his upbringing and education, the sound of his voice, his dry sense of humor, my emotional reactions to him, and so on; these are all present in the penumbra. A staggering amount of detailed information, as well as more general knowledge, is all there. This data is not necessarily expressed as an active representation, in terms of neurons firing away, but in a more passive form, as elevated calcium concentration or dendritic depolarization at pre- and post-synaptic terminals, that may or may not lead to postsynaptic spiking.

To handle this information efficiently, the brain has to symbolize it. This, in a nutshell, is the purpose of qualia. Qualia symbolize a vast repository of tacit and unarticulated data that must be present for a sufficient amount of time. Qualia, the elements of conscious experience, enable the brain to effortlessly manipulate this *simultaneous information*. The feeling associated with seeing purple is an explicit symbol for the rush of associations with other purple objects, such as the purple cloak of Imperial Rome, an amethyst, the Purple Heart military decoration, and so on.

In motion-induced blindness (page 14) you don't see the yellow disks for a while since they are suppressed by the perceptually dominant cloud of moving blue dots. In this state, the informational impact of the yellow disks is very low. Once you *see* them, the underlying neuronal coalition activates the penumbra for a sufficient amount of time that you become conscious of the yellow color. The symbol for this state, lasting some minimal amount of time, is the associated quale (I shall discuss different aspects of qualia in Section 18.3).

Given the large number of discrete attributes that make up any one percept and the even larger number of relevant relationships among them, phenome-

---

[14]Unconscious priming is likely to occur at the synapses linking the NCC with the penumbra. This means that the associated concepts may be easier to activate in the immediate future.

nal feelings have evolved to deal with the attendant complexities of handling all of this information in real time. Qualia are potent symbolic representations of a fiendish amount of simultaneous information associated with any one percept—its meaning. Qualia are a peculiar property of highly parallel, feedback networks, evolved to efficiently represent an onslaught of data. Out of the firing activity of the NCC for purple and the associated penumbra emerges the quale for this hue.

Why Do Qualia Feel Like Anything?

But why do these symbols feel like anything at all? Why can't the brain summarize and encode this information without any sensations, as in a conventional computer?

Chalmers has surmised (Section 1.2) that phenomenal states are a fundamental property of any information-processing system, a universal primitive, like mass or charge. On this account, a roundworm or even a single-celled *Paramecium* would be conscious (without necessarily being very intelligent or even self-conscious). This sort of exuberant panpsychism has a charming metaphysical appeal—since it would make experience ubiquitous—but seems impossible to verify. A more sober hypothesis is that subjective states are limited to information-processing systems possessing a particular computational architecture, range of behavior, or minimal complexity.[15] In any case, an answer as to why feelings are associated with these symbols may emerge out of an information-theoretical formulation of first- and third-person perspectives.

These are deep waters, with little agreement among scholars. Given today's limited ability to intervene in the brain in a delicate and directed manner, empirical means to verify or refute these ideas seem quite remote. For now, it is more profitable for my quest to focus on the NCC and not worry too much about these foundational issues.[16]

It is a thought-provoking exercise to speculate on the extent to which qualia are unique to brains. Can computers or robots have feelings? Is it possible that, for reasons beyond our current understanding, a serial machine, even if powerful, could never execute the relevant operations to represent all the different aspects of an object or event and all the possible relationships among them, in this fashion?

---

[15] See Chapter 8 in Chalmers (1996); Edelman and Tononi (2000); and Edelman (2003).

[16] Such a focus has worked well elsewhere. The inability to satisfactorily answer the question, "Why is there nothing rather than something?" has not measurably impeded the progress of physics.

Why Are Qualia Private?

Happily, not all aspects of the mind-body problem appear so daunting. Take the problem, often remarked upon by poets, of why it is impossible to convey an exact experience to somebody else. Why are feelings *private*? The answer, I believe, is straightforward and has two components.

First, the meaning of any one sensation depends on the genetic makeup of the individual and on his or her previous experiences and life history. Since these are never exactly alike in two individuals, it is not easy to reproduce a feeling in another brain.

Second, any subjective percept is encoded by multi-focal activity at essential nodes. If I want to tell you about my experience of seeing a glorious purple, the relevant information needs to be transmitted from these nodes to the parts of the brain involved in speech, and onward to the vocal cords and tongue. Given the massive sideways and feedback connections characteristic of the cortex, this information is, of necessity, re-encoded during the course of this transmission. The explicit information expressed by the motor neurons animating my speech muscles is therefore *related*, but not *identical*, to the explicit information at the essential node for color.

That's why I can't convey the exact nature of my color experience to you (even if we have the same set of wavelength-sensitive photoreceptors).[17]

It is, however, possible to convey the *difference* between percepts, such as the difference between orange and yellowish-red, because a difference in firing activity in the color area can still be associated with a difference in firing pattern in the motor stages.[18]

14.7 | WHAT DOES THIS IMPLY ABOUT THE LOCATION OF THE NCC?

In Section 14.1, I remarked that speculations about the biological usefulness of the NCC are only helpful insofar as they reveal something about its elusive nature. Let me expand upon this.

The front of the cortex is concerned with contemplating, planning, and executing voluntary motor outputs of one sort or another. By and large, premotor, prefrontal, and anterior cingulate cortices actively maintain sensory or memory information, help retrieve data from long-term memory, and manipulate all of this data for planning purposes. Evidence for this comes from careful

---

[17]This explanation does not rule out the possibility of a future technology that would allow an outside observer to directly tap into my essential nodes for color.

[18]It is probably a general rule that the nature of anything—Kant's famous *Das Ding an sich*—is never expressible, except in its relationship to other things.

observation of patients with lesions in the frontal lobes, and from fMRI experiments in normal subjects.[19]

If our executive summary hypothesis is valid, then the essential nodes that represent the sensory information in an explicit manner must have direct access to the planning modules of the brain—the prefrontal and anterior cingulate cortices, in particular. Given cortical neuroanatomy, it is unlikely that an indirect connection, involving one or more neuronal relays between these nodes and the planning stages, would suffice. Such an indirect link would be too weak, from a biophysical point of view, to efficiently and reliably drive the intended target neurons. The critical pathway must be monosynaptic—neuron-to-neuron.

Furthermore, the neurons at the essential nodes in the back of the cortex must receive reciprocal feedback from the front of the brain. Sustained spiking activity that circulates between select neuronal populations in the inferior temporal cortex (IT) or the medial temporal lobe and the prefrontal cortex (including direct connections between IT and the human speech area known as Broca's area[20]), could constitute the NCC for object perception. Similarly, reverberant activity between the cortical area MT and the frontal eye fields could be the NCC for seeing motion. Unless a visual area directly projects to the front part of the cortex, activities in that region can't directly enter awareness, because the activity of frontal areas is needed to help establish the coalition as *the* dominant player in the cortex.

It would follow from this hypothesis that a person with no prefrontal and premotor cortices could not be conscious. For now, this is difficult to test directly. I know of no patients who have lost all of these regions in both hemispheres and have survived.[21] And there are no techniques that can quickly, reversibly, and safely inactivate all of this tissue on both sides.

Some relevant experiments have been done, though. Following surgical removal of the limbic, parietal, and frontal cortices, monkeys are functionally quite blind, unable to exploit visual information. It seems that the ventral pathway can only influence behavior with the participation of nonvisual cortical regions.[22] There is also direct evidence of visual deficits in patients with

---

[19]For instance, frontal lobe patients are typically impaired when solving "brain teaser" type problems that require planning ahead, such as the "Tower of Hanoi" or the "Water Jug" tasks (Fuster, 2000; and Colvin, Dunbar, and Grafman, 2001).

[20]Monosynaptic, interhemispheric connections from IT in the right hemisphere into Broca's area in the left hemisphere have been traced in a human brain (Di Virgilio and Clarke, 1997).

[21]Even Dandy's famous patient (Brickner, 1936) retained Broca's area and continued to talk. For a review of frontal patients, the vast majority of whom have unilateral lesions, see Damasio and Anderson (2003).

[22]Nakamura and Mishkin (1980 and 1986). The massive destruction of nervous tissue needed for these experiments makes me wary about placing too much faith in such drastic interventions.

damage to the dorsolateral prefrontal cortex, well away from the regions at the back of the cortex.[23]

In general, prefrontal patients do not complain of severe losses in conscious perception. However, neither do patients whose brains have been severed along the midline (Chapter 17). Likewise, patients who lost color perception in part of their visual field do *not* report seeing the world in gray in that part and in color everywhere else (footnote 9 in Chapter 8). It is quite remarkable how often fairly dramatic deficits go unnoticed, a sad testament to the limited power of the human mind for veridical introspection.

The executive summary hypothesis has an interesting and nonintuitive corollary. The primary visual cortex in the macaque monkey has no direct projections past the central sulcus. V1 doesn't send its axons much beyond V4 and MT and certainly not into the premotor or prefrontal cortex.[24] Francis and I therefore concluded in 1995 that activity in V1 does not directly enter into consciousness—that the NCC for seeing can't be in V1, even though a functioning V1 (as well as intact retinae) is needed for normal seeing.

As explained in Chapter 6, V1 cells in the monkey fire exuberantly to things the monkey doesn't see. Aftereffects involving invisible stimuli implicate post-V1 stages as critical for perception. The only evidence that speaks against our thesis is fMRI data, which has been taken to show that human V1 does follow the subject's percept. However, this conclusion is based on one particular interpretation of the fMRI signal that is being questioned (see Section 16.2).

14.8 | RECAPITULATION

As consciousness is a property of highly evolved biological tissue, it must have one or more functions. This rather speculative chapter deals with this topic.

Francis and I proposed the executive summary hypothesis: The NCC are useful because they enable an organism to summarize the present state of affairs in the world, including its own body, and to make this terse summary accessible to the planning stages. It is the attributes of this summary that are labeled with subjective feelings. These qualia are the raw material out of which

---

[23] Barcelo, Suwazono, and Knight (2000).

[24] Almost nothing is known about the detailed pattern of cortico-cortical connections in humans, so all references here are to the brain of the macaque monkey. V1 has no direct projections to the frontal eye fields, or to the broad prefrontal region surrounding and including the principal sulcus (Felleman and Van Essen, 1991), or, as far as we know, to any other frontal area. Moreover, V1 does not project to the caudate nucleus of the basal ganglia (Saint-Cyr, Ungerleider, and Desimone, 1990), to the intralaminar nuclei of the thalamus, the claustrum (Sherk, 1986), or to the brainstem, with the exception of a small projection from the peripheral V1 to the pons (Fries, 1990). V1 does provide, however, the dominant visual input to most of the posterior visual cortical areas, including V2, V3, V4, and MT. Among subcortical targets, V1 projects to the superior colliculus, the LGN, and the pulvinar (Chapter 4).

conscious experience is built. They influence the general-purpose, flexible, and deliberate reasoning and decision-making machinery in the frontal lobes.

Research and common experience suggests that the *acquisition* of rapid, effortless zombie behaviors requires consciousness. This is particularly true of the ritualized sensory-motor activities humans love to engage in—rock-climbing, fencing, dancing, playing the violin or piano, and the like. Once a task is sufficiently rehearsed, conscious introspection interferes with its smooth execution. True mastery requires a surrendering of the mind, a letting go of the aim so ardently pursued, in order for the body and its senses to take over.

Could there be organisms like us but devoid of any conscious mental life? Possibly. But given the large array of sensors and the range of output effectors accessible to higher animals, evolving sensory-motor zombie agents to deal with all possible combinations of input-output arrangements for all possible behaviors is awkward. Far better to complement the army of rapid but limited sensory-motor agents with a somewhat slow, but flexible, strategy for summarizing what is out there and planning the future accordingly.

This account, however, is insufficient to explain why it should feel like anything to be conscious. One popular explanation is that these feelings, qualia, serve no useful purpose, that they are epiphenomenal. This appears questionable. Qualia are too structured to be an irrelevant byproduct of the brain. I favor the idea that qualia are closely tied up with meaning.

The NCC derive their meaning from their synaptic relationships with other groups of neurons that may or may not be active themselves. They encode the many concepts and experiences associated with any one conscious percept—its penumbra. Qualia are a potent symbolic representation of the vast storehouse of simultaneous information inherent in this meaning (a shorthand to codify all of these data). Qualia are a special property of massively parallel networks. This framework also explains why qualia are private and why their full content can't be communicated to others.

It follows from our executive summary hypothesis that the NCC must be intimately linked to the planning stages, located within the premotor, prefrontal, and anterior cingulate cortices. Francis and I therefore concluded that the NCC neurons must directly project into the front of the cortex. In the monkey, there are no direct connections from V1 to any frontal areas, so it seems reasonable to assert that the NCC can't be in V1 (as emphasized in Chapter 6).

Let me now return from the speculative realm to the more concrete. I will consider next the microstructure and dynamics of visual consciousness. Studying the evolution of an individual percept provides critical cues to the circuits that underlie consciousness.

CHAPTER FIFTEEN

On Time and Consciousness

"Well, then, what is time?" asked Hans Castorp, and bent the tip of his nose so far round that it became white and bloodless. "Can you answer me that? Space we perceive with our organs, with our senses of sight and touch. Good. But which is our organ of time—tell me that if you can. You see, that's where you stick. But how can we possibly measure anything about which we actually know nothing, not even a single one of its properties? We say of time that it passes. Very good, let it pass. But to be able to measure it—wait a minute: to be susceptible of being measured, time must flow evenly, but who ever said it did that? As far as our consciousness is concerned it doesn't, we only assume that it does, for the sake of convenience; and our units of measurement are purely arbitrary, sheer conventions—"

From *The Magic Mountain* by Thomas Mann

Only a dead brain is static, is quiet. A living brain is an astonishingly dynamic organ. Neurons discharge spontaneously (another way of saying that it is not clear why they fired at that point in time) in the absence of any obvious input. The EEG, too, reveals this dynamic character with unceasing episodes of more intense activity superimposed onto a highly fluctuating background that neuroscientists can't yet understand. All this vehement churning of chemical and electrical signals shows up at the phenomenological level, too. You know from introspection how difficult it is to focus your thoughts for long on any one topic. The content of your consciousness is shifting evermore: You look up from your computer to see the trees swaying outside, then hear the dogs bark, before you suddenly remember, unbidden, next week's project deadline. You need to make a concerted effort to concentrate on one thing.

With this in mind, let me address the dynamics of consciousness. A percept doesn't occur instantly. The brain processes that precede the NCC develop over an appreciable amount of time. How long does it take for a stimulus to be consciously perceived? How does this depend on the above-mentioned background processes? Does the underlying NCC arise gradually or abruptly? What happens if two images closely follow each other? How is it that the second one can erase the first one from sight? What does this reveal about the nature of the NCC? Does perception evolve continuously or in discrete intervals, like the frames in a movie? These topics are covered in this chapter.

15.1 │ HOW SWIFT IS VISION?

How long does it take to see something? One way to answer this is to measure *reaction times*: Flash a stimulus onto a screen and have subjects release a button as soon as they see it or as soon as they can reliably tell whether they saw a vertical or a horizontal bar. The trouble with such experiments is that the response times include not only the processing interval necessary to extract the relevant information from the retinal signals, but also the time it takes to generate the motor response and activate the fast twitch muscles of the fingers.

Simon Thorpe and his coworkers at the Centre de Recherche Cerveau et Cognition in Toulouse, France, measured visually evoked scalp potentials (Section 2.3) in a discrimination study. Subjects had to quickly decide whether or not an animal was present in colored photographs of natural environments (as in Figure 9.3) that were briefly flashed onto a monitor. This task was challenging, because subjects were given no *a priori* information about what animal to expect (e.g., a tiger in a jungle, parrots in a tree, or elephants in the savanna). As it turned out, people, whether trained or not, had no trouble with this task, with reaction times a tad faster than half a second.

The psychologists recorded the averaged evoked potential when pictures with animals were shown and compared it to the potential following animal-free images. The two wave-forms were indistinguishable in the first few moments after image onset, but started to diverge sharply after 150 msec. That is, some brain process encoded the answer ('animal' or 'no animal') at this remarkably early point in time.[1]

As the net-wave of light-induced activity leaves the retina, it reaches the magnocellular input layer of V1 (the coarse, fast pathway from the retina) within 35 msec. This leaves little more than 100 msec to activate the networks in and around the inferior temporal cortex (IT) and beyond, that have to extract one bit of information from each image (namely, "Is there an animal in

---

[1] The original study was described in Thorpe, Fize, and Marlot (1996). The median reaction time to release the button was 450 msec. Reaction times depend on the complexity of the sensory processing and on the type of motor response required (Luce, 1986) but can be as low as 350 msec (VanRullen and Thorpe, 2001). Control experiments proved that there was nothing special about animals, because detecting whether or not a vehicle was present in city or highway scenes took just as short a time.

this scene?"). With neuronal reaction times to synaptic input hovering around 5 to 10 msec, this does not leave time for many iterative computations.[2]

However, that the brain infers within 150 msec that an animal is present does not necessarily imply that this information is consciously accessible at this point in time. That may take much longer. Indeed, when the image is briefly flashed but is then immediately hidden from view by a second image, subjects detect the presence or absence of an animal only slightly less successfully (compared to the situation without the second, masking, image), even though often they are barely conscious of having seen anything, let alone an animal.[3] So, while this experiment shows that vision can act with great speed, it isn't immediately useful in timing the onset of the conscious percept.

15.2 | THE ALL-OR-NONE CHARACTER OF PERCEPTION

When lightning strikes during a thunderstorm, the world stands out in stark relief. Even though the electrical discharge is brief, enough photons reach the retina to provide a clear image. This and related experiences with flash bulbs demonstrate that we can perceive very brief events, even if the finite temporal dynamics of photoreceptors and neurons will smear out the brain's response to them.[4] What, however, is the time course of the percept itself? Does it gradually become more vivid until it peaks and then decays? Or, is the percept born fully formed, like Pallas Athena out of the head of Zeus, only to die equally abruptly? In either case, I expect its neuronal correlate to mirror the percept. So, if a feeling comes suddenly into being, the NCC should do likewise.

Talis Bachmann at the University of Estonia is a vigorous advocate of the *microgenetic* approach to consciousness.[5] It views the formation of any conscious percept as unfolding in time, similar to the process of developing a

---

[2]A remarkable difference between brains and computers is expressed by how long it takes an organism to achieve some task relative to the "switching speed" of the underlying processors (neurons versus transistors). This ratio is less than 100 when *you* recognize a face but is in the billions for a machine vision algorithm running on a state-of-the-art computer. The difference is a consequence of the massive parallel nature of brains (Koch, 1999).

[3]Subjects respond equally fast to images of simple geometric forms, whether or not they are aware of them. This shows that reaction times can be completely divorced from the time necessary to achieve consciousness (Taylor and McCloskey, 1990).

[4]*Bloch's law* states that for stimulus durations of less than a tenth of a second, perceived brightness depends on the product of the stimulus intensity and its duration. That is, the same brightness percept results if the stimulus is shown for half as long provided that the intensity of the stimulus is doubled.

[5]Bachmann (1994, 2000). Note that microgenetic here refers to the fine-grained temporal analysis of the origin (*genesis*) of perception rather than to any genetic, inheritable process. I warmly recommend Bachmann's (2000) book for its lucid, candid, and quite funny precis of the most popular psychological and biological theories of consciousness.

photograph. A multitude of distinct cognitive events are involved, all of which have their own temporal dynamics, culminating in the establishment of a percept. Arising within experimental psychology, the microgenetic paradigm maps quite naturally onto the multitude of distinct neurobiological mechanisms in the brain.

The earliest experiments to study the time course of perception date to the 19th century. A projector called a tachistoscope displayed images for short

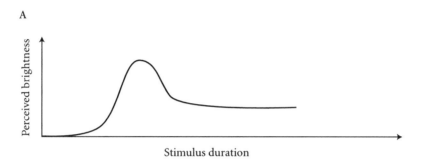

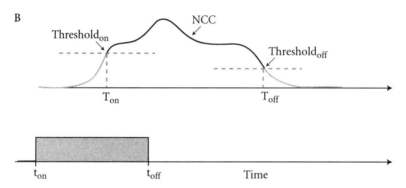

FIGURE 15.1 *Perceiving a Flash of Light* **A:** The perceived brightness of a flash of light of variable duration compared to the brightness of a constant reference light. For short presentation times, the perceived brightness is higher than for longer lasting stimuli. This curve does *not* imply that the time course of any one percept waxes and wanes. **B:** Hypothetical time course of the "critical" activity at the essential node for the brightness percept for a fixed stimulus duration, $t_{off} - t_{on}$. Once this exceeds Threshold$_{on}$, the neural activity is sustained enough to project widely throughout the cortex and the subject becomes conscious of the brightness. Awareness is expressed until the NCC drop below Threshold$_{off}$. Note that the entire curve in B corresponds to a single point in A.

times. The subject compared her sensation for the brightness of a flash of light of variable duration to the brightness of a steady light of the same luminosity. The resultant curve (Figure 15.1A) has been interpreted to mean that the observer fleetingly experienced a gradual increase in the sensation of brightness, rising from some baseline to a peak and then settling down to some equilibrium level for long-lasting stimuli.

The neuropsychologist Robert Efron, at the Veterans Hospital in Martinez, California, has pointed out that this is a common fallacy. Figure 15.1A does not illustrate the evolution of a percept in time, but rather graphs how brightness is experienced for flashes of different durations: A short flash is seen as dimmer than a longer one of the same intensity which, in turn, is seen as brighter than a steady light.[6] There is no evidence that the brightness of a flash of constant intensity is perceived as waxing and waning. This agrees with everyday experience when you see a light turn on and off abruptly.

On page 256, one of Efron's experiments is discussed in which a 10 msec flash of red is immediately followed by a 10 msec flash of green. Subjects never report that the red light changes into a green one, but see a constant yellowish light instead.

These observations are compatible with the idea that the NCC come into being abruptly, rather than gradually. Figure 15.1B illustrates the hypothetical events occurring at an essential node for brightness, probably somewhere in the extrastriate cortex. The critical activity, for instance, synchronized firing, builds up until it reaches some sort of threshold. At this point, possibly manifested by a rapid volley of spikes, the activity has sufficient strength to activate a coalition of neurons in distant regions of the visual hierarchy, including earlier areas and areas in the front of the cortex. This distributed activity in turn feeds back, amplifying local happenings until a stable equilibrium is reached. At that point, the explicit brightness information becomes widely available. The subject sees the light. Its perceived brightness depends on the details of the population code laid down across the neurons that make up the NCC.[7]

The percept is extinguished by a variety of means; the eyes may move, the input may disappear, and the synaptic and neuronal responses may adapt and become progressively smaller. Competition with other incipient percepts also helps quench the NCC, as the brain must exercise delicate control to prevent

---

[6]Broca and Sulzer (1902). For a thorough airing of the literature pertaining to the temporal evolution of sensation, see Efron (1967) and Bachmann (2000).

[7]Close inspection of the schematized NCC curve in Figure 15.1B reveals subtle temporal changes in the supra-threshold activity. Such changes might well be picked up by a post-synaptic readout mechanism and thereby might ultimately affect behavior. If the mechanism underlying the NCC is insensitive to the temporal gyrations in the firing activities at the essential node, however, the subject will continue to experience a constant percept.

one coalition from dominating too long.[8] Some direct or indirect remnants of the previous NCC activity, like glowing embers, remain for some time. Often, these vestiges can be detected by sensitive behavioral techniques such as priming (Section 11.3).

Measuring the confidence of a perceptual judgment is one way to assess the degree of consciousness.[9] Take the subject from the previous brightness experiment who pushes a button whenever she sees the light. You now ask her to rate how confident she is by assigning a number between 0 and 9 to her decision. If she is sure of her judgment, she should give an 8 or 9; if she is guessing, a 0 or 1 is appropriate. Intermediate numbers are reserved for intermediate degrees of confidence. All trials are finally sorted by confidence level. If performance on the task is plotted as a function of confidence, a rising curve is typically obtained: When guessing, performance is worse than when the subject is sure of her judgment. The more confident she is that on *this* one trial she saw the light, the more likely she is to be actually right. How does this continuous relationship square with the all-or-none stance I advocate?

Two things are going on here. Due to uncontrolled fluctuations in the person's attentional state and background brain processes, the threshold for seeing the light is exceeded on some trials but not on others. She either *sees* a light or doesn't. Her *confidence* is derived from a different aspect of the NCC, such as the lifetime of the associated coalition. The longer the coalition at the essential node stays above the threshold on any one trial, the easier it is to infer that the light did turn on. I make the idealized assumption that the probability for exceeding the threshold does not depend on the lifetime of the coalition. Both are independent, stochastic processes (in practice, they will be correlated to some extent). So, even if the threshold at the essential node for brightness is exceeded, other factors conspire to make the NCC duration shorter or longer (for instance, whether a light was seen on the last trial, whether the subject was

---

[8] A few technical digressions: Due to a phenomenon physicists refer to as *hysteresis*, the threshold for extinction is probably lower than the threshold for genesis (as in Figure 15.1B). Hysteresis alludes to the history-dependence of a system. When an input is increased, the firing activity increases steadily until it reaches a threshold, when it suddenly jumps to a much higher level. When the input is now decreased again, the jump back to the smaller level of activity does not take place until a much lower value of the input. Both on and off thresholds in Figure 15.1B are probably dynamic ones, susceptible to recalibration. Once the on threshold for sufficiency of a conscious percept is exceeded—a neuronal event that may be marked by a burst of spikes—it may take some minimal time for the neuronal assembly to dip below the off threshold. That is, the NCC may have a lower bound on its lifetime. Indeed, psychologists have claimed the existence of a *minimal perceptual moment* (e.g., Efron, 1970b, 1973a). From a mathematical point of view, the all-or-none character of perception may not be caused by a true threshold but may reflect a steep and self-amplifying portion of the response curve.

[9] See Kolb and Braun (1995) or Kunimoto, Miller, and Pashler (2001).

thinking of her boyfriend, or whether her eyes jittered). Under these conditions, a smoothly increasing relationship between confidence and performance would be expected. In cases of fleeting awareness, the threshold may only be exceeded so briefly that the subject is essentially guessing.

So far, I have only considered a percept with one attribute, brightness. Objects in the real world, however, have many attributes. A face is characterized by a location, an identity and a gender, hair, the hue of its skin, the angle of gaze of its eyes, imperfections such as scars or acne, and so on. These aspects are represented in an explicit manner at the associated essential nodes. Does the activity in these different loci have to cross threshold at the same time? This would demand some sort of tight synchronization, a requirement I discussed as part of the binding problem in Section 9.4. But what if no such synchronization existed? If the NCC activities at the different essential nodes came into being at different times, shouldn't the associated properties be perceived at different times?

Quite possibly! Consider the following remarkable observations by Semir Zeki, the intrepid explorer of the extrastriate cortex first encountered in Chapter 2. Zeki and his students carefully assessed the extent to which different attributes of a changing display are perceived simultaneously. They found that the perception of a change in color *preceded* the perception of a change in motion by about 75 msec. This is surprising, particularly because magnocellular neurons mediating motion respond more rapidly than neurons in the parvocellular pathway carrying wavelength information (Table 3.1).[10]

These findings prompted Zeki to conclude that the vaunted unity of awareness, emphasized by mystics and philosophers alike, may be illusory (at least for these short times). Perception, or a change in perception, may be asynchronous, with different regions generating microconsciousness for color, motion, form, and so on at different times.

Shouldn't such a glaring discrepancy—lasting on the order of a couple of movie frames—be noticeable? If I look at a speeding car, its motion doesn't appear to lag behind its color. Perhaps the question should be, "How could the brain notice such an asynchrony?" It couldn't, unless it had some mechanism that detected differences in the onset, offset, or duration of the NCC at different nodes and represented these differences explicitly at some other node. Without

---

[10]See Moutoussis and Zeki (1997a, b) and Zeki and Moutoussis (1997). Similar results have been reported by Arnold, Clifford, and Wenderoth (2001). The consequences for asynchronous perception are discussed by Zeki (1998) and Zeki and Bartels (1999). The generality of these findings has been called into question (Nishida and Johnston, 2002). When interpreting these data, one must be careful in exactly what is being compared. Asking subjects to judge whether changes in color occur at the same time as changes in the direction of motion is different from asking them whether one particular color is always paired with one particular motion. The discussion in Dennett and Kinsbourne (1992) is germane here.

such processes, the car and all its attributes will be experienced as occurring at the same time.

15.3 | MASKING WIPES A STIMULUS FROM CONSCIOUSNESS

So far, I've considered neural events in response to a single stimulus. What happens when one input rapidly succeeds another one? In discussing the effects of selective attention in Chapter 9, I took pains to emphasize that stimuli compete with each other when their associated activities overlap in the brain. It should not surprise you then to learn that the second image can profoundly alter the way the first one is seen. If both are briefly presented in close temporal and spatial proximity to each other, strange things can happen; distances can shrink, objects can appear distorted, or can disappear entirely. You've entered a *Twilight Zone*, where commonsense notions of space, time, and causality are violated in the privacy of your head.

For Short Presentation Times, Two Stimuli Blend into One

In one of Efron's experiments, a small red disk, shown for 10 msec on a monitor, was immediately followed by a green disk at the same location, also for 10 msec. Instead of seeing a red light turn into a green one, subjects saw a single yellow flash. Similarly, if a 20 msec blue light was followed by a 20 msec yellow light, a white flash was perceived, but never a sequence of two lights whose color changed.[11] These experiments demonstrate the existence of an *integration period*. Stimuli falling within the duration of this period are blended into a unitary, constant percept.

The extent of the integration period depends on stimulus intensity, saliency, and other parameters. How long the period lasts is unclear. If a 500 msec green light is followed by a 500 msec red one, subjects see a green light changing to red.[12] The critical duration is probably less than a quarter of a second.[13]

---

[11] Efron (1973b); Yund, Morgan, and Efron (1983); see also Herzog et al. (2003).

[12] The stimulus duration at which the temporal modulation disappears is proportional to the inverse of the *chromatic flicker fusion frequency*. This frequency is measured by continuously modulating the color of some stationary pattern in time. While the individual colors can be clearly made out when they change back and forth slowly, at some alternation rate they blur and only a single, hybrid, color is perceived (Gur and Snodderly, 1997; and Gowdy, Stromeyer, and Kronauer, 1999). In the auditory domain, distinguishing successive speech sounds (phonemes) forms the building blocks of language processing. Babies or children with language learning and literacy impairments, as in dyslexia, have grave difficulties in distinguishing and discriminating brief, successive auditory stimuli (Tallal et al., 1998; and Nagarajan et al., 1999). It may be possible that these individuals have generalized deficits in processing rapid signals.

[13] Blending doesn't always occur. In *feature inheritance*, the perceived object inherits features of a perceptually invisible earlier image (Herzog and Koch, 2001).

The Temporal Order of the Two Events Is Not Lost

This is not to say that the brain has no means of distinguishing these two brief sequences. A red-green flash has more of a greenish hue than a green-red flash. The brain can also distinguish which of two adjacent spots of light occurs earlier; when one flash is followed 5 msec later by a second flash of light at a neighboring location, you see the spot move from the first to the second location. When the temporal order is inverted, the sense of motion reverses, too.[14]

The auditory system does even better. If a click is delivered, via earphones, to the left ear and, a few hundred *microseconds* later, a second click is given to the right ear, you hear a single tone, originating somewhere inside the skull, toward the left ear. When the second click comes before the first click, the perceived source of the tone shifts toward the right.

In all three cases, the temporal order of events is transformed into a perceptual dimension. The seemingly paradoxical coexistence of such sensitive *order discrimination thresholds* with integration periods in the 100 msec range can be reconciled by postulating distinct mechanisms that underlie these different tasks. The moral is that many jobs, no matter how menial, are carried out by distinct neuronal processes. Each is limited in its domain and often does only one job, and not, as might be expected, two superficially similar jobs.

Masking Can Hide a Stimulus

Masking is a popular tool to probe perception (see Sections 6.2 and 11.3). It refers to the ability of one stimulus, the *mask*, to interfere with the processing of a second one, the *target*. Masking reveals that the kinship between events in the physical world and the way they are perceived can depart quite radically from naive realism, making it a rich medium for exploring the nature of consciousness.[15] The most common form is *backward masking*, in which the target is *followed* by the mask. The mask's action can be so powerful that the first image is totally hidden, is never seen. In *forward masking*, the reverse occurs and the target is preceded by the mask.

The French cognitive psychologist Stanislas Dehaene and his colleagues in Paris used masking to compare the effects of visible and invisible words on the brain. Volunteers lay inside a magnetic scanner while being bombarded by a stream of images that included slides with simple words, each one illuminated for 29 msec. Under one condition (Figure 15.2, left), the words were clearly

---

[14]Westheimer and McKee (1977) and Fahle (1993).

[15]Psychologists distinguish three main forms, *backward*, *forward*, and *metacontrast masking* (Breitmeyer, 1984; Bachmann, 1994 and 2000; Breitmeyer and Ögmen, 2000; and Enns and DiLollo, 2000). Philosophers (Dennett, 1991, and Flanagan, 1992) have explored the implications of masking for theories of the mind. In none of these cases is the stimulus ever physically obscured by the mask.

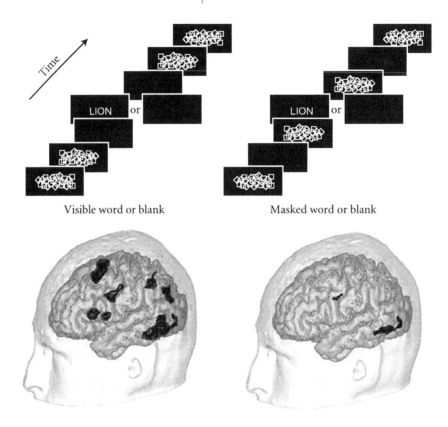

Visible word or blank   Masked word or blank

FIGURE 15.2 *The Effect of Visual Masking* The brain's response to seen and unseen words. Volunteers looked at a stream of images, with each word shown for 29 msec (all other frames were displayed for 71 msec). In one condition (right side), no words were seen, since each one was preceded and followed by a slide covered by random symbols, perceptually obscuring the letters. When these masks were removed (left side), subjects saw the words. Their brains were much more active, as measured with magnetic resonance imaging (the activity following the image sequence with words was compared to the sequences with blanks). Both seen and masked words activated regions in the left ventral pathway, but with vastly different amplitude. Conscious perception triggered additional widespread activation in the left parietal and prefrontal cortices. Modified from Dehaene et al. (2001).

legible. When each word slide was preceded and followed by a mask (a random jumble of letters and symbols), subjects didn't see any words (Figure 15.2, right).

Consider the striking difference in hemodynamic activity.[16] While the nonconscious stimulus did kindle some response in the left fusiform gyrus (part of

---

[16]Dehaene et al. (2001). Responses were sparse in the right hemisphere, compatible with hemispheric specialization for language.

the ventral stream), response magnitude was much larger when the words were consciously perceived. Word perception also evoked additional and widespread multi-focal activity in a plethora of left parietal and prefrontal regions.

Masking can be explained in terms of competition among stimuli that activate overlapping networks of neurons. Masking prevents the stimulus-triggered net-wave from penetrating as deeply into the cortex as would the net-wave of an unmasked stimulus.[17]

What is thought-provoking about backward masking is that one input can influence the percept triggered by an earlier one. How can this happen? How can the mask activity interfere with the NCC for a target that's always 29 msec ahead? In a network without any feedback connections, isn't the net-wave triggered by the mask forever chasing the target-induced net-wave? If the NCC relied on cortico-cortical or cortico-thalamic feedback loops, however, later input could affect processing of an earlier stimulus. How much this influence extended back into time would depend on the delay in this loop.

Behaviorally, the interval during which masking is effective can be extended up to 100 msec. That is, a mask that is not flashed onto the screen until a tenth of a second *after* the target first appeared can still impact target perception.

Backward masking might prevent the formation of a percept but may not eliminate subliminal processing, as when the subject feels she is guessing but still performs better than chance in detecting the light. Unconscious processing in masked trials probably relies primarily on feedforward activity.[18]

The *flash-lag illusion* provides further fodder for the hypothesis that awareness requires additional time, indicative of feedback circuits. A line or a spot of light, flashed at the instant another continuously moving line or spot arrives at the same location, appears to lag behind the moving object. That is, even though both objects are at the same position at the same time, the moving stimulus looks to be ahead of the flashed one. This effect has been interpreted to imply that awareness doesn't commit itself to a percept until about 80 msec (or later) after the event has occurred.[19]

---

[17]The neuronal correlates of masking in the monkey cortex are explored by Rolls and Tovee (1994); Macknik and Livingstone (1998); Thompson and Schall (1999); Macknik, Martinez-Conde, and Haglund (2000); and Keysers and Perrett (2002). Thompson and Schall (2000) use masking to characterize the NCC in frontal eye field neurons. Masking probably selectively interferes with either the leading or the trailing components of the stimulus-induced neuronal activity, signalling the onset and disappearance of the stimulus.

[18]This has been made plausible by VanRullen and Koch (2003b) for those trials in which masked—and perceptually invisible—images of letters are rapidly and correctly detected.

[19]The flash lag effect, first described by Gestalt psychologists, was re-discovered by Nijhawan (1994, 1997). The modern exploration of this illusion has turned into a gold mine of experimental insights (Sheth, Nijhawan, and Shimojo, 2000; Eagleman and Sejnowski, 2000; Krekelberg and Lappe, 2001; and Schlag and Schlag-Rey, 2002).

It Takes at Least a Quarter of a Second to See Something

Adding this 100-msec interval inferred from backward masking to the 150 msec necessary for the net-wave to propagate from the retina to higher visual regions in the ventral pathway (Section 15.1) yields an estimate of about a quarter of a second as the minimal time needed to *see* something.

Within the framework of Figure 15.1B, 250 msec is the interval between stimulus onset and the establishment of the associated NCC, $T_{on} - t_{on}$. Depending on stimulus properties, what was seen in the recent past, and depending on fluctuations in the activity in the cortex, this time can be longer, but probably not shorter.[20] Perception always trails reality by a fair bit, and events on the ground can change so rapidly that the NCC can't quite keep up, explaining many otherwise puzzling perceptual phenomena. Zombie agents, on the other hand, can act with more celerity.

Looking on the bright side, the integration period may permit the NCC to be based on more than just the immediate input. The additional processing time might serve to recall explicit memories or items circulating in the short-term buffer and incorporate them into the final percept. Or, if additional sensory information arriving within the past 100 msec contradicts the original information, a new, blended percept is created. When events are changing rapidly, it may be best to wait a while to find out how the situation develops before committing to one particular interpretation of what is out there.

Forward versus Feedback Activity

Backward masking reinforces the idea that nonconscious processing may be based on transient, forward activity, too ephemeral to engage the planning modules. This processing mode might mediate zombie behaviors without awareness. In contrast, conscious processing must involve feedback from the front of the cortex to the back.[21]

Consider a baseball player, waiting to strike the approaching ball. Its looming silhouette triggers a net-wave moving up the visual hierarchy, to V1, MT, and beyond. Somewhere along the line, a decision is made—to swing or not to swing the bat—and communicated to layer 5 pyramidal neurons that project

---

[20]This is not to say that the duration of the percept ($T_{off} - T_{on}$) is identical to the duration of the stimulus ($t_{off} - t_{on}$).

[21]This theme has been forcefully advocated by Cauller and Kulics (1991); Lamme and Roelfsema (2000); DiLollo, Enns, and Rensink (2000); Bullier (2001); Supèr, Spekreijse, and Lamme (2001); and Pollen (2003). None of this is to argue that any sort of feedback activity will, by itself, guarantee consciousness. If the Milner and Goodale two-visual-streams hypothesis is true (Section 12.2), it raises the question of why feedback in the dorsal pathway is insufficient to give rise to the NCC.

down to the basal ganglia, spinal cord, and the appropriate muscles. All of this happens without involving awareness. The batter's zombie acts faster than his conscious perception (Section 12.3).

He won't see the approaching ball until neurons in the front of his cortex with access to working memory and planning receive the visual information and, in turn, feed back onto cells in the upper parts of the visual hierarchy. These spikes reinforce the activity at the essential nodes in the back, which further strengthens frontal activity. This self-amplifying feedback loop may act so rapidly that it behaves to all intents and purposes like a threshold. Through its actions, it assembles and stabilizes a far-flung (as in Figure 15.2) quasi-stable coalition in posterior parietal, medial temporal, anterior cingulate, prefrontal, and premotor cortices. This coalition is *experienced* as a rapidly looming ball.[22] If you're a physicist, it might be helpful to think of this reverberatory activity as a standing wave in a nonlinear medium.[23]

Intermediate situations exist, too. While the batter is focusing on the pitcher, waiting for him to throw the ball, teammates and spectators in the background move about. These constantly changing images lead to the formation of very transient assemblies in V4, IT, and elsewhere (the proto-objects mentioned in Chapter 9). Unless the strength of these coalitions is boosted by attending to them, their activity quickly decays and new coalitions arise in their place. So, at best, the batter will only experience a fleeting level of awareness for the background events.

How can these ideas be evaluated? Cortico-cortical and cortico-thalamic feedback is excitatory, using glutamate as the neurotransmitter. It is almost certain that the synaptic *feedback* traffic involves different glutamate subtypes than the *forward* projections. Or that different proteins are associated with the synapses of these distinct pathways. Laboratories throughout the world are busy targeting such proteins for molecular interventions that would interfere with the function of one specific subtype of the glutamate receptor. Mice or monkeys could then be genetically engineered so that feedback connections could be briefly silenced, rendered inoperable, without affecting forward or sideways connections. Such zombie animals might still perform learned or instinctual behaviors, but not those requiring consciousness.

---

[22]The biophysical substrate of such facilitatory feedback interactions may be found in the apical tuft, the topmost portion of the dendritic tree of tall, layer 5, neocortical pyramidal neurons. Their strategic location—right in the termination zone of cortico-cortical feedback—and the complement of voltage-dependent currents found there, renders them highly susceptible to coincident synaptic input, more so than at the cell body (Williams and Stuart, 2002, 2003; see also Rhodes and Llinás, 2001). In other words, such a pyramidal neuron located somewhere in the visual cortex, will respond to synchronized input from several locations in the front of the cortex by generating a volley of spikes.

[23]Grossberg (1999) argues explicitly for such an analogy.

15.4 | INTEGRATION AND DIRECT BRAIN STIMULATION

Speculations about the existence of both a threshold and an integration period for perception are supported by neurosurgical experiments. In the 1960s, the neuropsychologist Benjamin Libet at the University of California School of Medicine in San Francisco carried out a research program on the timing of conscious experience.[24]

The setting was open-skull surgery in patients who suffered from Parkinson's disease or intractable pain. For clinical reasons, the neurosurgeon probed the exposed surface of the somatosensory and related cortices with an electrode that sent pulses of current into the underlying gray matter. Libet recorded the minimal current intensity, I_{min}, below which no sensation or feeling was produced, no matter how long the electrical stimulus was applied. The nature of the sensations, as reported spontaneously by the patients, varied with the site of the electrode and included tingling, pins and needles, prickling, vibrations, feelings of warmth and cold, touch, movement, and pressure.

Libet placed great emphasis on the all-or-nothing attribute of conscious perception: "A sensory experience either appeared after a sufficiently long activation even if very weak, or it was not present at all with a briefer activation."[25] Furthermore, Libet discovered that to obtain a minimal sensation, the amplitude of the current had to vary inversely with its duration (Figure 15.3). Thus, low intensity stimuli required longer stimulation times than bigger ones.

Libet used these observations as the cornerstone for his *time-on* theory. According to him, the transition from a nonconscious to a conscious event requires a sufficient increase in the duration of appropriate neuronal activities. When these persist for longer than a minimum time, they become sufficient for awareness.

When considering the curves in Figure 15.3, Francis and I hypothesized that they could be well fitted by a simple mathematical model that assumes that the electrical current causes some substance to accumulate until a threshold is reached and the NCC are born. The higher the current amplitude, the sooner this value is reached and the sooner the patient feels something.[26]

---

[24]Libet (1966, 1973, and 1993). Ongoing experiments have refined and extended Libet's observations (Ray et al., 1999; and Meador et al., 2000).

[25]Libet (1993).

[26]The model we had in mind was the *leaky integrate-and-fire* process (Koch, 1999). Think of a sustained current charging up a capacitance, building up the voltage across it. This increase is counteracted by current leaking away through a resistance, causing the potential to exponentially decay without any input. Once the voltage across the capacitance reaches a threshold, some action is triggered, the voltage is reset, and the process begins anew. If the amplitude of the current flowing onto the capacitance is small, the threshold is reached later; if the current is large, the threshold is reached sooner. For some minimal value of the input, the build-up of the voltage exactly matches the decay, so the threshold is never reached. With a time constant of around

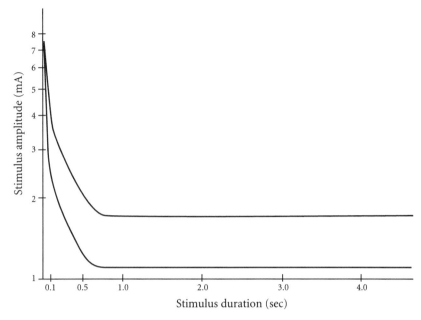

FIGURE 15.3 *Electrical Stimulation of the Somatosensory Cortex* Libet directly stimulated the exposed cortex of neurosurgery patients. The minimal stimulus amplitude necessary for his subjects to feel anything (usually a tingling, a touch, or a vibration) is plotted as a function of how long the current injection lasted (the electrode used to obtain the bottom curve had twice the pulse rate of the electrode in the top curve). The lower the intensity, the longer the artificial stimulus had to be applied to give rise to some sensation. Modified from Libet (1966).

The mechanistic implications of this fit are provocative. The stimulus electrode, lying on top of layer 1, excites many underlying neurons. Due to the indiscriminate nature of this artificial situation, both excitatory and inhibitory neurons discharge and their mutual effect is minor (because they partially cancel each other). As this occurs, adaptation builds up in the cells below the electrode. That is, the firing rates of these cells slowly decay—due, for instance, to an influx of calcium ions into their cell bodies. If the firing rate of inhibitory cells decreases more rapidly than that of excitatory ones, then inhibition might, at some point, cease to adequately keep excitation in check. When this occurs, excitation rapidly exceeds normal bounds and gives rise to an anomalous event

250 msec, the behavior of this model closely follows the curves in Figure 15.3. A stimulation study with intracranial electrodes implanted into the cortex in young epileptic patients bears out one prediction of this simple exercise—namely, even very brief pulses can trigger phenomenal sensations (Ray et al., 1999).

that the patient experiences. It is as if the surgeon's electrode caused a "micro-seizure" that triggered the NCC. Whether this process remains confined to a local neighborhood or whether it engages distributed activity at distal sites is unclear.

15.5 | IS PERCEPTION DISCRETE OR CONTINUOUS?

The implicit assumption up to this point has been that you and I experience the world in a continuous fashion; that the seamless nature of perceptual experience is reflected in the smooth waxing and waning of the NCC; that as the world changes, the NCC change likewise (within the limits imposed by the smearing out of fast signals).

This is not, however, the only possibility. Perception might well take place in discrete processing epochs, *perceptual moments*, *frames*, or *snapshots*. Your subjective life could be a ceaseless sequence of such frames, never ending, until the moment you fall into a deep sleep.[27]

Within one such moment, the perception of brightness, color, depth, and motion would be constant. Think of motion painted onto each snapshot (Figure 15.4). Motion is not experienced because of a change in position between two consecutive snapshots, as in the movies or by the motion-blind patient L.M. (Section 8.3), but is represented within a single snapshot.

If a new input arrives, say because the eyes just moved, it triggers a net-wave whose spikes are superimposed onto the ongoing background processes in the brain. Activity at the essential node for some attribute would build up until a dominant coalition established itself and the NCC came into being. If the subject continued to attend to the stimulus, the dynamics of the system would have to be such that with some degree of regularity the NCC turn off and on again, constant within one perceptual moment but changing from one to the next before reaching a new quasi steady-state. Since the majority of neuronal processes would evolve in a more continuous manner, such on-and-off processing would be a tell-tale sign of the NCC.

Plenty of psychological data favors discrete perception, with the duration of each snapshot being quite variable, lasting anywhere between 20 and 200 msec. Whether this large variability (a factor of ten) reflects the inadequate nature of the tools used to probe the brain, a plurality of quantized processes with a spectrum of processing periods, a single process with a very flexible integration interval, or something else, is not clear. The most compelling hints are

---

[27]This is an old idea that has been around, in one guise or another, since at least the 19th century (Stroud, 1956; White, 1963; Harter, 1967; Pöppel, 1978; and Geissler, Schebera, and Kompass, 1999).

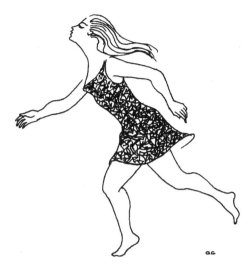

FIGURE 15.4 *Discrete Perception of Motion* The snapshot hypothesis proposes that the conscious perception of motion is represented by the (near) constant activity of some NCC at the essential nodes for motion. The figure, drawn by Odile Crick, provides a helpful analogy. It shows how a static picture can suggest motion, similar to a Frank Gehry building.

periodicities in reaction times[28] and an astounding motion illusion in which regularly spaced objects are, on occasion, seen to move opposite to the direction of physical motion.[29]

A key property of discrete processing periods is that events that fall within one bin would be treated as simultaneous. If two events occurred in two consecutive frames, they would be experienced as taking place one after the other. There have been some ingenious tests of this hypothesis using two flashes of light that on some trials are seen as one, and on others as two consecutive flashes.[30] The minimal interstimulus interval for which two successive events

---

[28]Venables (1960); White and Harter (1969); Pöppel and Logothetis (1986); and Dehaene (1993). VanRullen and Koch (2003c) survey and summarize the relevant findings.

[29]This variant of the *wagon wheel illusion* is seen under steady light (Purves, Paydarfar, and Andrews, 1996). It is only seen intermittently and is different from the usual wagon wheel effect, which is caused by the inherent temporal quantization of television and movies.

[30]For some particular value of the interstimulus interval between the two lights, flashed one after the other, the subject is as likely to *see* a single light as two consecutive ones (Wertheimer, 1912). The proposal by Gho and Varela (1988) that the determining factor is the phase of the alpha rhythm relative to the onset of the two flashes could not be experimentally verified by either Rufin VanRullen or David Eagleman (personal communication) in independent experiments.

were consistently perceived as simultaneous varied between 20 and 120 msec.[31] As discussed above, these long times are compatible with the existence of specialized circuits that can resolve tiny temporal differences.

Perceptual moments have often been linked to brain waves in the α (8 to 12 Hz) range, whose rhythm is supposed to underlie discrete temporal processing. Furthermore, the phase of the α wave is thought to be reset by an external input triggering the onset of a new integration period.[32]

After Francis and I published these observations, we received an amazing account from the neurologist Oliver Sacks concerning what he labels *cinematographic vision*. This rare neurological disturbance can manifest itself during visual migraine. Sacks has experienced such an attack firsthand. I can do no better than quote from his evocative depiction:

> I asked her to look at the picture, talk, gesture, make faces, anything, so long as she moved. And now, to my mixed delight and disquiet, I realized that time was fractured, no less than space, for I did not see her movements as continuous, but, instead as a succession of "stills," a succession of different configurations and positions, but without any movement in-between, like the flickering of a film (the "flicks") run too slow. She seemed to be transfixed in this odd mosaic-cinematic state, which was essentially shattered, incoherent, atomized.

Presciently, Sacks had ventured, "The term cinematographic vision denotes the nature of visual experience when the illusion of motion has been lost." Similar time-garbled episodes, radical departures from the continuously flowing physicist's time, can occur under other pathological conditions. Patients compare these to films run too slowly.[33] The migraine may have temporarily inactivated the cortical motion areas, thereby depriving Sacks and his patients of the illusion of motion. What remains are temporally shattered percepts. It would be exciting if such a state could be reversibly induced in volunteers with the help of TMS or some other harmless technique.

---

[31] Kristofferson (1967); Hirsh and Sherrick (1961); Lichtenstein (1961); White and Harter (1969); and Efron (1970a).

[32] Modern signal analysis methods permitted Makeig et al. (2002; see also Varela et al., 2001) to analyze conventional EEG data on a trial-per-trial basis. This analysis revealed a stimulus-induced phase-resetting of the α rhythm. On the basis of local intracranial electrode recordings in patients, Rizzuto et al. (2003) concluded likewise that the phase of oscillations in the 7–16 Hz range were shifted or reset following randomly timed stimuli. See Sanford (1971) for a review of the older literature.

[33] The offset quote is from Sacks (1984). Flickering in these migraines occurs at a rate of 6 to 12 per second. The quote in the text comes from Sacks (1970). See also the case history of H.Y., a post-encephalitic patient, in *Awakenings* (Sacks, 1973).

If conscious perception takes place in discrete moments, then perception of the *passage of time* may well relate to the rate at which snapshots occur. If the duration of individual moments becomes longer, there will be fewer of them in one second. Therefore, a given external event will appear to last a shorter time; time has sped up. Conversely, if the duration of a snapshot becomes shorter, more of them will occur per unit time and the same one-second interval will now be subdivided into more snapshots and will feel like it has passed much more slowly.[34]

This last phenomenon is known as *protracted duration* and is frequently commented upon in the context of accidents, natural catastrophes, and other violent events in which time appears to slow down considerably. Phrases such as "when I fell, I saw my life flash before me," or "it took him ages to lift the gun and aim at me" are commonly used. Indeed, it is now conventional for movies to portray such scenes through slow-motion cinematography; they use more frames for some events, such as bullets dropping from a gun chamber, reflecting first-person experience than for the rest of the film. Does protracted, top-down attention, as would occur in these situations, reduce the duration of individual snapshots?[35]

How does the temporal relationship between stimulus onset and the phase of the snapshot influence processing? If they occur randomly with respect to each other, it might explain the ever-present variability in reaction times. If the input is timed to arrive at the same moment relative to the onset of a snapshot, might this jitter be reduced?[36] Can periodic sounds or lights entrain the perceptual moments?[37]

If quantized processing is limited to a minority of neurons involved with the NCC, it will be difficult to detect with EEG, MEG, or fMRI techniques, all of which rely on bulk tissue measurements. Even microelectrodes that record multiple neurons won't pick up such quantized processing unless they are properly targeted at the relevant coalitions and not just blindly inserted into

---

[34]A numerical example may be helpful. Say that the duration of a frame is normally about 100 msec and the passage of 10 frames is experienced as one second. If the frame duration increases to 200 msec, then 1 second in real, physical time, amounting to 5 frames, will be experienced as half a second. Perceived duration is halved; time speeds up. Conversely, if the frame interval shrinks to 50 msec, 20 frames occur in the same second, which is now experienced as two seconds; time slows down.

[35]There is an extensive literature on the phenomenology of perceived time (Dennett and Kinsbourne, 1992; Pastor and Artieda, 1996; and Pöppel, 1978, 1997). Of most relevance to the present purpose is the monograph by Flaherty (1999).

[36]Fries et al. (2001a) characterized spontaneous but coherent fluctuations in spiking activity among adjacent cells in the visual cortex that might influence task performance.

[37]Burle and Bonnet (1997, 1999) reported that visual reaction times could be paced by a series of irrelevant audible clicks.

the tissue. What is needed are reliable optical or electrical means to identify and simultaneously record from hundreds or more of cortical and thalamic neurons throughout the brain to characterize any periodic firing patters.

15.6 | RECAPITULATION

The visual brain is fast. It can distinguish animal pictures from nonanimal ones in 150 msec and act on this information within less than half a second. It takes longer to consciously see the animal—probably at least 250 msec.

Conscious perception is likely all-or-none. This implies that the NCC at any one location come into being abruptly, by exceeding some sort of threshold.

Brief stimuli are not perceived as evolving in time. When two short events follow each other, the brain melds them into a single, constant percept. In backward masking, one image can completely interfere with a previous one, preventing it from being seen. This can most easily be explained by postulating that some critical activity at an essential node exceeds a threshold—and thereby becomes sufficient for a conscious percept—only with help from feedback from the front of the brain. The additional processing time, about 100 msec, implies that perception is revisionist, trailing reality.

These two vital clues about the NCC, that their genesis require *feedback activity* to exceed a *threshold*, were reinforced by Libet's brain stimulation experiments.

I discussed the tantalizing possibility that perception, and the NCC do not evolve continuously, as the world does, but discontinuously. Any perceptual attribute is constant within one processing period, one snapshot. What you experience at any given point in time is static (with motion "painted" onto the snapshot), even if the stimulus is changing. Some data from the psychological, clinical, and EEG literature argues in favor of this supposition. It would also help to answer some puzzling observations concerning the perceived passage of time.

Let me now come to the experiments at the heart of the inchoate science of consciousness. These help to pinpoint the NCC neurons for object perception in the inferior temporal cortex and beyond.

CHAPTER SIXTEEN

When the Mind Flips: Following the Footprints of Consciousness

A single thought is enough to occupy us:
We cannot think of two things at once.

From *Pensées* by Blaise Pascal

Let me come to the most direct means of localizing the neuronal correlates of consciousness, the NCC. Given the nature of the organ that generates consciousness, research aimed at demystifying this enigma must query the relevant microscopic variables—the spiking responses of individual neurons. Center stage are physiological and psychophysical experiments in which the relationship between what's in the world and what's in the mind is not one-to-one but one-to-many. For lack of a better term, I call these phenomena *perceptual stimuli*.

The hallmark of a perceptual stimulus is that one and the same input can be associated with different phenomenal states. Which state is experienced depends on many factors, such as any previous exposure to this stimulus, the attentional state of the subject, or fluctuations in various brain variables.

Consider the twelve lines making up the *Necker cube* (Figure 16.1). Due to the inherent ambiguity of inferring its three-dimensional shape from a two-dimensional drawing, the lines of the cube can be interpreted two ways, differing only in their orientation in space. Without perspective and shading cues, you are as likely to see one as the other. The physical stimulus—the line drawing—doesn't change, yet conscious perception flips back and forth between these two interpretations, in what is a paradigmatic example of a *bistable percept*.[1]

---

[1]Gregory (1997) provides a popular account of the psychology of bistable and ambiguous figures. For a compendium of these and many other illusions, see Seckel (2000, 2002).

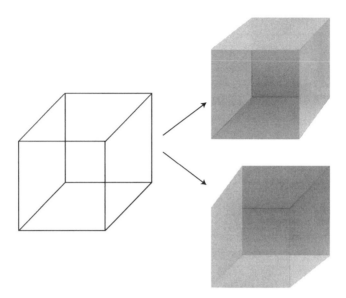

FIGURE 16.1 *The Bistable Necker Cube* The line drawing on the left can be seen in one of two ways, shown on the right. Without any other cue, your mind flips back and forth between them. You never see a combination of the two.

You never see the cube suspended in a position halfway between the inside and the outside configurations, nor do you see an amalgamation of the two. Your mind can't simultaneously visualize both shapes. Instead, each configuration vies for *perceptual dominance*. This is but one manifestation of a general phenomenon, that in the presence of ambiguity, the mind doesn't supply multiple solutions but prefers a single interpretation that may change with time. This aspect of experience is sometimes referred to as the *unity of consciousness*.[2]

Motion-induced blindness (see page 14) is another perceptual stimulus that underscores the multifarious nature of consciousness.[3] The perceptual stimuli most popular with brain scientists, however, are *binocular rivalry* and *flash suppression*. Both permit the astute observer with the right tools to distinguish neurons that slavishly follow the physical input from those that correlate with the subjective percept. Think of it as tracking the neural footprints of consciousness.

---

[2] See Bayne and Chalmers (2003) and the volume edited by Cleeremans (2003) on this theme.

[3] An even simpler one-to-many stimulus is the sequence of two lights discussed in footnote 30 on page 265. On some occasions you see the stimulus as a single flash of light, and on others as two flashes.

Given everything that is known about the retina, it is unlikely that its activity changes when the conscious percept does. A ganglion cell in your eye reacts automatically to a patch of light or a corner of the cube whether you perceive it in one orientation or the other. Put differently, the same retinal state can be associated with two, distinct phenomenal states. Somewhere in the corridors of your forebrain, however, are neurons whose activity mirrors the waxing and waning of your conscious percept. Such cells—candidates for the NCC—have been discovered in monkeys and humans, and are the topic of this chapter.

16.1 | BINOCULAR RIVALRY: WHEN THE TWO EYES DISAGREE

In the course of everyday life, your two eyes are constantly presented with similar, though not identical, views of the world. The brain can extract sufficient cues from the small discrepancies between these two images to discern depth.

What happens, though, if corresponding parts of your left and right eyes see two quite distinct images, something that can easily be arranged using mirrors and a partition in front of your nose? Suppose your left eye sees vertical stripes whereas your right eye sees horizontal ones. Quite plausibly you might expect to see a plaid pattern—a superposition of the horizontal and vertical stripes. And, indeed, this sometimes happens. Under the right circumstances, though, a far more tantalizing phenomenon occurs: You perceive just one of the two patterns, say the vertical stripes that stimulate your left eye. After a few seconds, this image begins to fade, and patches of the image from the right eye appear, until after a transition period, only the horizontal stripes are visible (the vertical ones have disappeared). The two percepts can alternate in this manner indefinitely, even though both eyes remain continuously open. Psychologists call this phenomenon *binocular rivalry* because one image perceptually suppresses and dominates the other (Figure 16.2).[4]

The extent to which any pair of patterns compete—such as a face and a moving grating, or a smiling girl and a car—depends on their relative contrast, spatial frequency content, and familiarity. If the two images are equally salient, then each one is usually visible for about the same amount of time. The duration of these *dominance periods*—how long either one is visible—varies con-

---

[4]The phenomenological aspects of binocular rivalry are well described in Yang, Rose, and Blake (1992). Blake and Logothetis (2002) summarize the pertinent psychological and physiological observations. Lee and Blake (1999) investigate whether binocular perception arises out of competition between inputs from the two eyes or between two patterns that happen to originate in separate eyes. Andrews and Purves (1997) argue compellingly that binocular rivalry occurs more often in real life than previously realized.

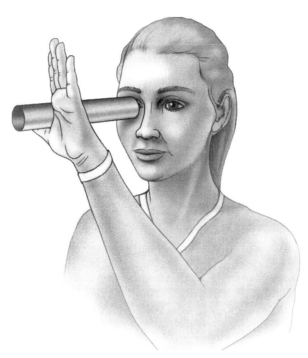

FIGURE 16.2 *There is a Hole in My Hand* You can observe something akin to rivalry with the aid of a piece of paper. Roll it tightly into a small tube and hold this cylinder with your left hand in front of your right eye in the manner drawn. You should see a hole in your left hand! Point the tube at a dark background and hold it steady. After a while you'll see the back of your left hand. This percept will alternate with the sight of the hole and whatever you are pointing it at. If your left eye dominates, reverse 'left' and 'right' in these instructions.

siderably across subjects and trials.[5] Even if one of the rivalry-inducing images is fainter or less salient than the other, the weak one will dominate the stronger one at some point, though usually only for a short time. Binocular rivalry can be thought of as a reflexive alternation between percepts that can be influenced, though not completely abolished, by sensory or cognitive factors.

---

[5] If the frequency with which each dominance period occurs is plotted in a histogram, a smooth function emerges (Levelt, 1965). In other words, the duration of dominance is unpredictable on a case-by-case basis, but is governed by a stochastic process with some degree of regularity, with the duration of one phase of dominance statistically independent of the duration of the following pattern. Mood disorders, such as depression, are associated with a dramatic lengthening of dominance times (Pettigrew and Miller, 1998). The duration of dominance of one pattern can be influenced by selectively attending to it.

Rivalry can be induced most easily with small images. Unless these are carefully designed, rivalry with larger pictures results in a piecemeal percept, in which the two images dominate in different parts of the visual field, fractionating it into a mosaic-like collage, not unlike a quilt. Locally, though, the percept is still constructed from one or the other picture and not from the superposition of the two.

At the neuronal level, rivalry was long believed to be due to reciprocal inhibition between populations of cells representing input from the left and from the right eyes. One coalition fires away, preventing the other from responding. As this inhibition fatigues, the other group eventually dominates. It's a bit like presidential elections in the United States, where the voters, with a fair degree of regularity, alternate between sending a Democrat and a Republican to the White House.

Recent psychological and imaging evidence has suggested that this automatic switching is complemented by active processes linked to attention. Mechanisms located in prefrontal and parietal areas can bias the system toward one or the other coalition. This enables the chosen coalition to build up sufficient strength to dominate and to widely distribute its informational content, bringing that image to consciousness.[6]

16.2 | WHERE DOES PERCEPTUAL SUPPRESSION OCCUR?

Where in the brain does the fight for dominance occur? Retinal neurons are not influenced by the percept; they are driven exclusively by the photoreceptor input. Perceptual modulation could occur as early as the lateral geniculate nucleus, halfway between the retina and primary visual cortex. However, recordings from geniculate neurons have shown that their firing rate is indifferent to whether a monkey saw a rivalrous or a nonrivalrous stimulus.[7] The interplay between dominant and suppressed stimuli, therefore, occurs in the cortex.

Early Cortical Areas Mostly Follow the Stimulus

The cortical sites underlying binocular rivalry in monkeys have been explored in a brilliant, decade-long effort by Nikos Logothetis—from his early work

---

[6]The arguments for rivalry as reciprocal inhibition among neurons in the early visual stages are well summarized by Blake (1989). The view that rivalry is the expression of exploratory behavior under the control of high-level cognitive processes in the frontal lobe, is forcefully expressed in Leopold and Logothetis (1999); see also Lumer and Rees (1999). The ideas regarding the causes of rivalry—low-level, sensory-driven versus higher-level, mental operations—and their reception in the scientific community have themselves waxed and waned over the past 200 years.

[7]These experiments involved awake and fixating monkeys (Lehky and Maunsell, 1996).

with Jeffrey Schall at the Massachusetts Institute of Technology, to the subsequent refinement of his experimental paradigm with David Sheinberg and David Leopold at Baylor College of Medicine in Houston, and now at the Max Planck Institute for Biological Cybernetics in Tübingen, Germany.[8]

Recording spiking activity in behaving animals is notoriously difficult for any number of technical reasons. An additional challenge lies in the very nature of bistable perception, which precludes an external observer from knowing the subject's experience. In a rivalry experiment, paid volunteers, usually undergraduate students, provide a verbal report of their percept or, for a better parallel with animal studies, signal their percept by pressing the appropriate buttons. Electrophysiologists can train monkeys on the same task and carry out a variety of tests to confirm that the monkeys' response profiles are similar to those of the humans. This assures skeptics that the animals report their perceptual experience in roughly the same manner as people do.[9]

The principle behind these experiments is straightforward, but the practice is more complicated, so I'll have to simplify a bit. In one example, the monkey was taught to hold one lever whenever it saw a stylized sunburst, and another lever when it saw any of a variety of other images—people, faces, butterflies, man-made objects, and so on. The animal was then placed into the binocular rivalry setup, which projected the sunburst pattern into one eye and a second image into the other eye. The monkey indicated which picture it saw by pressing the appropriate lever (the animal was taught not to respond during transition periods). Once training was complete, an electrode was lowered into the brain of the animal and was positioned next to a spiking neuron, and the search for a "preferred" stimulus that excited this cell commenced. That is, the neuroscientists were searching through a photo library to find an image that, when shown by itself to the monkey, evoked a reliable and strong response.

During the rivalry phase of the experiment, this effective stimulus was projected into one eye while the sunburst pattern, which evoked only a feeble response in this cell, was projected into the other. While the animal signaled

---

[8]Binocular rivalry in monkeys was pioneered by Myerson, Miezin, and Allman (1981). The corpus of Logothetis's work on the neurophysiology and psychophysics of bistable percepts in humans and monkeys is considerable and includes Logothetis and Schall (1989); Logothetis, Leopold, and Sheinberg (1996); Sheinberg and Logothetis (1997); Leopold and Logothetis (1999); and Leopold et al. (2002). For reviews, see Logothetis (1998) and Blake and Logothetis (2002).

[9]Monkeys and humans have similar dominance distribution times during rivalry and are affected in the same way by varying stimulus contrast (Leopold and Logothetis, 1996). Logothetis uses additional controls to make sure the monkeys are faithfully reporting their perception.

which of the two stimuli it was seeing, the activity of the neuron was continuously monitored. And now the million-dollar question:[10] Will the cell's discharge rate reflect the constant retinal input or the varying conscious percept?

The majority of cells in primary and secondary visual cortices fired with little regard for the ebb and flow of perception. By and large, a neuron increased its activity to the stimulus in one eye no matter what the monkey saw. Only six out of 33 cells were somewhat modulated by perception; when the animal did not see the preferred stimulus, the neuron's firing rate was reduced compared to those episodes when it saw the stimulus.[11] The majority of V1 cells fire no matter whether the monkey sees one or the other stimuli. These data reinforce an important point I've made before—namely, exuberant cortical activity does not guarantee a conscious percept. Not just any cortical activity contributes to consciousness.

The lack of a significant perceptual influence on the firing activity of V1 neurons explains why aftereffects that depend on these neurons are little affected by perceptual suppression. Recall from Section 6.2 that orientation-dependent aftereffects can be induced by invisible stimuli. The ability of unseen things to affect vision was first demonstrated in the context of binocular rivalry; even though a pattern in one eye is suppressed, it still causes an orientation-dependent or a motion-dependent aftereffect.[12] These results are compatible with our hypothesis that the NCC are not found among V1 cells (Chapter 6).

One source of ongoing controversy is a pair of fMRI studies of binocular rivalry in human V1. One experiment reported a consistent modulation of V1 hemodynamic activity with rivalry. The hemodynamic signal associated with the visible image was stronger than the signal of the suppressed

---

[10]A million dollars is not far removed from the actual cost of carrying out these demanding experiments in several monkeys over the course of a few years. They require highly trained scientists and staff and lots of specialized equipment and facilities.

[11]These negative results are compatible with the lack of powerful, intereye inhibition in binocular V1 neurons (Macknik and Martinez-Conde, 2004). Gail, Brinksmeyer, and Eckhorn (2004) recorded local field potentials (LFP) together with the joint spiking activity of many neurons in V1 of monkeys trained to signal their percept during binocular rivalry. Like Leopold and Logothetis (1996), they saw no significant change in the spiking discharge as the animal signals one or the other percept. Curiously though, the LFP was modulated at frequencies below 30 Hz by the perceptual state of the monkey. Fries and his colleagues (Fries et al., 1997 and 2001c) reported that rivalry in squinting cats did not influence the mean rate of V1 neurons. Instead, Fries and colleagues found that dominance was signaled by the degree of spike synchrony in the 30 to 70 Hz frequency band. Feline V1 neurons that coded for the dominant stimulus had a higher spike coherency compared to neurons representing the suppressed image. What causal effect, if any, the perceptual changes in the different frequency bands have on the cortex outside of V1 is not clear.

[12]Blake and Fox (1974) and Blake (1998).

image.[13] The second experiment used the ingenious strategy of tracking the brain's response in the cortical representation of the blind spot (see Figure 4.2). These researchers found that the signal in this region was as strongly modulated by rivalry as it was when the perceptually suppressed stimulus was simply turned on and off. They concluded that rivalry was completely resolved in V1.[14]

The conclusion that who wins and who loses in the competition for rivalry is decided in V1 is questionable, because it assumes that the sluggish hemodynamic signal is directly correlated to the very brisk spiking activity in projection neurons. Sometimes the opposite is true.[15] Increases in blood flow and oxygenation levels that underlie the fMRI signal are strongly coupled to synaptic activity—the release and uptake of neurotransmitter and to electrical processing in local circuits. Synaptic input may or may not initiate action potentials that travel down the axon, depending on the relative amount of excitation and inhibition. This biophysically more informed reading of the fMRI data suggests that feedback from higher areas reaches down to V1 and triggers synaptic input there, without necessarily changing the firing rate of neurons that project out of V1. Research efforts over the next few years should resolve this discrepancy between single cell electrophysiology and fMRI techniques.

Are Intermediate Regions the Site of Competition?

The neuronal response patterns in areas V4 and MT are more varied than those in V1.[16] About 40% of V4 cells are correlated with the animal's behavior, that is, with its (assumed) perception. Curiously, a third of these modulated neurons increase their firing rate when the monkey sees the preferred stimulus, while the remaining cells respond best when their preferred stimulus is suppressed. MT recordings with moving gratings reveal a qualitatively similar picture. Forty percent of neurons modulate their firing rate with the perception of the animal. Half of these fire when their preferred direction is perceptually

---

[13] Polonsky et al. (2000).

[14] Tong and Engel (2001).

[15] In one spectacular experiment, Logothetis (2004) inhibited pyramidal neurons in V1 by the local infusion of a chemical agent. He used electrical recodings to confirm that these cells were silenced while simultaneously measuring hemodynamic activity in the anesthetized monkey. Remarkably, the amplitude of the local field potential and of the magnetic resonance signal triggered by visual input was basically unaffected. In other words, the sensory-evoked synaptic release required metabolic energy that was picked up by the fMRI technique, even though no action potentials were generated by the cells that must convey the result to other brain regions. For more information, see footnote 2 on page 135.

[16] Leopold and Logothetis (1996).

suppressed. Thus, in both regions, some groups of cells actively signal when their preferred stimulus is invisible—a sort of unconscious "Freudian" representation of a suppressed stimulus.

The firing profile of many V4 and MT cells indicates that they change their output primarily during transitions when the percept changes over from one image to the other. One plausible conclusion is that the coalitions in these intermediate areas are competing against each other, attempting to resolve the ambiguity imposed by the two disparate images. At some point a winner is established, and its identity (and probably also that of the loser) is signaled to the next stages.

16.3 | THE FOOTPRINTS OF CONSCIOUSNESS LEAD TO THE INFERIOR TEMPORAL CORTEX

When Sheinberg and Logothetis recorded from cells in the inferior temporal cortex (IT) and in the lower bank of the superior temporal sulcus (STS) that delimits IT on its upper side, they found that the competition between the rivalrous stimuli was resolved. Nine out of ten cells fired in congruence with the monkey's percept. Whenever the monkey saw the preferred stimulus of the neuron, the cell fired. When the other image dominated, the cell's response was muted. Unlike the situation in V4 and MT, no IT cells signaled the suppressed and invisible stimulus.[17]

Let me illustrate these results for the neuron depicted in Figure 16.3. The experimentalists first established that the cell fired more strongly to the sight of a monkey's face than to a sunburst pattern. During the period indicated in gray, the animal looked at both images under binocular conditions, reporting which one it saw. As the monkey's mind changed, the neuron did likewise. Although the retinal input remained constant, the neuron's response was stronger when the monkey saw the face than when it saw the sunburst.

The echoes of this titanic clash between coalitions of neurons can be picked up by imaging human brain activity. The visual psychologist Nancy Kanwisher at the Massachusetts Institute of Technology had previously shown that the fMRI signal in the fusiform face area (Section 8.5) responds more vigorously to faces than to the sight of houses, places, and landmark buildings. The converse is true for the parahippocampal place area: Here, the fMRI signal is stronger for pictures of houses and places than it is for faces. This differential sensitivity allowed her and her collaborators to compare hemodynamic activity in these two areas, high up in the visual hierarchy, while volunteers were lying

---

[17] Sheinberg and Logothetis (1997) and Logothetis (1998).

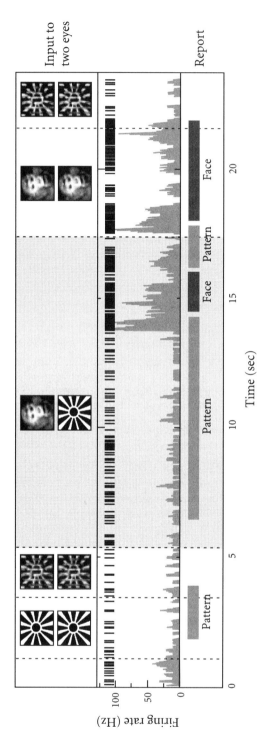

FIGURE 16.3 *Binocular Rivalry in a Neuron in the Inferior Temporal Cortex.* A fraction of a minute in the life of a typical IT cell. The upper row indicates the retinal input, with dotted vertical lines marking stimulus transitions. The second row shows the individual spikes from one trial, the third the smoothed firing rate over many trials, and the bottom row the monkey's percept. It was taught to press a lever only when it saw either one or the other image, but not to a superposition of both. The cell responded weakly to either the lone sunburst pattern or when this picture was superimposed onto the image of a monkey's face (around 5 sec). During binocular rivalry (gray zone), the monkey's perception vacillated back and forth between seeing the face and seeing the sunburst. Perception of the face was consistently accompanied (and preceded) by a strong increase in firing rate. From N. Logothetis (private communication).

inside a magnetic scanner, experiencing rivalry between images of faces and houses. Consistent with the single-cell data, the hemodynamic signal in these two areas, high up in the visual hierarchy, mirrored the subjective percept. Indeed, the signal was sensitive enough to predict whether the subject saw, during the preceding period, a face or a house, a limited form of mind reading.[18]

To hammer home the point that neurons in and around the inferotemporal cortex may be members of the coalition sufficient for conscious, visual experiences, consider the *flash suppression* illusion. Discovered by Jeremy Wolfe as part of his Ph.D. research at the Massachusetts Institute of Technology, flash suppression exploits binocular suppression, with the percept more easily controlled than in free-running rivalry. Suppose you are looking with one eye at an image. After a while, a different picture is flashed into your other eye. If the two images fall onto corresponding parts of the two retinae, you will see the newly flashed picture, but not the old one, even though it is still there, right in front of you. The second image, due to its novelty, is more salient than the older one and eliminates the older picture from sight.[19]

Monkeys act as if they experience something similar. Analogous to their rivalry experiments, Sheinberg and Logothetis trained animals to indicate their perception by pushing one of two levers while electrodes monitored individual neurons. A photo of a young orangutan's face, by itself, evoked a vigorous response (left panel in Figure 16.4). Flashing the sunburst pattern into the opposite eye wiped out the perception of the face; at the neuronal level, the cell's response was rapidly and almost completely extinguished, even though the cell's preferred image remained in one eye. Cells in lower regions did not shut down in this dramatic fashion to a nonperceived stimulus. The right panel in Figure 16.4 portrays the opposite scenario. The sunburst by itself evokes no spikes. After the picture of the ape's face was projected into the other eye, the cell abruptly increased its firing rate and the animal indicated that it saw the face. Physically, the input was the same in both cases. The perceptual experience was quite different, however, and this neuron expressed this difference.[20]

---

[18]Tong et al. (1998). See also Epstein and Kanwisher (1998).

[19]Wolfe (1984), who studied the psychology of flash suppression in people, demonstrated that this effect was not due to forward masking, light adaptation, or any other mechanism that reduced the visibility of the first image. A short blank offset could be introduced between the monocular presentation and the flash without affecting the outcome.

[20]When listening to the crackle of an IT or STS neuron as its amplified spikes are fed into a loudspeaker, one has the distinct feeling of being able to tell which lever the monkey will pull. This has been confirmed by a rigorous statistical procedure in which the temporal modulation of the firing rate of almost any IT and STS cell reliably forecasts the animal's behavior (Sheinberg and Logothetis, 1997). IT and STS are far removed from output regions, ruling out the possibility that the physiologists were listening to the motor stages preparing to move one or the other hand.

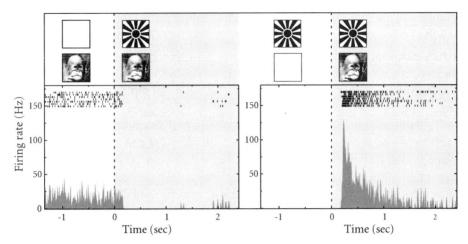

FIGURE 16.4 *A Neuron that Follows the Subject's Percept* The picture of a young ape evokes a vigorous response from this neuron in the superior temporal sulcus (leftmost portion of the left panel). When the picture of a sunburst is flashed into the other eye, the monkey signals that it sees this pattern and that the image of the young ape has disappeared. Although the ape's face is the cell's preferred stimulus, the cell's response drops to zero. Conversely, if the monkey fixates the sunburst pattern for a while, and the image of the ape's face is flashed on, the subject sees the face and the cell fires strongly (right panel). Neurons in earlier areas are largely unaffected by such perceptual changes. Modified from Sheinberg and Logothetis (1997).

The majority of IT and STS cells behaved in this manner. When the cell's preferred stimulus is perceived by the monkey, the cell responds. If the image is perceptually suppressed, the cell falls silent, even though legions of V1 neurons fire away vigorously to the sight of it.[21] None of this furious activity contributes to perception, however, which is *prima facie* evidence for our hypothesis that the NCC are not in V1.

Recall from footnote 14 on page 29 that the neurosurgeon Itzhak Fried implanted depth electrodes into the medial temporal and frontal lobes of epileptic patients to localize the seizure focus. Gabriel Kreiman, a graduate student in my laboratory, took advantage of this unique situation to record from microelectrodes that piggy-backed onto the bigger depth probes while the patients were experiencing flash suppression in their bed in the clinic. This experiment became possible after Kreiman discovered cells in the medial temporal lobe (MTL) that fired to specific image categories, such as animals or well-known individuals (see Figure 2.2). We found that about two-thirds of all responsive MTL cells followed the percept. That is, the cell fired when the

---

[21] D. Leopold and N. Logothetis, private communication.

patient consciously saw the picture, but its firing rate was reduced to baseline level when the image was invisible, yet still present in one eye. Indeed, none of the cells responded to a perceptually suppressed stimulus, so there was no hint of an unconscious representation in these parts of the brain.[22] It is reassuring that the single neuron data from humans who had no previous experience with such stimuli are similar to the recordings from highly trained monkeys.

16.4 | OPEN QUESTIONS AND FUTURE EXPERIMENTS

The exploration of the neurobiological basis of perceptual stimuli is in full swing. Every available technique is being pressed into service to delve ever deeper into the mechanisms underlying switches in the content of consciousness. Like any productive research program, the neuronal exploration of bistable percepts opens the door for further probing into the nature of the NCC.

One question that remains unanswered concerns the role of spike synchronization among neurons coding for the perceptually dominant pattern. Is spike synchrony among IT cells a signature event for the NCC? Asked differently, is a high degree of synchrony necessary to form a dominant coalition that corresponds to a specific percept?[23]

Another question concerns the extent to which the firing activity of (some of) these cells merely covaries with the animal's percept or whether these cells *are* the NCC for this percept. How tight is the link between the exact onset and strength of firing and the animal's behavior on a trial-to-trial basis?[24]

Neurobiology is not only an observational science, but also increasingly one where the nervous system can be perturbed in quantifiable ways to influence the organism's behavior. Such invasive experiments can help to bridge the gap between correlation and causation.

The easiest way to interfere is to microstimulate parts of the brain. Can dominance times during rivalry be biased by exciting groups of cells in IT or in the

---

[22]The flash suppression experiments recorded the activity of individual neurons in the amygdala, entorhinal cortex, hippocampus, and parahippocampal gyrus of untrained and conscious patients (Kreiman, Fried, and Koch, 2002). In the macaque monkey, there are strong connections between IT and the MTL.

[23]Singer and his colleagues argue that action potentials of V1 cells coding for the perceptually dominant image are more synchronized than those associated with the suppressed one (Engel et al., 1999, and Engel and Singer, 2001; see also footnote 11 in this chapter). Multi-electrode recordings in the behaving monkey have not resolved this issue. Murayama, Leopold, and Logothetis (2000) did find that synchrony among V1, V2, and V4 neurons is substantially higher when both eyes view the same image compared to when the two eyes are stimulated by different pictures.

[24]Gold and Shadlen (2002); and Parker and Krug (2003).

MTL that follow the percept? As mentioned in Section 8.5, the cellular representation for faces is clustered within the inferior temporal cortex. Injecting bipolar pulses of current from an intracortical electrode into a patch of IT cells may extend the dominance or shorten the suppression period of a face percept when it is competing with some other picture.

Other interventions that are rapidly becoming feasible involve silencing genetically identified cellular communities, such as neurons in the superficial layers of IT (see below) that project to the frontal lobes. Is an animal, deprived of these cells that communicate to the front of the cortex, still conscious? Will it still signal perceptual transitions?

What Cell Types Are Involved?

It is implausible that all of the storied IT and STS neurons that follow the percept express its phenomenological attributes directly. Some must be involved in the underlying winner-take-all operations; others must relay the winner's identity to the motor centers to initiate behavior or to short-term memory for future recall; some must carry a transient signal indicative of a perceptual switch; and still others might represent the same information but in a delayed manner.

When considering the temporal profile of cellular responses in these areas, I am struck by their extreme heterogeneity. An entire menagerie of distinct patterns can be observed. Some cells fire in a transient manner whereas others respond in a more sustained fashion. Some fire in bursts, some show a pronounced, rhythmic discharge in the 4 to 6 Hz range, while others (as in the right-hand side of Figure 16.4) peak early before settling down to a more sedate and sustained pace of firing. Do these reflect discrete cell types with discrete functions and connectivity patterns? This will be important to know.[25]

The search for the NCC can be refined by mapping the temporal evolution of the percept's visibility, brightness and other attributes onto specific classes of spike patterns. Is the percept encoded by the amplitude of the sustained discharge after a fraction of a second, or by the degree of synchrony among neighboring neurons? One experiment that might give the game away is to record during flash suppression before and after the induction of a rapidly acting anesthesia. What is the effect of putting the monkey to sleep? Whatever the NCC are, they should be abolished after this manipulation.

---

[25] A hint that specific cell classes might be involved comes from the incidental observation that almost all MT cells that modulated their firing rate with the percept of the moving grating were located in the deep layers (Logothetis and Schall, 1989).

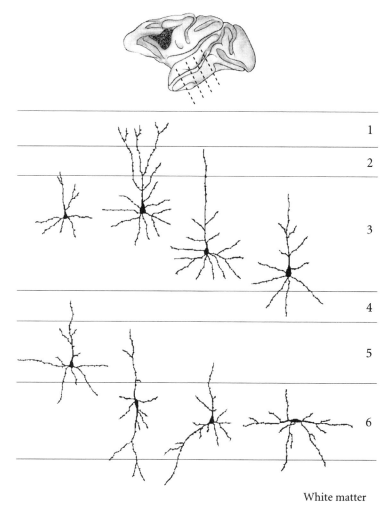

FIGURE 16.5 *The Cellular Substrate for the NCC?* A collage of neurons in the infero-temporal cortex of the monkey (taken from the four slices indicated with dashed lines) that project to a limited portion of the prefrontal cortex (stippled area in the inset). Modified from de Lima et al. (1990).

Neuroanatomy is critical to further delve into what goes on in IT. In a landmark study, John Morrison and his colleagues at the Salk Institute in La Jolla, California, visualized IT neurons that targeted regions around the principal sulcus in the prefrontal cortex (inset in Figure 16.5).[26] Their cell bodies were

---

[26] See de Lima, Voigt, and Morrison (1990). These researchers injected one tracer near the principal sulcus in the prefrontal cortex of four monkeys. The substance was taken up by axons

found in superficial layer 3 and in deep layers 5 and 6. Based on the cell's dendritic tree morphology and laminar position, the anatomists differentiated eight cell types (Figure 16.5). As a group, these pyramidal neurons and their dendrites spanned the entire depth of the cortex, although each cell type covered only a limited vertical extent.

Some of these projection neurons may form part of the NCC, but which ones? In what layers of the prefrontal cortex do their axons terminate? Do they branch to innervate other cortical regions? What is the relationship between these anatomically defined classes and the distinct spike patterns that I mentioned on page 282? Do any of these cells receive synaptic input from the same neurons in the prefrontal cortex to which they project, thus forming direct loops? Do they bond in special ways with their postsynaptic targets? Do they have a unique molecular signature that can be exploited in a clever way to rapidly, delicately, and reversibly shut them off for a brief time?

No molecular biologist would be satisfied to know that *some* fraction of all kinase enzymes, or of all proteins associated with the structural specializations at the synapse, change during synaptic plasticity. Instead, biologists seek to identify *which* of the hundreds of proteins necessary for synaptic function are up-regulated and which ones are down-regulated, how these are linked, which ones are located within the membrane and which ones within the cytosol, and so on. Why should brain scientists be satisfied with anything less specific regarding perception?

Perceptual Dominance and the Prefrontal Cortex

The inferior temporal cortex and neighboring regions not only project to the prefrontal cortex but also receive input from it. What is the role of this feedback in rivalry and related phenomena? I argued in Chapter 14 that the NCC require communication with the planning centers in the front of the brain. This must be a two-way street, with feedforward activity in IT reinforced by feedback from frontal regions. Without these regions (say, because they have been cooled or otherwise shut down), conscious perception would be lost, even though some sort of automatic cycling between the two stimuli could still take place during binocular rivalry. IT neurons may still show some degree of mod-

---

and transported in a retrograde direction from the synapses back to the cell body. After a few weeks, the animals were sacrificed and sections of the inferior temporal gyrus were examined to look for the telltale signs of the tracers in neurons. These weakly labeled cells were then injected intracellularly with a second dye that rapidly filled the entire dendritic tree and soma, allowing their detailed anatomy to be reconstructed. Morrison and his students recovered more than 400 cells in this manner, all of which were covered with spines, indicative of excitatory cells. Photodynamic staining techniques might be able to speed up this very labor-intensive work (Dacey et al., 2003).

ulation with these changes, but much less crisply than in a neurologically intact subject. Such predictions can soon be directly tested.

An innovative fMRI study by Erik Lumer and Geraint Rees at University College in London contrasted rivalry-induced switches with purely retina-driven ones (that is, when one or the other image was actually removed from that eye). They concluded that fronto-parietal regions were active whenever dominance switched from one to the other percept.[27] This hypothesis is supported by the clinical observation that patients with prefrontal lesions typically have abnormal transitions in bistable perception.[28]

If these areas help decide when to flip, they should have access to attributes of the currently suppressed image. Recall from Section 11.3 that cells in and around the principal sulcus in the prefrontal cortex act as short-term memory. As shown in Figure 16.5, IT projects to these regions. Are these prefrontal cells, encoding the previously seen but now suppressed image, responsible for its reemergence into consciousness during the next cycle?[29]

16.5 | RECAPITULATION

Like the Rosetta stone, perceptual stimuli allow the intrepid researcher to translate among three distinct languages—the subjective idiom of sensation and phenomenal experience, the objective language of behavioral psychology, and the mechanistic language of brain science, expressed in terms of spikes and assemblies of neurons. They offer the best hope of discovering the NCC.

Binocular rivalry and flash suppression are popular examples of one-to-many perceptual stimuli that are vivid and easy to control. Two images are projected into the eyes, but only one is seen while the other is suppressed. During rivalry, the two enter and depart from consciousness in a never-ending dance. What you see is not a superposition of the two images, but only one—the result of a ruthless competition in which the "winner takes all." Flash suppression is similar to binocular rivalry but more predictable, since the new image always trumps the older one.

---

[27]Lumer and Rees (1999); see also Lumer, Friston, and Rees (1998). Similar parietal and frontal regions are active during perceptual transitions occurring while viewing a range of bistable figures (such as the Necker cube and Rubin's face/vase figure; see Kleinschmidt et al., 1998).

[28]Patients with lesions in the right frontal lobe have difficulty switching from one percept to the other when viewing bistable stimuli (Wilkins, Shallice, and McCarthy, 1987; Ricci and Blundo, 1990; and Meenan and Miller, 1994).

[29]If so, this suggests that working memory and perceptual dominance are interrelated. Could some of the considerable variability in the dominance periods across individuals be due to variability in their working memory?

Neurophysiological evidence from trained monkeys demonstrates that only a small minority of cells in V1 and V2 (and none in the LGN) change their firing rate with perception. These modulations are modest compared to the all-or-none perceptual changes experienced during rivalry. Almost all V1 cells fire independently of the subject's conscious perception, which explains why some aftereffects can be reliably evoked by suppressed, and therefore invisible, stimuli.

More than one-third of the neurons in areas V4 and MT correlate with the percept. Many encode the dominant stimulus, while a significant fraction represent the invisible pattern.

The majority of IT and STS neurons follow the animal's behavior. None represent the suppressed stimulus. Single cell recordings from the human medial temporal lobe tell the same story—most selective cells follow the percept and none signal the invisible image. This effect is so strong and consistent that their firing rates can be used with high fidelity to infer the subject's behavior.

In this upper region of the ventral, vision-for-perception pathway, the victorious neuronal coalition rules supreme. Some of its members are the most promising candidates for the NCC. To further investigate this claim, it will be necessary to correlate the microstructure of conscious perception with the dynamic firing behavior of these neurons and to establish a causal link between the two by perturbing neurons in these areas appropriately.

The neurophysiological exploration of perceptual stimuli has yielded a treasure trove of insights into the mind-body interface. Another source of information about the neurology of the NCC is surgical interventions in the human brain. I will discuss this next.

CHAPTER SEVENTEEN

Splitting the Brain
Splits Consciousness

It was as if there were two minds within me arguing the toss. The 'voice'
was clean and sharp and commanding. It was always right, and I listened
to it when it spoke and acted on its decisions. The other mind rambled
out a disconnected series of images, and memories and hopes, which I
attended to in a daydream state as I set about obeying the orders of the
'voice'. I had to get to the glacier. I would crawl on the glacier, but I didn't
think that far ahead. If my perspectives had sharpened, so too had they
narrowed, until I thought only in terms of achieving predetermined aims
and no further. Reaching the glacier was my aim. The 'voice' told me
exactly how to go about it, and I obeyed while my other mind jumped
abstractly from one idea to another.

From *Touching the Void* by Joe Simpson

$\mathbf{I}$f consciousness resides in one sector
of the brain, couldn't it be split by slicing this region in two? While this sounds
silly, something not unlike this thought experiment has been performed.

The brain has a highly symmetrical structure, with two cerebral hemispheres, two thalami, two sets of basal ganglia, and so on. This symmetry is
one of its most noticeable features. Because consciousness in regular folk is
experienced singularly, you might conclude that its neuronal underpinning
must therefore be expressed in a single physical structure. For if the NCC were
localized in both the left and right hemispheres, where would the experience
of unity come from? This train of thought persuaded Descartes in the 17th
century that the pineal gland, one of the few structures that exists in a single
copy along the midline, is the seat of the soul.[1]

---

[1] See article 32 in Descartes' *Les Passions de L'Ame*, published in 1649. Descartes's reasoning was
supported by the erroneous observation that people didn't survive without a pineal gland. The
other major structure that is not duplicated is the pituitary gland.

What happens if the two cerebral hemispheres, like Siamese twins, are separated? Assuming that animals or people can survive such an ordeal, how badly off are they afterward? Will they experience a split in their perception of the world?

17.1 | ON THE DIFFICULTY OF FINDING SOMETHING IF YOU DON'T KNOW WHAT TO LOOK FOR

The *corpus callosum* is by far the largest collection of fibers that directly link one cortical hemisphere to the other (Figure 17.1). A smaller connecting bundle is the *anterior commissure*. It is an important landmark, the zero point of the most popular three-dimensional coordinate system used in brain imaging.[2]

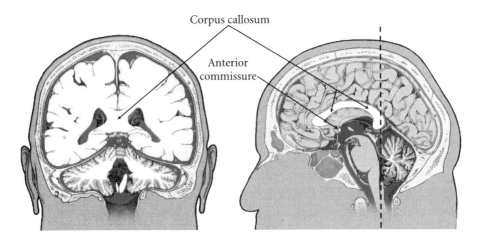

Corpus callosum

Anterior commissure

FIGURE 17.1 *The Corpus Callosum* This mass of 200 million axons, together with the much smaller anterior commissure, connects the two cerebral hemispheres. Sensory or symbolic information is relayed from one side to the other. In a complete split-brain procedure, both fiber bundles are cut. Modified from Kretschmann and Weinrich (1992).

---

[2]The axons in the corpus callosum, most of which are myelinated, originate among layer 2 and layer 3 pyramidal cells and project into layer 4 of their target region in the opposite hemisphere (Aboitiz et al., 1992). The two other cortical interhemispheric pathways are the anterior and the hippocampal commissures. Lower down are the intertectal commissure between the two colliculi, the posterior commissure linking the midbrain, and other connections at the level of the brainstem.

In certain cases of intractable epileptic seizures, part or all of these inter-hemispheric pathways are surgically cut as a last resort, preventing aberrant electrical activity from spreading from one hemisphere to the other and thereby causing generalized convulsions. This operation, first performed in the early 1940s and still occasionally carried out today, works as intended and does alleviate seizures. What is most remarkable about these *split-brain* patients, once they've recovered from the surgery, is their innocuousness in everyday life. They appear no different from their preoperative persona. They see, hear, and smell as before, they move about, talk, and interact appropriately with other people. They have their usual sense of self and report no obvious alterations to their perception of the world (e.g., their left visual field doesn't disappear). Clinicians were greatly puzzled by this lack of clear symptoms.

The moral for neuroscientists is that the brain is highly adaptive. If damaged, it compensates and obtains the information it needs in an enormously resourceful manner, by cross-cueing or by other tricks. Unless you have some idea of what could be wrong, what deficits to expect, you can completely miss them. This is an important strategic lesson to remember when chasing down the NCC.

The situation changed dramatically with Roger Sperry's pioneering research carried out in the 1950s and 1960s at my home institution, the California Institute of Technology, work for which he was awarded the 1981 Nobel Prize in Physiology or Medicine. By carefully observing frogs, rodents, cats, monkeys, and great apes whose cortical interhemispheric connections had been cut, Sperry and his collaborators showed that these animals effectively possessed two separate minds.[3] One hemisphere can be taught one response, while the other hemisphere learns another, even a conflicting, response to the same situation.

Joe Bogen, a neurosurgeon working at Loma Linda University Medical School in Los Angeles, together with Sperry and his student Michael Gazzaniga (now at Dartmouth College in New Hampshire and a founding figure of the field of *Cognitive Neuroscience*), tested the predictions from these animal experiments in his patients.[4] Ironically—in light of the previous difficulty of finding out what is wrong with these patients—it turns out to be rather easy to show that there is something seriously amiss with these patients.

---

[3]Complete sectioning is critical to elicit the full range of split-brain deficits. In particular, the anterior commissure needs to be cut, too, because it contains fibers linking the temporal and frontal cortical areas that mediate specific visual information. For more details, see Sperry (1961).

[4]Bogen, Fisher, and Vogel (1965), and Bogen and Gazzaniga (1965). For a magisterial overview of the neurology of split-brain patients, see Bogen (1993). Consult Akelaitis (1941, 1944) and Bogen (1997b) for the history of this procedure.

17.2 | THE TWO CEREBRAL HEMISPHERES DO NOT
SUBSERVE THE SAME FUNCTIONS

Knowledge about hemispheric specialization derives not only from observing split-brain patients but also by injecting the rapidly-acting barbiturate sodium amytal (the so-called "truth serum") into the left or right carotid artery. The circulating drug puts the hemisphere supplied by that artery to sleep for a few minutes, so that the behavior of the opposite, awake hemisphere can be tested.

The single most dramatic finding from these investigations is that the ability to speak, and to a lesser extent to comprehend language, is limited to one, the *dominant*, hemisphere. In more than nine out of ten patients it is the left cortical hemisphere that speaks, communicates through writing, and deals with other aspects of language with ease. The right hemisphere has only limited language comprehension and can't talk (although it can sing).[5] When a split-brain patient talks, it is his or her dominant hemisphere that is in control. The nondominant hemisphere is mute. It can still signal, however, by nodding the head or making meaningful signs with the fingers of the opposite hand.

Today, functional imaging offers a convenient and safe way to visualize hemispheric specialization in healthy volunteers directly. This confirms the inferences made from the clinic. In most people, the left hemisphere—Broca's area in the prefrontal cortex and Wernicke's area in the temporal lobe—are responsible for linguistic processing (Figure 15.2). For the remainder of this chapter I will assume that the left hemisphere is the dominant one.[6]

The right hemisphere is better at tasks requiring spatial cognition and relations, visual attention (recall from Section 10.3 that spatial neglect or extinction typically follows damage to the right parietal lobe), and visual perception, such as face recognition and imagery. Indeed, the fusiform face area in normal subjects (as circumscribed by functional brain imaging; Section 8.5) is much larger in the right than in the left fusiform gyrus.

Differences between the left and right hemispheres have become the stuff of folklore and cartoons. These findings have spawned a cottage industry of self-help books claiming that training one or the other hemisphere can increase creativity and thinking skills and tap into unused parts of the brain, all based on the flimsiest of evidence.

---

[5]Bogen and Gordon (1970; Gordon and Bogen, 1974) report on singing split-brain patients. Gazzaniga (1995) provides an excellent survey on the principles of human brain organization derived from split-brain studies. Geschwind and Galaburda (1987) discuss the biological mechanisms of cerebral lateralization in animals and people.

[6]In almost all right-handed subjects, the dominant, speaking hemisphere is the left one. Things are a bit more complicated for left-handed people. The spectrum extends from complete left dominance to complete right dominance with a minority showing no laterality at all.

17.3 | TWO CONSCIOUS MINDS IN ONE BODY

To understand the following, remember that sensory information from the left visual field or the left side of the body is represented in the right cerebral hemisphere, and vice versa. A typical split-brain patient is quite capable of calling a knife a knife if it is placed, out of sight (or with eyes closed), into his right hand—whose touch receptors project into the left somatosensory cortex, on the same side where his speech centers are located. When grasping the knife with his left hand—whose tactile information is sent into the silent, right hemisphere—he's at a loss to say what it is. If he is now given a picture chart, he can point at the drawing of a knife with his left, but not his right, hand. If asked why he chose that particular image, he doesn't know since his left, speaking, hemisphere has no information on what his left hand is grasping (in this test the patient must not look at the object). Instead of remaining silent, however, the patient often confabulates and invents some explanation to cover up the fact that he has no idea why his left hand did what it did.

One half of the brain quite literally does not know what the other half does, which can lead to situations somewhere between tragedy and farce. Victor Mark, a neurologist at the University of North Dakota, videotaped an interview with a complete split-brain patient. When asked how many seizures she had recently experienced, her right hand held up two fingers. Her left hand then reached over and forced the fingers on her right hand down. After trying several times to tally her seizures, she paused and then simultaneously displayed three fingers with her right hand and one with her left. When Mark pointed out this discrepancy, the patient commented that her left hand frequently did things on its own. A fight ensued between the two hands that looked like some sort of slapstick routine. Only when the patient grew so frustrated that she burst into tears was one reminded of the sad nature of her situation.[7]

Other clinical anecdotes involve patients that unbutton their shirt or blouse with one hand and close it with the other. These examples of hemispheric rivalry usually disappear a few weeks after the operation.

In a visual search task (as in Figure 9.2), split-brain patients appear to deploy two independent attentional searchlights to scan an array, one for the left and

---

[7]In this unusual patient, both hemispheres had the ability to speak. This led to frequent back-and-forth between them, as when Mark echoed one of her statements that she did not have feelings in her left hand. She then insisted that her hand was not numb, followed by a torrent of alternating Yes's and No's, ending with a despairing "I don't know!" For the details consult Mark (1996).

one for the right field of view.[8] With the corpus callosum intact, competition between the two hemispheres reduces the effective search rate, manifesting itself in a single, spatial focus of attention.

Any connections remaining after complete sectioning of the corpus callosum and the anterior commissure are incapable of relaying specific sensory or symbolic information, such as "a red vertical bar in the upper left visual field." However, they can communicate more diffuse emotional states, such as anger, happiness, or embarrassment. For instance, if one hemisphere is shown pictures of a sexual nature that cause the patient to blush, the other side is aware of the emotion without knowing why.

The intellectual abilities of the left hemisphere is close to that of the general population. Or, put differently, the intellect of the normal, entire brain is not much different from that of one of its halves (the dominant one). This explains the seeming lack of deficits in most split-brain patients, particularly when they are asked how they feel (because it is the left hemisphere that does the talking).

Yet the cognitive and motor capabilities of both sides, while not the same, have the same general character. The right hemisphere can access explicit memory and symbolic processing, something beyond the abilities of zombie systems. It certainly passes the delay test for consciousness introduced in Section 13.6.[9]

Because both the speaking *and* the mute hemispheres carry out complex, planned behaviors, both hemispheres will have conscious percepts, even though the character and content of their feelings may not be the same. The two minds have autonomous but shared experiences in one body, as emphasized by Sperry:

> Although some authorities have been reluctant to credit the disconnected minor hemisphere even with being conscious, it is our own interpretation based on a large number and variety of nonverbal tests, that the minor hemisphere is indeed a conscious system in its own right, perceiving, thinking, remembering, reasoning, willing and emoting, all at a characteristically human level, and that both the left and the right hemisphere may be conscious simultaneously in different, even in mutually conflicting, mental experiences that run along in parallel.[10]

---

[8]The reaction times of four split-brain patients shows that their search rates for a target hidden among a field of distractors spread across the entire field of view were approximately twice as fast as search rates when the target and distractors were limited to one hemifield only. This pronounced difference was not present in a group of normal control subjects (Luck et al., 1989 and 1994).

[9]For instance, if the left hand of a blindfolded split-brain patient can palm momentarily a star-shaped object, the left—but not the right hand—can later retrieve it in a bag filled with other objects (Bogen, 1997c).

[10]See Sperry (1974). The idea that bi-hemispheric brain organization must be reflected in a duality of the mind goes back to at least the middle of the 19th century (Wigan, 1844).

This independence has been confirmed within the context of binocular rivalry (as treated in the previous chapter). Both hemispheres show the pattern of dominance and suppression expected of two (more or less) independent brains.[11]

How does it *feel* to be the mute hemisphere, permanently encased in one skull in the company of a dominant sibling that does all of the talking? Given the right's inability to speak, is it less self-conscious than its twin? Is its content of consciousness more closely related to that of great apes and monkeys that can't talk? Imagine the silent storms raging across the remaining interbrain connections, giving control of this or that part of the body to one or the other hemisphere.[12] Will some future technology permit direct access to the right hemisphere and its conscious mind?

In split-brain patients, the NCC must exist, at least semi-independently, in the left and the right cortical hemispheres (without denying that some classes of percepts might be unique to one or the other). How, then, is integration achieved in the intact brain? The NCC must employ the callosal fibers to establish a single, dominant coalition throughout the forebrain, sufficient for a single conscious sensation, rather than two.

But is integration truly always achieved? Can echoes of the two hemispheres arguing with each other be found in everyday life? Read again the chapter epigraph from the harrowing account of Simpson's fall into a crevasse, on the verge of death, and his subsequent crawl onto a glacier with a broken leg. Sounds like the "voice" might come from his left hemisphere, urging him to get off the mountain, while the right cortex isn't much use except for distracting him with suggestive images. During a workout, have you ever experienced the unvoiced conflict raging in your head between the "better" self that insists on running yet another mile or adding more weights to the bar and your "inner wimp" that invents reason after reason for why enough is enough? Are these the reflections of the two hemispheres? Do they have distinct attributes, characteristic of the more linguistic and the more visual hemispheres? Are split-brain patients, or those people who live with but a single cortical hemisphere, devoid of such conflicting streams of consciousness?[13]

---

[11] O'Shea and Corballis (2001) report on binocular rivalry in split-brain observers. Their data argue against the tantalizing, but unlikely, hypothesis that in binocular rivalry the two hemispheres are competing against each other, with the left hemisphere preferring one percept and the right one the other (Pettigrew and Miller, 1998; and Miller et al., 2000).

[12] Marchiafava-Bignami disease, a rare complication of chronic alcoholism, is characterized by necrosis and subsequent atrophy of the corpus callosum and the anterior commissure (Kohler et al., 2000). The philosopher Puccetti (1973) wrote a fictionalized court case of such a patient, whose right hemisphere killed his wife in a particularly lurid manner. The jury found the husband—more precisely, his language-dominant hemisphere—not guilty. As far as I know, nobody has taken up the challenge of writing an account of the mental life of split-brain patients from the point of view of one or the other hemisphere (but see Schiffer, 2000).

[13] Bogen (1986).

17.4 | RECAPITULATION

At the macroscopic level, the brain—like the body—is a structure with a remarkable degree of bilateral symmetry. The mind, however, has but a single stream of consciousness, not two. Under ordinary conditions, the two hundred million callosal axons, with the help of the anterior commissure and other minor fiber bundles, integrate neural activity in the two halves of the forebrain, such that only a single dominant coalition forms, sufficient for a percept.

In split-brain patients, these pathways have been severed to prevent epileptic seizures from spreading from one cortical hemisphere to the other. Remarkably, after recovery, these patients act, speak, and feel no different than before. They do not complain of a loss of half their visual field or of other dramatic deficits. Upon closer inspection, however, a persistent and profound disconnection syndrome can be observed. If specific information is provided to one or the other hemisphere, the information is not shared with its twin.

This clinical experience, fortified by fMRI studies in volunteers, proves that in most people, regions in the left cortex are specialized for linguistic processing (including reading and writing). The right hemisphere, by itself, is mute but can communicate by pointing, nodding the head, or singing. As if to compensate, the right cortical hemisphere specializes in aspects of visual attention and perception, such as face recognition.

It seems that split-brain patients harbor two conscious minds in their two brain halves. In these patients, the NCC must be present, independently, on each side. In the intact brain, activity in the two hemispheres competes and only one coalition survives, sufficient for a single conscious percept.

Can the members of this dominant coalition that subserve consciousness be recruited throughout the front of the brain, seat of the highest mental faculties, or are some of these regions excluded from awareness and subjective feelings? This is the topic of the next chapter, once again a more speculative one.

CHAPTER EIGHTEEN

Further Speculations on Thoughts and the Nonconscious Homunculus

I don't know if it has happened to you at all, but a thing I've noticed with myself is that, when I'm confronted by a problem which seems for the moment to stump and baffle, a good sleep will often bring the solution in the morning. The nibs who study these matters claim, I believe, that this has something to do with the subconscious mind, and very possibly they may be right. I wouldn't have said off-hand that I had a subconscious mind, but I suppose I must without knowing it, and no doubt it was there, sweating away diligently at the old stand, all the while the corporeal Wooster was getting his eight hours.

From *Right Ho, Jeeves* by P.G. Wodehouse

Aren't you conscious of your innermost thoughts, plans, and intentions? Most people would reflexively answer yes. Most would assign consciousness to the top of the processing pyramid that starts with the eyes, ears, nose, and other sensors and ends with the "conscious me" as the endpoint of all perception and memory. Here, at the apex of the information processing hierarchy, is the ultimate arbiter for any and all executive functions and motor control.

I think that this view is wrong, that it's a cherished chimera. In this chapter, toward the end of the book, I permit myself the luxury of, once again, speculating on a view of which Francis and I have grown fond, that is, a cognitive architecture in which the NCC reside between a representation of the outer world of physical objects and events and an inner, hidden world of thoughts and concepts. This view has some surprising consequences.

18.1 | THE INTERMEDIATE-LEVEL THEORY OF CONSCIOUSNESS

Qualia are the elements that make up conscious experience. Qualia are what I am aware of: the sight of the valley floor far below me, the heat of the sun's rays on my back, the tension in my hands as I grip the rock, and a juxtaposition of fear and exhilaration peculiar to climbing on exposed walls within me. These are all subjective feelings. I argued in Section 14.1 that the function of these is to summarize the current state of affairs in the world and to forward this executive summary to the planning stages.

Nothing in the aforementioned implies that consciousness has access to this inner sanctum, to the regions where different courses of action are considered, decisions are made and long-term goals are evaluated and updated.

Indeed, a long-standing stance in psychology is based on the seemingly paradoxical idea that you are *not* directly conscious of your thoughts. By "thoughts" I mean all sorts of manipulations of sensory or more symbolic data and patterns. An example is the transformation needed to tell whether two gloves on a table are the same or are a left-right pair. The claim then is that you are only conscious of a representation of thoughts in sensory terms. The thoughts themselves, here the operations that try to match one glove to the other, remain beyond the pale of awareness. The great, uninterrupted stream of consciousness that is your mental life is but the reflection of your thoughts, not the thoughts themselves.

Let me expound upon this by referring to the writings of the cognitive scientist Ray Jackendoff from Brandeis University outside Boston. In his 1987 book *Consciousness and the Computational Mind*, Jackendoff defends the *intermediate-level theory of consciousness*. His arguments are grounded in a deep knowledge of linguistics and music, though he also makes some suggestions about visual perception.[1]

Jackendoff's analysis is based on a tripartite division of the mind-body into the physical brain, the computational mind, and the phenomenological mind. The brain includes the familiar territory of synapses, neurons, and their activities. The computational mind takes the sensory input, performs a series of operations on it, changes the internal state of the organism, and generates some motor output. It acts, in principle, no differently than a robot equipped with similar input and output sensors might. The phenomenological mind is the one that feels, that experiences qualia. Jackendoff confesses he has no idea how these experiences arise out of computation, echoing Chalmers's Hard Problem (Section 14.4). Nor is Jackendoff concerned with the NCC, but rather with what type of computations have qualia associated with them.

---

[1] Jackendoff (1987 and 1996).

Common sense suggests that awareness and thought are inseparable and that introspection reveals the contents of the mind. Jackendoff argues at length that both these beliefs are untrue. Thinking, the manipulation of concepts, sensory data, or more abstract patterns, is largely not conscious. What is conscious about thoughts are images, tones, silent speech, and, to a lesser degree, other bodily feelings associated with intermediate-level sensory representations.[2] Neither the process of thought nor its content is knowable by consciousness. You are not directly conscious of your inner world, although you have the persistent illusion that you are!

An example may make this clearer. A bilingual person can express a thought in either language, but the thought that underlies the words remains hidden. It manifests itself to consciousness only by suggestive imagery or unspoken speech, or by externalizing it. Hence the stock phrase, "How do I know what I think 'till I hear what I say?"

This idea, which dates back at least to the philosopher Immanuel Kant, is quite appealing to us, although it has attracted rather little attention from other brain scientists. Freud proposed something similar, based on his extensive studies of disturbed patients. Consider this quotation:

> In psycho-analysis there is no choice but for us to assert that mental processes are in themselves unconscious, and to liken the perception of them by means of consciousness to the perception of the external world by means of sense-organs.[3]

A related idea was advanced by Karl Lashley, an influential American neuroscientist from the middle of the last century:

> *No activity of mind is ever conscious* [Lashley's italics]. This sounds like a paradox, but it is nonetheless true. There are order and arrangement, but there is no experience of the creation of that order. I could give numberless examples, for there is no exception to the rule. A couple of illustrations should suffice. Look at a complicated scene. It consists of a number of objects standing out against an indistinct background: desk, chairs, faces. Each consists of a number of lesser sensations combined in the object, but there is no experience of putting them together. The objects are immediately present. When we think in words, the thoughts come in grammatical form with subject, verb, object, and modifying clauses falling into place without our having the slightest perception of how the sentence structure is produced.... Experience clearly gives no clue as to the means by which it is organized.[4]

---

[2]Of course, there are disenting views from Jackendoff's (1987) position that all thoughts are expressed in sensory terms (Strawson, 1996; Siewert, 1998; and many of the commentators in Crick and Koch, 2000).

[3]From his essay on *The Unconscious* (Freud, 1915).

[4]Lashley (1956).

Both authors arrived at broadly the same conclusion from significantly different perspectives and research traditions.[5]

You are only conscious, then, of representations of external objects (including your own body) or internal events by proxy. You are not directly conscious of something in the world, say a chair, but only of its visual and tactile representation in the cortex. The chair is out there; your only direct knowledge of it is derived from explicit, but *intermediate*, representations of your senses in your brain that leave out many fine details, like the chiaroscuro patterns of changing brightness, the exact wavelength distribution of the incoming light, and other minutiae that retinal neurons are susceptible to. Likewise with recalled or imagined things. By and large, these are mapped onto visual, auditory, olfactory, gustatory, vestibular, tactile, and propioceptive representations. A subset of these, the NCC, are experienced as qualia. These involve one or more (Section 18.3) dominant coalitions stretching between cortical regions in the back and more frontal ones.

18.2 | THE NONCONSCIOUS HOMUNCULUS

The intermediate-level theory of consciousness accounts well for a widely shared and persistent feeling: That there is a little person, a *homunculus*, inside my head who perceives the world through the senses, who thinks, and who plans and carries out voluntary actions. Frequently ridiculed in science and philosophy, the idea of a homunculus is, nevertheless, profoundly appealing because it resonates with the everyday experience of who "I" am.

This overwhelming sense of the way things are may reflect the neuroanatomy of the forebrain. Indeed, Francis and I believe[6] that somewhere in the confines of the frontal lobe are neuronal networks that act to all intents and purposes like a homunculus. This is a nonconscious homunculus who receives massive sensory input from the back of the cortex (olfaction is an exception to this rule), makes decisions, and feeds these to the relevant motor stages. Crudely put, the homunculus "looks at" the back of the cortex; neuroanatomically this means that it receives a strong, driving projection from there into its input layer (Section 7.4) while the connections in the reverse direction look quite different.

The psychologist Fred Attneave cites two kinds of objections to a homunculus.[7] The first is an aversion to dualism, because it might involve "a fluffy kind

---

[5]Stevens (1997) has expressed similar ideas in a different idiom. For a philosophical perspective on all of this, see Metzinger (1995).

[6]Crick and Koch (2000 and 2003).

[7]See Attneave's 1961 essay entitled *In Defense of Homunculi*. He tentatively locates the homunculus in a subcortical region, such as the reticular formation. Attneave considers it to be conscious. His basic idea is otherwise similar to the one discussed here.

of nonmatter. . .quite beyond the pale of scientific investigation." This criticism does not apply here since the homunculus corresponds to the action of a real physical system, situated in the frontal lobe and closely associated structures, such as the basal ganglia. The second challenge has to do with the supposed regressive nature of the concept. Who, after all, is looking at the brain states of the homunculus? Wouldn't this require another homunculus inside the first one, to control and plan its actions? Like a never-ending set of ever-smaller Russian dolls, one stacked inside the other, this leads to an infinite regress with each homunculus being controlled by another, even smaller one. However, in our case there is no infinite regress because the homunculus is not meant to explain qualia (Section 14.6). Our homunculus acts more like a computational entity.

The concept of the nonconscious homunculus is not trivial. As discussed in the previous section, it is responsible for many complex operations, such as thoughts, concept formation, intentions, and so on. Indeed, I am tempted to label all such operations as *supramental*, given their location in the mind's processing hierarchy. Supramental processing is beyond conscious perception; this stands in contrast to the *submental* domain concerned with the more primitive processing stages that likewise escape conscious access.

The nonconscious homunculus proposal throws new light on certain other open questions, such as that of creativity, problem solving, and insight. It has long been asserted that much of creativity is not conscious. The French mathematician Jacques Hadamard queried famous scientists and fellow mathematicians about the origin of their innovative ideas. They reported that a long period of intense engagement with the problem, a sort of incubation, followed by a good night's sleep or a few day's diversions, preceded the crucial insight that just "popped into their head." The cognitive inaccessibility of insights has been confirmed by more recent studies of problem solving.[8]

I have had similar experiences. Let me tell you about an eerie one. I am usually a sound sleeper, but a few years ago I suddenly woke up in the middle of the night knowing I was going to die: not right there and then, but someday. I did not have any premonition of accidents about to happen, cancer, or so on—just the gut realization that my life was going to end, sooner or later. I have no idea why I woke up and why I was suddenly pondering eternity. I had experienced a close death in my family ten years earlier, but had spent little time thinking about it since then. Judging from this haunting incident, which remains with me to this day, my nonconscious homunculus must have been occupied with death for quite some time.

---

[8] See Hadamard (1945) as well as Poincaré's (1952) famous account. Cognitive science has supported the hypothesis that creativity involves nonreportable (that is, nonconscious) processes (Schooler, Ohlsson, and Brooks, 1993; and Schooler and Melcher, 1995).

18.3 | THE NATURE OF QUALIA

In Section 14.6 I argued that qualia are symbols, a peculiar property of highly parallel feedback networks that stand for an enormous amount of explicit and implicit information. The explicit information is expressed by the NCC at the various essential nodes, while the implicit information is distributed across a large population of neurons that make up the NCC's penumbra.

Just as there are different types of artificial symbols—letters, numbers, hieroglyphs, traffic signs—there are distinct neuronal symbols with their trademark qualia. In the case of qualia, these differ not only in their content but also in their time course, intensity, and whether they are elemental or composites.

A bright red light triggers a simple color quale, while looking at a dog or a face leads to a much richer and detailed percept. All three arise rapidly and can disappear equally quickly. Conversely, the quale associated with the feeling of *déjà vu* or being angry takes a lot longer to develop and subside and may have fewer associations.

As a class, the phenomenal feelings associated with imagination and memory tend to be less vivid than those generated by an external stimulus, although people's ability to conjure up mental images varies considerably.[9] Consider the tan Husky-Shepherd mix lying at my feet as I write this. I can clearly see her snout, pointed ears, attentive eyes tracking my every movement, and gorgeous coat of fur. If I close my eyes and try to recall her, the image of the dog is hazy and vague. The associated qualia are much weaker, less intense, and less life-like, with fewer details.[10]

I believe that the degree of vividness manifests itself at the neuronal level as the extent of the coalition representing the NCC. The more widespread the neuronal membership of the winning coalition, the more details and aspects are consciously expressed and the more vivid the percept.

As pointed out in Section 5.4, single neuron recordings in patients and functional brain imaging of volunteers demonstrate that the response in the upper stages of the vision-for-perception processing hierarchy to imagined pictures is as selective and almost as strong as it is to pictures that are seen.[11] It is likely

---

[9]Sacks (2003) discusses this variability in imagery. He mentions his mother, a surgeon and anatomist, who would gaze intently at a lizard's skeleton for a minute and then, without referring to the animal again, sketch a number of drawings, each one rotated by thirty degrees. Sacks compares this to his own faint and evanescent attempts at imagery.

[10]Some classes of percepts, in particular those associated with smells and, mercifully, pain, are difficult to imagine or recall. This might be due to a lack of cortico-cortical feedback projections into the olfactory and insular cortices responsible for these percepts.

[11]The single-cell data on imagery are described in Kreiman, Koch, and Fried (2000b) and the fMRI studies in Kosslyn, Thompson, and Alpert (1997); O'Craven and Kanwisher (2000); and

that cells in the early stages of the visual cortex, in V1, V2 and V3, are less strongly activated during imagery than during retinal stimulation. In other words, the further down the visual hierarchy a given area is, the less it participates in imagery and the less vivid the perceived picture in the mind's eye. The feedback pathways from the front of the cortex reaching back, into the far end of the brain, may not have the spatial selectivity necessary to influence the firing activity there in a precise enough manner. The result is a less compelling sense of seeing with your mind's eye. This can be a good thing, for otherwise you might not be able to tell reality from a delusion.

One class of conscious feelings has a rather different character from straightforward sensory percepts. Examples include feelings of familiarity, novelty, having a name on the tip of the tongue, the sudden rush of understanding a sentence or argument, and the various emotions. The feeling of consciously willing an act, referred to as the feeling of *authorship*, also falls into this category. This percept mediates the sense of being the agent who voluntarily initiated some motor action, such as lifting a hand or squeezing a lever.[12] Whether the qualia associated with these feelings, more diffuse and less detailed than sensory percepts, exist in their own right or are mixtures or modifications of various bodily sensations, is unclear.

Chapter 16 summarizes the compelling evidence that the NCC for visual percepts involve coalitions based in the higher regions of the ventral pathway. I argued in Chapters 14 and 15 that feedback from the frontal lobes is probably necessary to consolidate the winner. Such a coalition would stretch from higher visual cortices to the prefrontal cortex. Would a winning coalition whose membership is primarily recruited from the frontal lobes have a fundamentally different character, explaining the different classes of qualia? Might the distinction between crisp and rapid sensory qualia, and less vivid, more diffuse, and lingering abstract qualia correspond to different kinds of coalitions in the back and the front of the brain? These questions cannot be answered without a much better understanding of the anatomy and physiology of the prefrontal and anterior singulate cortices. We don't even know whether this sector of the brain is organized along hierarchical lines, as is the sensory cortex.

Kosslyn, Ganis, and Thompson (2001). For an elegant monkey study implicating the prefrontal cortex as the source of recalled information, consult Tomita et al. (1999).

[12] Wegner (2002) provides both real-life and laboratory examples in which the feeling of authorship does not correspond to the actual course of events. In some cases, the subject believes that she was responsible for an action that was, in reality, triggered by another person; in others, the converse situation occurred and the subject denied being responsible for some action when she, undoubtedly, did cause it. It appears that some part of the brain is responsible for generating the feeling, the percept, of being the initiating agent of some motor action. Is the NCC for authorship percepts to be found in the motor or premotor regions of the cortex?

18.4 | RECAPITULATION

In this chapter I introduced Jackendoff's intermediate-level theory of consciousness, which postulates that the inner world of thoughts and concepts is forever hidden from consciousness, as is the external, physical world, including the body.

One consequence of this hypothesis is that many aspects of high-level cognition, such as decision-making, planning, and creativity, are beyond the pale of awareness. These operations are carried out by the nonconscious homunculus residing in the front of the forebrain, receiving information from the sensory regions in the back, and relaying its output to the motor system.

A further consequence is that you are not directly conscious of your thoughts. You are conscious only of a re-representation of these in terms of sensory qualities, particularly visual imagery, and inner speech.

Let me put this differently. The bulk of nervous tissue is given over to submental processing that transforms sensory inputs into motor outputs. Some fraction of neurons that access explicit representations of the external world are sufficient for specific conscious percepts. Supramental processing—thoughts and other complex manipulations of sensory or abstract data and patterns—occurs in the upper stages, the habitat of the nonconscious homunculus. Its content is not directly knowable by consciousness, which arises at the interface between the representations of the outer and inner worlds.

Real, physical stimuli usually give rise to much more intense and complex qualia than imaginary ones. This is probably because the cortico-cortical feedback connections from the front of the cortex back into the relevant sensory regions are, without help from a sensory input, unable to recruit the large coalition needed to fully express the sundry aspects of an object or event. It may be possible that qualia associated with the winning coalition in the front of the brain have a different character than those associated with the back.

The picture that emerges from all of this is quite elegant in its symmetry. You can never directly know the outer world. Instead, you are conscious of the results of some of the computations performed by your nervous system on one or more representations of the world. In a similar way, you can't know your innermost thoughts. Instead, you are aware only of the sensory representations associated with these mental activities. If true, this has profound implications for the age-old project of Western philosophy, encapsulated in the adage *Know Thyself.*

What remains is the sobering realization that the subjective world of qualia—what distinguishes you and me from zombies and fills our life with color, music, smells, gusto, and zest—depends crucially on the subtle, flickering spiking patterns of a set of neurons, located strategically between these outer and inner worlds.

CHAPTER NINETEEN

A Framework for Consciousness

Only those who risk going too far
can possibly find out how far one can go.

T.S. Eliot

The last seventeen chapters dealt with the biological and psychological foundations of consciousness in great detail. I here pull all these threads together and present them in a unified fashion. Francis's and my ultimate aim has been to map all the concepts in the vicinity of consciousness onto the properties of synapses, action potentials, neurons, and their coalitions. Our program has been to concentrate on the neuronal correlates of consciousness, the NCC. As explained in Chapter 5, we are less concerned with the enabling factors necessary for any conscious state to occur, than we are to discover the chain of neuronal events that leads up to any one specific sensation.

No matter their philosophical or religious proclivities, scholars who think about these matters agree that there are material correlates of consciousness in the brain and that their properties can be analyzed using the scientific method. And many—though not all—students of the mind agree that discovering the NCC will be profitable for any final theory of consciousness.

Surveying the state of the brain sciences in a 1979 article in *Scientific American*, Francis Crick opined that "What is conspicuously lacking is a broad framework of ideas within which to interpret all these different approaches." In the intervening years, he and I have constructed such a framework for thinking about the conscious mind.

We decided to distill our approach into nine working hypotheses that explicitly articulate our assumptions and published these in *Nature Neuroscience* in 2003.[1] It seems appropriate to finish the book by listing and discussing this broad set of connected ideas. Our framework is not a set of crisply formulated

---

[1] Crick and Koch (2003). In this chapter, I added a tenth assumption that emerges naturally from my treatment of the penumbra, meaning, and qualia in Chapter 14.

propositions, but rather a suggested point of view for an attack on a most difficult scientific problem. Unlike physics, biology has few ironclad principles and
laws. Natural selection produces a hierarchy of mechanisms, so there are few
rules in biology that do not have exceptions. A good framework is one that is
reasonably plausible—relative to the available scientific data—and that turns
out to be largely correct. It is unlikely to be correct in all details.

19.1 | TEN WORKING ASSUMPTIONS TO UNDERSTAND THE MIND-BODY PROBLEM

First, a few of my philosophical background assumptions.

Philosophical Background Assumptions

I have been careful to avoid taking a rigid ideological position on the exact
nature of the kinship between objective brain events and subjective conscious
ones. In the face of more than two millennia of scholastic dispute, not enough
is known at this stage to make any firm pronouncements.

Our approach is to focus on the empirically most accessible aspects of the
mind-body problem, perceptual awareness or consciousness. This makes the
problem more tractable since the neuronal mechanisms underlying perception are quite accessible in animals. We neglect for now the contributions that
emotions, moods, and language make toward perceptual awareness.

We do assume that any phenomenological state—seeing a dog, having pain,
and so on—depends on a brain state. The neuronal correlates of consciousness
are the minimal set of neuronal events jointly sufficient for a specific conscious
phenomenal state (given the appropriate background enabling conditions; see
Section 5.1). Every percept is accompanied by some NCC.

At the core of the mind-body problem are qualia, the elements of consciousness. Francis and I seek to explain how these arise from, or out of, the action
of the nervous system.

Assumption 1: The Nonconscious Homunculus

A convenient way to think of the overall behavior of the cerebral cortex is
that the front of the cortex is looking at the back. By this I mean that the
long-distance, forward projections from the back are strong connections (Section 7.4), sufficient to drive their postsynaptic targets in layer 4 of the recipient
frontal area. This view is in accordance with the way most people think of
themselves: as a homunculus, sitting inside the head, and looking out at the
world.

The NCC involve one coalition of forebrain neurons (or perhaps a few; Sections 2.1 and 11.3). The NCC may not have direct access to regions of the forebrain involved in decision-making, planning, and other aspects of high-level cognition. That is, consciousness may be limited to the intermediate levels of the brain (Section 18.1). In that sense, the proverbial homunculus in the frontal lobe is largely not conscious. This division of labor does not lead to an infinite regress, since the qualia are not generated by the homunculus itself (Section 18.2).

Thoughts are not consciously accessible either (Chapter 18). It is only their sensory reflection and re-representation in inner speech and imagery that are directly knowable.

Assumption 2: Zombie Agents and Consciousness

Many, if not most, motor actions in response to external events are rapid, transient, stereotyped, and nonconscious. These are mediated by highly specialized and trained zombie agents that are not, by themselves, associated with conscious awareness. They can be thought of as generalized, cortical reflexes (Chapters 12 and 13).

Consciousness deals with broader, less commonplace, and more taxing aspects of the world or a reflection of these in imagery (Chapter 14). Consciousness is necessary for planning and choice among multiple courses of action. Otherwise, a vast army of zombie agents would have to deal with all possible contingencies encountered in the real world. The function of consciousness is to summarize the current state of the world in a compact representation and make this "executive summary" accessible to the planning stages of the brain (Section 14.1), which includes the nonconscious homunculus. The content of this summary is the content of consciousness.

The slower, conscious system may interfere somewhat with simultaneously active zombie agents. By means of sufficient repetition, specific sensory-motor behaviors that initially require consciousness, such as hitting a backhand in tennis, can eventually be carried out effortlessly by an automatic zombie agent (Section 14.2).

It is likely that a net-wave of action potentials, sweeping in from the sensory periphery in a feedforward manner, through more central structures and onward to the muscles, can trigger zombie behaviors without being sufficient for conscious awareness (Sections 12.3 and 15.3).

Assumption 3: Coalitions of Neurons

The forebrain is a highly interconnected and fiendishly complex tapestry of neuronal networks. Any one percept, real or imagined, corresponds to a coalition of neurons. A coalition reinforces the firing activity of its member neurons, probably by synchronizing their spiking discharge, and suppresses competing ones. The dynamics of coalitions will not be easy to understand, though it is clear that winner-take-all competition plays a key role.

At any one moment, the winning coalition, expressing the actual content of consciousness, is somewhat sustained. A very short-lived coalition corresponds to a fleeting form of consciousness (Section 9.3). A useful metaphor is the hustle and bustle underlying the electoral process in a democracy (Section 2.1).

Coalitions vary in size and character. Consider, for example, the difference between seeing a scene and imagining it later, with your eyes closed. The coalitions that are sufficient for imagery—less vivid a percept than that arising from normal seeing—are likely to be less widespread than the coalitions produced by external input, and may not reach down to the lower tiers of the cortical processing hierarchy (Section 18.3).

Given the all-or-none character of conscious perception (Section 15.2), the neural activity representing some feature has to exceed a threshold (which might differ from one attribute to the next). It is unlikely to do so unless it is, or is becoming, part of a successful coalition. The neural activity sufficient for the conscious perception of this attribute, the NCC, is maintained above threshold for a while, probably with the aid of feedback from frontal structures, such as the anterior cingulate and the prefrontal cortex. Some aspects of the NCC may be binary; for instance, they may take on one of two different firing rate values—and may also show hysteresis, that is, the activity may stay there longer than its support warrants. Different conscious aspects of a percept may exceed thresholds at slightly different times, reflecting the fact that the unity of consciousness breaks down at these short times.

Assumption 4: Explicit Representations and Essential Nodes

An explicit representation of some stimulus attribute is a set of neurons that "detects" that feature without much further processing (Section 2.2). If no such neurons exist or if they are destroyed, the subject is unable to consciously perceive that aspect directly. Underlying every direct and conscious perception is an explicit representation (the "activity principle"; Figure 2.5). Explicit coding is a property of individual neurons.

The cerebral cortex, at least its sensory regions, can be thought of as having nodes. Each node expresses one aspect of any one percept. An aspect cannot become conscious unless there is an essential node for it (Section 2.2). This is a necessary but not sufficient condition for the NCC. There are other necessary conditions, such as projecting to the front of the brain and receiving appropriate feedback that exceeds some threshold for some time (Sections 12.3 and

15.3). If the essential node for some aspect, such as color, is destroyed, the subject loses *that* aspect of conscious perception, but not others.

A node, all by itself, cannot produce consciousness. Even if the neurons in that node were firing away, this would yield little effect if their output synapses were inactivated. A node is part of a network. Any one conscious percept is associated with a coalition, consisting of multi-focal activity at numerous essential nodes, each one representing one particular attribute.

The neuronal substrate for the twin concepts of explicit coding and essential nodes is likely to be the columnar organization of information in the cortex (Section 2.2). A column can be envisioned as the smallest useful node. The receptive field property common to most cells in a column is made explicit there. This column will (usually) be part of the essential node for that property.

Assumption 5: The Higher Levels First

Following an eye movement that brings a new part of the visual scene into view, the neural activity, the net-wave, moves rapidly, in a forward manner, up the visual hierarchy all the way to the prefrontal cortex and to the relevant motor structures. Such forward activity is the basis for at least some nonconscious zombie behaviors (Sections 12.3 and 15.3).

After reaching the prefrontal cortex, signals travel backward down the hierarchy, so that the first stages contributing to the content of consciousness are the higher levels. This signal is then relayed back to the prefrontal areas, followed by corresponding activity at successively lower levels. Neuronal representations for the gist of a scene in higher areas mediate the vivid sense of perceiving an entire scene at once, of seeing everything—a compelling illusion (Section 9.3).

How far up the hierarchy the initial net-wave travels depends upon expectation and selective attention.

The upper stages of the ventral, vision-for-perception pathway (Figure 7.3), in and around the inferior temporal cortex and its postsynaptic structures, are the most likely hunting grounds for neurons that correlate with visual consciousness (Section 16.3). NCC cells are unlikely to be found in the primary visual cortex (Chapter 6) or earlier. The dorsal pathway is not essential for conscious perception of form, shape, color, and object identity.

Assumption 6: Driving and Modulatory Connections

When considering the dynamics of coalitions, it is essential to understand the nature of neuronal connections. The systematic arrangement of neuronal (synaptic) inputs into discrete classes is still quite primitive.

Excitatory cells can be initially classified as driving or modulating their target structures (Section 7.4). Forward projections are driving, because they can trigger a vigorous action potential discharge, while feedback acts to modulate the cellular response. The majority of connections from the back of the cortex to the front are likely to be driving. This is why it seems as though the front of the brain is looking at the back. Conversely, the reverse connections, from the front to the back, are largely modulatory. This classification of driving and modulatory connections also applies to the thalamus (Section 7.3). *Strong* loops of driving connections do not normally occur within the confines of the cortico-cortical or cortico-thalamic networks.

Assumption 7: Snapshots

Perceptual awareness may correspond to a series of static snapshots, with motion "painted on" to them (Section 15.5). That is, perception may occur in discrete epochs of variable duration (between 20 and 200 msec). This bears a striking resemblance to a movie in which the illusion of movement and life is created by rapidly flipping through a series of stationary scenes.

Unlike the clock period in computers, the duration of successive snapshots varies and probably depends on the saliency of the input, eye movements, habituation, expectancy, and so on. Furthermore, the time of a snapshot for one attribute may not exactly coincide with that for another attribute.

The challenge is to understand how temporally discontinuous snapshots emerge out of meta-stable coalitions of neurons whose firing activities evolve continuously in time.

Assumption 8: Attention and Binding

Selective attention can be divided into at least two forms—one which is bottom-up and saliency-driven, and another which is top-down and volitionally controlled. Bottom-up attention is rapid and automatic. Dominated by the input stream, bottom-up attention expresses the saliency of some feature or object relative to features in its vicinity. Top-down attention depends on the task at hand and can be directed to a location in space, to a particular attribute throughout the field of view, or to an object (Sections 9.1 and 9.2).

These psychological concepts can all be expressed in terms of the relevant neuronal networks. More than one object or event can be perceived simultaneously, provided that their representations don't overlap in the relevant thalamic and cortical networks. If they do overlap, bottom-up attention favors the most salient one. If their saliency is comparable, top-down attention is needed to boost the neuronal representation of the attended stimulus at the expense of the neglected stimulus. That is, attention biases the competition among rival coalitions, especially during their formation (Sections 10.1 and 10.2).

Without such overlap, top-down attention may not be strictly necessary to perceive an object (Section 9.3). For instance, a single, familiar, isolated object can be consciously perceived when top-down attention is occupied elsewhere. Gist perception is likely to bypass attentional selection mechanisms.

Based on the aforementioned, attention is closely allied to consciousness yet is likely to be implemented by a distinct neuronal process. Therefore, there may not always be a one-to-one relationship between the focus of attention and the current content of consciousness.

The various attributes of any one object—its color, motion, the sounds it makes, and so on—are represented in an explicit manner by essential nodes throughout the cortex. How this information is combined to yield a single, unitary percept constitutes one facet of the binding problem (Section 9.4); another is how information from multiple objects is kept distinct.

Three types of binding mechanisms need to be distinguished. Groups of cells can be specified epigenetically to respond to particular combinations of inputs, such as location and orientation in V1. Neurons can also be wired up through experience to encode an object, such as the face, voice, and mannerisms of a familiar or famous individual. Both of these forms of binding may be independent of top-down attention. A third type of binding deals with novel or rarely encountered objects or events. In this case, top-down, selective attention is probably necessary to bind the activities of separate essential nodes (coding for the various attributes of the perceived object) together.

Assumption 9: Styles of Firing

Synchronized and rhythmic action potential discharge (in particular, in the 30 to 60 Hz band) may increase the postsynaptic impact of neurons—their punch—without necessarily altering their average firing rate (Section 2.3). One likely purpose is to assist a nascent coalition in its competition with other newly forming coalitions. Attention may bias the competition between coalitions by modulating the degree of synchrony among neurons within a coalition, boosting the group's postsynaptic impact.

Synchronization of spiking activity among neurons may not be needed once a successful coalition has reached consciousness, because it may be able to maintain itself, without the assistance of synchrony, at least for a while.

Firing rhythms in the 4 to 12 Hz bands may correspond to the discrete snapshot processing.

Assumption 10: Penumbra, Meaning, and Qualia

The winning coalition recruits its members in the cortex, thalamus, basal ganglia, and other closely allied networks. This coalition will influence a large number of neurons that are not part of the NCC—their penumbra. The penumbra includes the neural substrate of past associations, the expected consequences of the NCC, the cognitive background, and future plans. The penumbra is outside of the NCC proper, although some of its elements may become part of the NCC as the NCC shift. The penumbra provides the brain with the meaning of the relevant essential nodes—their aboutness (Section 14.5).

It is unclear whether mere synaptic activation of the penumbra is sufficient for meaning or whether the NCC need to trigger action potentials within the cells making up the penumbra. The answer probably depends on the extent to which projections from the penumbra back to the NCC support or maintain the NCC.

Qualia are a symbolic form of representation of all of this vast ocean of explicit and implicit information associated with the NCC. They come to stand for the penumbra. Qualia are a property of parallel feedback networks in the brain whose activity lasts for a minimal amount of time.

Why qualia *feel* the way they do remains an enigma.

19.2 | RELATIONSHIP TO THE WORK OF OTHERS

The last twenty years have seen a steady stream of biologically-flavored proposals regarding the NCC. These are noteworthy for the refreshing directness with which they attack this problem, which elicited snickers among the cognoscenti only a few years earlier.[2] I have already referred to many of the individual ideas in the relevant chapters. A few of these scholars have conceptualized the problem in terms that are amenable to the type of sustained, neurobiological approach at the cellular level that I advocate. How does our body of work relate to these?

As I pointed out in Chapter 5, Edelman by himself, as well as jointly with Tononi, has built over the years a sophisticated framework for naturalizing consciousness.[3] Starting from the twin observations that consciousness is experienced as integrated (the unity of consciousness) and as highly differentiated (an astronomically large number of phenomenal states are possible), Edelman and Tononi have inferred the existence of a large cluster of thalamocortical neurons organized as a unified neuronal process of high complexity, the *dynamic core*. This coalition of neurons underlies conscious experience. It is stabilized for hundreds of milliseconds by massive feedback (what Edelman

---

[2] Besides those cited earlier or in the main text, I would like to mention Greenfield (1995); Cotterill (1998); Calvin (1998); Llinas et al. (1998); Jaspers (1998); and Taylor (1998).
[3] Edelman (1989, 2003); Tononi and Edelman (1998); and Edelman and Tononi (2000).

calls reentrant signaling loops) and is defined by the functional requirement that core members interact more strongly with each other than with the rest of the brain. The dynamic core is not that different from our conception of the NCC as the dominant coalition of neurons stretching halfway across the cortex.

Edelman and Tononi deny that local, intrinsic properties of neurons, of defined neuronal circuits, or of cortical areas play any privileged role in the neuronal roots of consciousness. They stress the import of global features of the dynamic core, in particular the abilities of groups of neurons to form a sheer limitless number of subassemblies of high network complexity. A sobering drawback of any such holistic theory is the inherent difficulty of subjecting it to empirical validation and of explaining why so much brain activity and behavior can occur without conscious sensation.

The edifice closest to ours in spirit is the one by Dehaene (Section 15.3) and the eminent molecular biologist Jean-Pierre Changeux of the Institut Pasteur in Paris.[4] In their thinking, backed up by a computer model of the neural events accompanying visual attentional selection and deselection, the primary correlate of consciousness is a sudden, self-amplifying surge in activity, nurtured by feedback activity from prefrontal, cingulate, and parietal cortices. Once this activity exceeds a threshold, it is powerful enough to access a global network of reciprocally connected, long-range projection neurons that provide access to working memory, and to other cognitive resources such as planning. This is a neuronal instantiation of Baars's global workspace (see footnote 26 on page 98). Competition within this network prevents more than one neuronal coalition surviving at any one moment. Bottom-up and top-down attentional signals influence access to the global workspace.

There are obviously many commonalities between their proposal and ours. Where we differ most decisively is in our arguments concerning explicit coding, essential nodes, and the exclusion of the NCC from certain regions—such as the primary visual cortex and parts of the prefrontal cortex, the habitat of the nonconscious homunculus.

I am encouraged that, on the whole, many of these proposals converge on concepts that are not too dissimilar (though often expressed in different idioms).

There is one marked difference between the ideas expressed in this book and those of others. Most scholars emphasize how the collective, Gestalt-like traits of the brain and its networks are critical to understanding consciousness. While there is no doubt that many global aspects will be absolutely of the essence for the genesis of consciousness, this should not come at the expense of neglect-

---

[4]Changeux (1983); Dehaene and Naccache (2001); Dehaene, Sergent, and Changeux (2003); and Dehaene and Changeux (2004).

ing the attributes of synapses, neurons, and their particular arrangements. As molecular biology has demonstrated so convincingly, it is the specific inter-actions among individual molecules that permits them to encode and copy information over the lifetime of the organism. Our approach tries to synthe-size both local and holistic aspects of consciousness to arrive at a new view of a very ancient problem.

19.3 | WHERE DO WE GO FROM HERE?

I want to conclude this chapter by venturing some guesses about the meth-ods and experiments that will be needed to bring the quest for the nature of consciousness to a successful conclusion.

It is essential to develop a principled understanding of the properties of small and large coalitions of forebrain neurons using electrical or optical recordings of their spike trains in appropriately trained animals. Deciphering, displaying, and understanding the gigabytes of data obtained from even a single experiment of this type will require new computational methods and algorithms.

It has now become possible to monitor the simultaneous spiking activity from many neurons at numerous stages in the visual hierarchy and in the front of the cortex while a monkey is experiencing binocular rivalry, flash suppres-sion, motion-induced blindness, or other perceptual stimuli in which one and the same physical stimulus can give rise to different percepts (Chapter 16). Modern anesthetic technology permits the monkey to be rapidly and reversibly put to sleep while the electrodes stay in place. This should allow for a direct comparison between conscious and nonconscious states and might uncover crucial clues that illuminate the NCC.

Occasionally, multiple electrodes are chronically implanted into alert patients. With their consent, this can provide sparse but critical data about the behavior of neurons during conscious perception or imagery. It would be invaluable if cortical tissue could be stimulated appropriately with such electrodes to generate specific percepts, thoughts, or actions.[5]

Magnetic resonance imaging techniques need to be further refined. While lacking the spatio-temporal resolution of microelectrodes, they allow metabolic, hemodynamic, or neuronal activity throughout the entire brain to be moni-tored. The use of sophisticated MR dyes that track increased levels of intra-cellular calcium, or gene products in animals, are particularly noteworthy.[6] Invasive methods that detect early-immediate genes (such as c-fos), considered

---

[5]Fried et al. (1998); and Graziano, Taylor and Moore (2002).
[6]Li et al. (2002); and Alauddin et al. (2003).

to be a marker of neuronal activity, are immensely useful since they permit individual active neurons to be pinpointed in rodents or other animals with small brains.[7]

The critical role of neuroanatomy as the essential backdrop for this research cannot be overemphasized. It is analogous to the insight the human genome project provided for molecular biology. The knowledge of detailed connectivity patterns within the cerebral cortex and the thalamus needs to be greatly expanded, in particular to characterize the many different types of pyramidal cells in any particular cortical area. What do they look like, where do they project and, eventually, does each have a set of characteristic genetic markers? Are there types of pyramidal cells that do not occur in all cortical areas? When recording spiking activity from a neuron, it would be helpful to know what cell type it is and to where it projects. An understanding of the geography of the frontal lobe, now in its infancy, is badly needed. Is there a hierarchy, or possibly a reverse hierarchy there, as there is in the visual system (Section 7.2)?

As I have emphasized throughout the book, neurons are not just stereotyped machines that transduce synaptic input into trains of action potentials for their output. They have unique identities; in particular, their axons project to different locations and connect with different classes of cells. It is very likely that their message differs, too, depending on the nature of the recipients. When monitoring the output of a neuron with the help of a nearby electrode, it is imperative to know the target audience of *this particular cell*. Anonymous recordings, as they are widely practiced today, will never be sufficient to help dissect the circuits responsible for any percept. Relevant techniques (e.g., antidromic stimulation, photoactivation) need to be developed and enhanced so that they can be routinely applied to behaving animals. Having the complete inventory of projection neurons for any one region would help this task enormously.

The true potential of molecular biology to uncover and dissect brain circuits is just beginning to be exploited. Methods are currently under development that deliberately, selectively, transiently, and reversibly silence genetically identified populations of mammalian neurons.[8] These tools permit many of the ideas outlined in this book to be tested by dissecting the relevant circuits. For example, imagine that some types of cortico-cortical feedback connections could be turned off and on again, by briefly interrupting the appropriate synapses, without interfering with forward pathways. This would allow the importance of top-down feedback signals for selective attention and consciousness to be directly assessed. To fully realize the immense promise of

---

[7]Though these methods are rather laborious. Dragunow and Faull (1989); and Han et al. (2003).
[8]Lechner, Lein, and Callaway (2002); Slimko et al. (2002); and Yamamoto et al. (2003).

these molecular techniques, assays for attention and consciousness that work in mice and simpler organisms, such as fruitflies, must be developed. These tests should be robust and practical enough that they allow large-scale screening for behavioral mutants.

19.4 | RECAPITULATION

All the conceptual spade work Francis and I have engaged in over the years is summarized in this chapter in the form of ten working assumptions. This provisional framework is a guide to constructing more detailed hypotheses, so that they can be tested against already existing evidence. Furthermore, the framework should suggest new experiments. As the coming years accumulate to decades, a more rigorous theoretical edifice will replace our tentative scaffolding.

Francis and I aim to explain all aspects of the first-person perspective of consciousness in terms of the activity of identified nerve cells, their interconnectivities, and the dynamics of coalitions of neurons. This is a bit like playing three-dimensional chess: You must keep simultaneous track of the phenomenology of consciousness, the behavior of the organism, and the underlying neuronal events. It won't be easy, but then no truly worthwhile task ever is.

We live at a unique point in the history of science. The technology to discover and characterize how the subjective mind emerges out of the objective brain is within reach. The next years will prove decisive.

CHAPTER TWENTY

An Interview

"Would you tell me, please," said Alice, "what that means?"

"Now, you talk like a reasonable child," said Humpty Dumpty, looking
very much pleased. "I meant by 'impenetrability' that we've had enough
of that subject, and it would be just as well if you'd mention what you
mean to do next, as I suppose you don't mean to stop here all the rest of
your life."

From *Through the Looking Glass* by Lewis Carroll

What does all of this amount to in the
grand scheme of things? Thinking about consciousness naturally gives rise to
a host of questions about meaning, animal experimentation, free will, the possibility of machine awareness, and so on. In this coda, I address some of these
topics in a format more conducive to speculation, a fictitious interview.

Interviewer: Let's start at the beginning. What is the overall strategy that you
are pursuing in tackling this problem?

Christof: First, I take consciousness seriously, as a brute fact that needs to
be explained. The first-person perspective, feelings, qualia, awareness, phenomenal experiences—call it what you want—are real phenomena that arise
out of certain privileged brain processes. They make up the landscape of
conscious life: the deep red of a sunset over the Pacific Ocean, the fragrance
of a rose, the searing anger that wells up at seeing an abused dog, the memory of the exploding space shuttle *Challenger* on live TV. Science's ability to
comprehend the universe will be limited unless and until it can explain how
certain physical systems can be sufficient for such subjective states.

Second, I argue for putting aside, for now, the difficult problems that
philosophers debate—in particular the question of why is it that it feels
like something to see, hear, or to be me—and concentrate on a scientific
exploration of the molecular and neuronal correlates of consciousness
(NCC). The question I focus on is, *What are the minimal neuronal mechanisms jointly sufficient for a specific conscious percept?* Given the amazing

technologies that brain scientists have at their disposal—engineering the mammalian genome, simultaneously recording from hundreds of neurons in a monkey, imaging the living human brain—the search for the neuronal correlates of consciousness, the NCC, is tractable, clearly defined, and will yield to a concerted scientific attack.

I: Do you mean to imply that discovering the NCC will solve the mystery of consciousness?

C: No, no, no! Ultimately, what is needed is a principled account explaining why and under what circumstances certain types of very complex biological entities have subjective experiences and why these experiences appear the way they do. The past two thousand years are littered with attempts to solve these mysteries, so they truly are hard problems.

Remember how much the elucidation of the double-helical structure of DNA revealed about molecular replication? The two complementary chains of sugar, phosphate, and amine bases, linked by weak hydrogen bonds, immediately suggested a mechanism whereby genetic information could be represented, copied, and passed on to the next generation. The architecture of the DNA molecule led to an understanding of heredity that was simply beyond the capabilities of the previous generations of chemists and biologists. By analogy, knowing where the neurons that mediate a specific conscious percept are located, where they project to and receive input from, their firing pattern, their developmental pedigree from birth to adulthood, and so on, might provide a similar breakthrough on the way to a complete theory of consciousness.

I: A fond dream.

C: Perhaps so, but there is no credible alternative to understanding consciousness by searching for the NCC. Experience has shown that logical argumentation and introspection, the preferred methods of scholars throughout all but the past two centuries, are simply not powerful enough to crack this problem. You can't reason your way to an explanation of consciousness. Brains are too complicated, and are conditioned on too many random events and accidents of evolutionary history, for such armchair methods to successfully illuminate the truth. Instead, you have to find out the facts. How specific is the tapestry woven by axons among neurons? Does synchronized firing play a critical role in the genesis of consciousness? How crucial are the feedback pathways criss-crossing cortex and thalamus? Are there special neuronal cell types that underlie the NCC?

I: What, then, is the role of philosophers in your quest for a scientific theory of consciousness?

C: Historically, philosophy does not have an impressive track record of *answering* questions about the natural world in a decisive manner, whether it's the origin and evolution of the cosmos, the origin of life, the nature of the mind, or the nature-versus-nurture debate. This failure is rarely talked about in polite, academic company. Philosophers, however, excel at *asking* conceptual questions from a point of view that scientists don't usually consider. Notions of the Hard versus the Easy Problem of consciousness, phenomenal versus access consciousness, the content of consciousness versus consciousness as such, the unity of consciousness, the causal conditions for consciousness to occur, and so on, are fascinating issues that scientists should ponder more often. So, listen to the questions posed by philosophers but don't be distracted by their answers. A case in point is the philosopher's zombie.

I: Zombies? Cursed, dead people walking around with outstretched arms?

C: Well, no. People like you and me but with no conscious feelings at all. David Chalmers and other philosophers use these soulless, fictitious creatures to argue that consciousness does not follow from the physical laws of the universe; that knowing about physics, biology, and psychology won't help one iota in understanding how and why experience enters the universe. Something more is required.

This radical, imaginary zombie doesn't strike me as a very useful concept; but there is a more modest and restricted version. Therefore, Francis and I co-opted this catchy term for the set of rapid, stereotyped sensory-motor behaviors that are insufficient, by themselves, for conscious sensations. The classic example is motor control. When you want to run along a trail, you "just do it." Proprioceptive sensors, neurons, and the muscular-skeletal system take care of the rest, and you're on your way. Try to introspect and you'll be confronted with a blank wall. Consciousness has no access to the amazingly complex sequence of computations and actions that underlie such a seemingly simple behavior.

I: So zombie behaviors are reflexes, only more complex?

C: Yes. Think of them as cortical reflexes. Reaching for a glass of water by extending your arm and automatically opening the hand to grasp it constitutes a zombie action that requires visual input to control the arm and hand. You carry out thousands of these actions daily. You can "see" the glass, of course, but only because neural activity in a different system is responsible for the conscious percept.

I: You imply that unconscious, zombie systems co-exist with conscious ones in normal, healthy folks.

C: Exactly. A disconcertingly large fraction of your everyday behavior is zombie-like: You drive to work on autopilot, move your eyes, brush your teeth, tie your shoelaces, greet your colleagues in the hall, and perform all the other myriad chores that constitute daily life. Any sufficiently well-rehearsed activity, such as rock climbing, dancing, martial arts, or tennis is best performed without conscious, deliberate thought. Reflecting too much about any one action will interfere with its seamless execution.

I: Why, then, is consciousness necessary at all? Why couldn't I be a zombie?

C: Well, I know of no logical reason why you couldn't, although life would be pretty boring without any sensations (of course, you wouldn't feel any ennui as a zombie). However, evolution took a different turn on this planet.

Some simple creatures may be nothing but bundles of zombie agents. Thus, it might not feel like anything to be a snail or a roundworm.

If, however, you happen to be an organism with plenty of input sensors and output effectors, say, a mammal, devoting a zombie system to each and every possible input-output combination became too expensive. It would have taken up too much room in the skull. Instead, evolution chose a different path, evolving a powerful and flexible system whose primary responsibility is to deal with the unexpected and to plan for the future. The NCC represent selected aspects of the environment—the ones you are currently aware of—in a compact manner. This information is made accessible to the planning stages of the brain, with the help of some form of immediate memory.

In computer lingo, the current content of awareness corresponds to the state of cache memory on the CPU. As your stream of consciousness flitters from a visual percept to a memory to a voice out there, the content of the cache fluctuates, too.

I: I see. The function of consciousness, therefore, is to handle those special situations for which no automatic procedures are available. Sounds reasonable. But why should this go hand-in-hand with subjective feelings?

C: Aye, there is the rub. Right now, there are no set answers. Or, to be more precise, there is a cacophony of answers, none of them persuasive or widely accepted. Francis and I suspect that meaning plays a critical role.

I: As in the meaning of a word?

C: No, not in any linguistic sense. The objects I feel, see, or hear out there in the world are not meaningless symbols but come with rich associations. The bluish tinge of a fine porcelain cup brings back childhood memories. I know I can grab the cup and pour tea into it. If it falls to the ground it will shatter. These associations don't have to be made explicit. They are built up from countless sensory-motor interactions with the world over a lifetime of experiences. This elusive meaning corresponds to the sum total of all synaptic interactions of the neurons representing the porcelain cup with neurons expressing other concepts and memories. All the vast information is symbolized, in a shorthand way, by the qualia associated with the percept of the cup. That's what you experience.

Leaving that aside for now, what is so important in this field, which has been plagued by hundreds of years of unsubstantiated speculations, is that our framework leads to tests for consciousness. Zombie agents operate in the here and now, so they have no need for short-term memory. You see an outstretched hand, so you reach out and shake it with your own hand. A zombie could not handle a delay between the sight of the hand and the motor action; it didn't evolve to deal with that. The more powerful, albeit slower, consciousness system would have to take over.

These different behaviors can be shaped into a simple operationalized test for consciousness in animals, babies, or patients that can't easily communicate their experiences. Force the organism to make a choice, such as inhibiting an instinctual behavior, following a delay of a few seconds. If the creature can do so without extensive learning, it must make use of a planning module that, at least in humans, is closely linked to consciousness. If the NCC underlying this action is destroyed (or rendered inoperable for some time) by some external means, the delayed response shouldn't happen anymore.

I: This is hardly very rigorous.

C: At this point in the game it is too early for formal definitions. Think back to the 1950's. How far would molecular biologists have gotten if they had worried about what exactly they meant by a gene? Even today, this is no easy matter. Think of it as a sort of Turing test, except it is not meant for intelligence but for consciousness. It is good enough to be applied to sleepwalkers, monkeys, mice, and flies, and that's what counts.

I: Wait. Are you saying that insects may be conscious?

C: Many scholars believe that consciousness requires language and a representation of the self as a basis for introspection. While there is no doubt that humans can recursively think about themselves, this is just the latest elaboration of a more basic biological phenomenon that evolved a long time ago.

Consciousness can be associated with quite elemental feelings. You see purple or have pain. Why should these sensations require language or a highly developed notion of the self? Even severely autistic children or patients with massive self-delusions and depersonalization syndromes don't lack basic perceptual awareness—the ability to see, hear, or smell the world.

The pre-linguistic origin of perceptual consciousness, the type of consciousness I study, raises the question of how far down the evolutionary ladder it extends. At what point in time did the *Ur*-NCC first appear? Given the close evolutionary kinship among mammals, and the structural similarity of their brains, I assume that monkeys, dogs, and cats can be aware of what they see, hear, or smell.

I: What about mice, the most popular mammal in biological and medical laboratories?

C: Given the comparative ease of manipulating the mouse genome, of inserting new genes or knocking out existing ones, applying the anti-zombie delay test to mice in some practical manner would give molecular neuroscientists a powerful model to study the basis of the NCC. My laboratory and others are developing such a mouse model of attention and awareness using classical Pavlovian conditioning.

I: Wait. Why did you say "awareness" instead of "consciousness"? Do they refer to different concepts?

C: No. It is more of a social convention. Consciousness—the C word—evokes powerful aversive reactions in some colleagues; so you're better off with some other word in grant applications and journal submissions. "Awareness" usually slips under the radar.

Continuing with animal consciousness, why stop at mice or, indeed, at mammals? Why be a cortical chauvinist? Do we really know that the cerebral cortex and its satellites are necessary for perceptual consciousness? Why not squids? Or bees? Endowed with one million neurons, bees can perform complicated actions, including amazing feats of visual pattern matching. For all I know, a hundred thousand neurons may be sufficient to see, to smell, and to feel pain! Maybe even fruitflies are conscious, to a very limited extent. Today we just don't know.

I: Sounds like unsubstantiated speculations to me.

C: For now, yes. But behavioral and physiological experiments bring these speculations into the realm of the empirical. And this is new. We were not in a position to think about such litmus tests until recently.

I: Could these tests be applied to machines to assess whether they are conscious?

C: I'm not only a member of the Biology faculty at Caltech, but also a Professor in the Division of Engineering and Applied Science, so I do think about artificial consciousness, based on an analogy to neurobiology. Any organism capable of behaviors that go beyond the instinctual and that has some way to express the meaning of symbols is a candidate for sentience.

The Internet taken as a whole is a tantalizing example of an emergent system with millions of computers acting as nodes in a distributed, but highly interconnected network. While there are file swapping programs that link large numbers of computers, or algorithms that solve mathematically intractable problems by distributing them over thousands of machines, these assemblies bear little relationship to the coalitions of neurons that excite and inhibit each other in the brain. There are no collective behaviors of the entire World Wide Web to speak of. I've never witnessed the spontaneous appearance of any purposeful, large-scale action not designed into the software. It doesn't make any sense to speak of the conscious Web unless it displays such behaviors on its own—by directing electrical power allocation, controlling airline traffic, or manipulating financial markets in a manner unintended by its makers. With the emergence of autonomous computer viruses and worms, this may change in the future, though.

I: What about a robot endowed with reflex-like behaviors—to avoid running into obstacles, to prevent its battery from draining, to communicate with other robots, and so on—in addition to a general planning module. Could that be conscious?

C: Well, suppose the planner was powerful enough to represent the machine's current sensory environment, including its own body and some of the information retrieved from its memory banks that is germane to the present situation, so that it would be capable of independent and purposeful behaviors. Assume, moreover, that your robot could learn to relate sensory events to positive and negative goal states so as to guide its behavior. A high ambient temperature, for example, might cause a drop in the machine's supply voltage—something it would want to avoid at all costs. An elevated temperature wouldn't be an abstract number anymore but would be intimately connected to the organism's well-being. Such a robot *might* have some level of proto-consciousness.

I: That seems like quite a primitive notion of meaning.

C: Sure, but I doubt that at your birth you were conscious of much more than pain and pleasure. There are other sources of meaning, though. Imagine that the robot establishes sensory-motor representations by some unsupervised learning algorithm. It would stumble and fumble its way around the world and would learn, by trial and error, that its actions lead to predictable consequences. At the same time, more abstract representations could be built up by comparing information from two or more sensory modalities (e.g., that moving lips and particular staccato sound patterns often go together). *The* *more explicit representations there are, the more meaningful any one concept is.*

To establish these meanings, it would be easiest if the machine designers could replicate the developmental phases of childhood for the robot.

I: Just like HAL, the paranoid computer in the movie *2001*! But you haven't answered my earlier question yet. Would your delay test distinguish a truly conscious machine from a fake that is just pretending to be conscious?

C: Just because this exercise distinguishes reflexive systems from conscious ones in biological organisms doesn't imply that it will do the same for machines.

It makes sense to grant at least some animal species sentience due to their evolutionary, behavioral, and structural similarity to humans, based on an argument of the form "since I am conscious, the more similar other organisms are to me, the more likely they are to have feelings." This argument loses its power, though, in the face of the radically different design, origin, and form of machines.

I: Let's leave this topic and look back to your earlier ideas about the neuronal correlates of consciousness. What did you and Francis propose?

C: In our first publication on the topic in 1990, we put forth the idea that one form of consciousness involves dynamic binding of neural activity across multiple cortical areas.

I: Wait, wait. What's binding?

C: Think of a red Ferrari zooming past. This triggers nervous activity at myriad locations throughout the brain, yet you see a single red object in the shape of a car, moving in a certain direction, and emitting a lot of noise. The integrated percept has to combine the activity of neurons that encode for the motion with neurons that represent red and others that encode the shape and the sounds. At the same time, you notice a pedestrian with a dog walking past. This also has to be expressed neuronally without confusing it with the representation for the Ferrari.

At the time of our 1990 paper, two German groups, led by Wolf Singer and Reinhardt Eckhorn, respectively, had discovered that neurons in the cat visual cortex, under certain conditions, would synchronize their discharge patterns. Often, this would occur periodically, giving rise to the famous 40 Hz oscillations. We argued that this was one of the neuronal signatures of consciousness.

I: What does the evidence look like now?

C: The neuroscience community remains deeply divided on the topic of oscillations and synchronization. A scientific journal will publish evidence in favor of their functional relevance, while a contribution in the following issue pooh-poohs the entire concept. Unlike cold fusion, which has no credible evidence in its favor, the basic existence of neuronal oscillations in the 20 to 70 Hz frequency range and synchronized discharges is accepted. There is a great deal more, however, that remains contentious. Our reading of the data is that synchronized and oscillatory firing helps one coalition—representing one percept—overcome the others in the competition for dominance. Such a mechanism might be particularly important during attentional biasing. We no longer believe that 40 Hz oscillations are *necessary* for consciousness to occur.

This uncertainty is symptomatic of the inadequacy of existing tools to probe the neuronal networks that underlie the mind. In a cortex of billions of cells, state-of-the-art electrophysiological techniques can listen to the pulses emanating from a hundred neurons. That's a dilution of one out of one hundred million. What is needed is the record of the simultaneous activity of ten thousand or one hundred thousand brain cells.

I: So, if the NCC are based on a coalition of cells, their existence could easily be missed among the din of those billions of neurons chattering to each other.

C: Precisely. It's like trying to learn something meaningful about an upcoming presidential election by recording the everyday conversations of two or three randomly chosen people.

I: I see. Let's move on to your next step.

C: This came in 1995 and pertained to the function of consciousness, which we had ignored up to that point. We hypothesized that a major function of consciousness was to plan for the future, allowing the organism to rapidly deal with many contingencies. This, by itself, was not so different from what other scholars had proposed. We took this argument a step further and asked about its neuroanatomical consequences. Because the planning parts of the brain are located in the frontal lobe, the NCC must have direct access to these brain regions. It turns out that in the monkey, none of the neurons within the primary visual cortex, V1, at the back of the brain, send their output to the front of the brain. We therefore concluded that V1 neurons are not sufficient for visual perception, that visual consciousness requires higher cortical regions.

That's not to say that an intact V1 isn't necessary for seeing. Just as the neural activity in your eyes does not correspond to visual perception—since otherwise you would see a gray disk of nothingness at the blind spot where the optic nerve leaves the eye and no photoreceptors exist—V1 activity is necessary but insufficient for sight. V1 is probably not necessary for visual imagery or for experiencing visual dreams.

I: I don't see why you make such a big deal out of this. So what if the NCC aren't in V1?

C: Well, if true—and the current evidence is quite encouraging—our hypothesis represents a modest but measurable step forward. This is emboldening because it demonstrates that, with the right approach, science can make progress in uncovering the material basis of consciousness. Our hypothesis also implies that not all cortical activity is expressed consciously.

I: So where, among the vast fields of the cortex, are the NCC?

C: Look within the ventral, "vision-for-perception," pathway if you're concerned with visual consciousness. Coalitions of neurons in and around the inferior temporal cortex, supported by feedback activity from cells in the cingulate and frontal cortices, is essential. By way of this reverberatory feedback activity, the coalition can win out over its competitors. The echoes of this conflict can be picked up by EEG or functional brain imaging.

Ongoing electrophysiological explorations of these brain regions continue apace. A popular strategy exploits visual illusions in which the relationship between an image and its associated percept is not one-to-one. Although the input is continuously present, sometimes you see it one way and sometimes in another. Such bistable percepts—the Necker cube is the classical example—are used to track the footprints of consciousness among the different neuronal cell types in the forebrain.

I: Why invoke a loop from the sensory regions of the cortex to the more frontal ones?

C: As I just mentioned, this is one of the pivotal roles of consciousness in the life of an organism—to plan for multi-contingency situations that can't be dealt with by the nonconscious sensory-motor agents. It is probably the projections to and from the frontal lobes, responsible for planning, thought, and reasoning and the seat of the self, that create the powerful feeling that there is a homunculus inside my head, the true "me." The little person—the original meaning of the term homunculus—is part of the front of the cortex observing the back. Or, in anatomical terms, the anterior cingulate, prefrontal, and premotor cortices are receiving a strong, driving synaptic input from the back of the cortex.

I: But who is, in turn, inside the homunculus's head? Don't you end up with an infinite loop?

C: Not if the homunculus is, itself, unconscious or has a reduced functional role compared to that of the conscious mind.

I: Can the homunculus freely initiate actions?

C: You must sharply distinguish the perception of will from the force of will. See, I can raise my hand and I certainly feel that "I" am willing this action. Nobody told me to and I didn't even think about this until a few seconds ago. Perception of control, of authorship—the sense that I am in charge—is essential to my survival, enabling my brain to label these actions as mine (this perception of authorship will have its own NCC, of course). The neuropsychologist Daniel Wegner points out that the belief "I can initiate actions" is a form of optimism. It lets me accomplish things with confidence and exuberance that a pessimist might never attempt.

I: But was your raised hand completely determined by prior events or was it freely willed?

C: You mean, do the laws of physics leave room for a will that is free in the metaphysical sense? Everybody has opinions on this age-old problem, but there are no generally accepted answers. I do know of many instances of a dissociation between an individual's action and her intentions. You can observe these slip-ups in your own life. When "you want" to climb above a ledge, for example, but your body doesn't follow because it's too scared. Or, when running in the mountains and your will slackens but your legs just keep on going. There are many extreme forms of dissociations between action and the experience of willing an action, including hypnosis, table turning, automatic writing, facilitated communications, spirit possession, deindividuation in crowds, and clinical dissociative identity disorders. But whether raising my hand was truly free, as free as Siegfried's destruction of the world order of the Gods in Wagner's *Der Ring des Nibelungen*, I doubt it.

I: From your answer I gather, in any case, that you think your quest for the NCC can be divorced from the question of free will.

C: Yes. Whether or not free will exists, you still have to explain the puzzle of experience, of sensation.

I: What will be the consequences of discovering the NCC?

C: The most obvious ones will be of a practical nature, such as techniques to track the status of the NCC. Such a conscious-ometer will enable medical personnel to monitor the presence of consciousness in premature babies and young infants, in patients whose minds are afflicted with severe autism, or senile dementia, and in patients who are too injured to speak or even to signal. It will permit anesthesiologists to better practice their craft. Understanding the brain basis of consciousness will allow scientists to determine which species are sentient. Do all primates experience the sights and sounds of the world? All mammals? All multi-cellular organisms? This discovery should profoundly affect the animal rights debate.

I: How so?

C: Species without NCC can be thought of as bundles of stereotyped sensory-motor loops, without subjective experience, zombies. Such organisms could be accorded less protection than animals that do show NCCs under some conditions.

I: So, you would not want to experiment with animals that can feel pain?

C: In the ideal world, no. However, one of my daughters died 8 weeks after birth from sudden infant death syndrome; my father wasted away over a period of twelve years from Parkinson's' disease compounded at the end by Alzheimer's disease; and a good friend killed herself in the throws of a florid episode of schizophrenia. Eliminating these and other neuronal maladies afflicting humanity requires animal experimentation—carried out with care and compassion and, whenever possible, with the animal's cooperation (as in the vast bulk of the monkey research described in this book).

I: What about implications for ethics and religion?

C: What matters from a metaphysical point of view is whether neuroscience can successfully move beyond correlation to causation. Science seeks a causal chain of events that leads from neural activity to subjective percept; a theory that accounts for *what organisms* under *what conditions* generate subjective feelings, *what purpose* these serve, and *how* they come about.

 If such a theory can be formulated—a big if—without resorting to new ontological entities that can't be objectively defined and measured, then the scientific endeavor, dating back to the Renaissance, will have risen to its last great challenge. Humanity will have a closed-form, quantitative account of how mind arises out of matter. This is bound to have significant consequences for ethics, including a new conception of humans that might radically contradict the traditional images that men and women have made of themselves throughout the ages and cultures.

I: Not everybody will be enthralled by this. Many will argue that this success marks the nadir of science's relentless, dehumanizing drive to deprive the universe of meaning and significance.

C: But why? Why should knowledge lessen my appreciation of the world around me? I am in awe that everything I see, smell, taste, or touch is made out of 92 elements, including you, me, this book, the air we breathe, the earth we stand on, the stars in the sky. And these elements can be arranged in a periodic kingdom. This, in turn, rests on an even more fundamental triad of protons, neutrons, and electrons. What secret form of cabbalistic knowledge provides greater satisfaction? And none of this intellectual understanding lessens my love of life and the people, dogs, nature, books, and music around me by one bit.

I: What about religion? Most people on the planet believe in some sort of immortal soul that lives on after the body has died. What do you have to say to them?

C: Well, many of these beliefs can't be reconciled with our current scientific world view. What is clear is that every conscious act or intention has some physical correlate. With the end of life, consciousness ceases, for without brain, there is no mind. Still, these irrevocable facts do not exclude some beliefs about the soul, resurrection, and God.

I: Now that your five-year-ordeal of writing this book is over and your children have left for college, what are you going to do?

C: As Maurice Herzog famously pealed at the end of *Annapurna*, his account of the first ascent of the eponymous Himalaya mountain, "There are other Annapurnas in the lives of men."

Glossary

40 Hz Oscillations: See oscillations.

Acetylcholine: A very important neurotransmitter excreted by synapses. In the peripheral nervous system, it transduces action potentials in motorneurons into muscle action. In the brain itself, the release of acetylcholine, known as cholinergic transmission, acts both rapidly, to directly excite its postsynaptic targets, as well as more slowly, to up- or down-regulate their excitability. Increasing activity of cholinergic neurons correlates with increasing arousal levels (Figure 5.1).

Achromatopsia: A specific deficit in the perception of colors due to localized damage to parts of the fusiform gyrus (Section 8.2).

Action Potential: All-or-none, pulse-like change in the electrical potential across the neuronal membrane, about 100 mV in amplitude and 0.5-1 msec in width. Action potentials, or spikes (also referred to as spiking discharge or firing activity) are the primary means of rapidly communicating specific information between neurons and from neurons to muscles (Section 2.3).

Activity Principle: A hypothesis according to which there will be one or more groups of neurons that explicitly represent the different attributes of every direct percept—seeing red, smelling wet moss, the feeling of initiating an action (see explicit coding; Figure 2.5).

Aftereffect: Prolonged exposure to a stimulus attribute causes a short-lived deficit in the ability to detect that attribute (as in the orientation-dependent aftereffect; Section 6.2). In some cases, the opposite attribute is seen, as in the motion aftereffect where the observer sees upward motion after being habituated to downward motion (also known as the waterfall illusion; Section 8.3) or in color afterimages. Aftereffects are thought to be caused by a recalibration or adaptation of the underlying neurons.

Akinetopsia: A specific deficit in the perception of visual motion due to a cortical lesion in and around area MT (Section 8.3).

Anterior cingulate cortex (ACC): Part of the central executive in the frontal lobe that may be key to the NCC (front endpages; Section 7.6). It is made up of Brodmann's areas 24, 25, 32, and 33 (Figure 7.1). The ACC monitors complex behaviors and is particularly active during cognitive conflicts and errors.

Arousal or gating system: A set of upper brainstem (mesencephalic reticular formation; Figure 5.1), hypothalamic and midline thalamic structures (intralaminar nuclei and reticular nuclei) that mediate arousal states (wakefulness and sleep). Bilateral damage to these causes coma. A functioning arousal system is a necessary condition for any conscious content to occur. Its neuronal correlates are part of the NCC$_e$ (Section 5.1).

Attention: The ability to concentrate on a particular stimulus, event, or thought while excluding competing ones. Selective attention is necessary for most forms of conscious perception. Two broad forms of selective attention can be distinguished, top-down and bottom-up attention (Chapter 9).

Attentional searchlight: See top-down attention.

Awareness: I use this term interchangeably with consciousness (see footnote 2 on page 2).

Back of the cortex: A shorthand for all cortical regions that lie behind the central sulcus, including all purely sensory regions (with the notable exception of olfaction). This definition is the complement of the front of the cortex.

Basal ganglia: A collection of nuclei buried below the cerebral cortex that are involved in the regulation of voluntary movement, procedural and sequence learning, and related behaviors. They receive input from throughout the cortex and the intralaminar nuclei of the thalamus and project back, via the thalamus, to the frontal lobes (Section 7.6). Many neurodegenerative diseases, such as Huntington's or Parkinson's disease, attack neurons in the basal ganglia.

Binding problem: How distinct attributes of one or several objects in the world, represented by neural activity at many distributed sites, are combined into unitary percepts is known as the binding problem (Section 9.4). For instance, how are the color, motion, and sounds of a red Ferrari, zooming past at high speed, combined into a single percept when their underlying neural activity is distributed across many cortical sites? And how is this activity kept apart from the neural representation of a simultaneously perceived motorcycle?

Binocular disparity: The relative separation of the image of an object in the two eyes. Disparity can be used to extract the distance between this object and the head, its depth (Section 4.4).

Binocular neurons: Visual neurons that can be driven by an input from either eye. Binocular neurons first occur in the primary visual cortex (Section 4.4). Monocular neurons only respond to input from one eye.

BINOCULAR RIVALRY: One example of a PERCEPTUAL STIMULUS, in which one picture is projected into the left eye and a different one to corresponding locations in the right eye. These stimuli are not seen superimposed, but are perceived one after the other. This provides a vivid illustration of the WINNER-TAKE-ALL dynamics of COALITIONS of neurons, comletely suppressing a competing percept (Chapter 16).

BISTABLE ILLUSIONS: A constant sensory input that can be perceived in one of two, mutually incompatible, ways. Two examples are the Necker cube (Figure 16.1), and BINOCULAR RIVALRY. See PERCEPTUAL STIMULI.

BLINDSIGHT: Residual visual-motor behavior without any visual experience. Patients profess to be blind in part of their field of view yet can respond appropriately to simple stimuli. This is but one example of a selective dissociation between behavior and consciousness (Section 13.2).

BOLD SIGNAL: See fMRI.

BOTTOM-UP ATTENTION: A rapid and automatic form of selective attention, that only depends on intrinsic qualities in the input (exogenous attention). In the visual domain, it is known as saliency-based attention. The more salient a location or object in the image, the more likely it will be noticed (Table 9.1).

BRAINSTEM: A division of the brain that includes the midbrain, pons, and medulla (front endpages).

CAUSATION: An event A can be said to cause another event B if (i) the onset of A precedes the onset of B and (ii) preventing A eliminates B. This definition must be suitably extended if *either* A *or* C can cause B. Given the highly interwoven, redundant, and adaptive networks in molecular-, cell- and neurobiology, moving from correlation to causation is not easy.

CENTER-SURROUND ORGANIZATION: The RECEPTIVE FIELD of a retinal neuron, that is, the region in visual space from which it can receive visual input (colloquially, "what it can see"), includes a quasi-circular region at the center, surrounded by an annulus-shaped region. Its response profile is opposite to that of the center. For example, an on-cell fires vigorously if a spot of light falls onto its central region. Its discharge is inhibited when an annulus of light stimulates its surround (Figure 3.4).

CEREBRAL CORTEX: Often simply called the cortex. A pair of large folded sheets of nervous tissue, a few millimeters in thickness and of variable extent on top of the brain. In humans, one cortical sheet is the size of a large pizza, about 1,000 square centimeters. The cortex is highly laminated (see LAMINAR POSITION) and is subdivided into the neocortex—characteristic of mammals—and older regions, such as the olfactory cortex and the hippocampus (Section 4.2).

CHANGE BLINDNESS: The inability to notice large changes in images or scenes (Figure 9.1), even though subjects have the (illusory) perception that they see everything at a glance.

CHOLINERGIC TRANSMISSION: See ACETYLCHOLINE.

CLASSICAL RECEPTIVE FIELD: See RECEPTIVE FIELD.

COALITION OF NEURONS: A group of mono- or poly-synaptically coupled FOREBRAIN neurons that encode one percept, event, or concept. Coalitions are born and die at the time scale of a fraction of a second or longer. Members of a coalition reinforce each other and suppress members of competing coalitions. Attention biases these competitive interactions. Synchronized and oscillatory firing plays an important role in strengthening one coalition at the expense of others, by bolstering its cohesiveness. Underlying every conscious percept must be a coalition of neurons *explicitly* expressing the perceived attributes (Section 2.1).

COLUMNAR ORGANIZATION: A (near) universal design feature of the cortex whereby most neurons under a patch of the cortex, within a column (extending across all layers), encode one or more features in common (e.g., vertical orientation). Columnar organizations have been found for visual orientation in V1 (Figure 4.4) and for the direction of motion in MT (Figure 8.3). I argue in Section 2.2 that the attribute represented in this columnar fashion is made explicit there (see EXPLICIT CODING).

COMA: A clinically-defined condition in which the patient cannot be aroused and shows no evidence of conscious sensation or nonreflexive behavior (Section 5.1). The comatose state can turn, within a few weeks, into a vegetative state with cyclical arousal (e.g., wakeful eye opening alternating with periods of closed eyes) but no evidence of awareness. If these symptoms remain unchanged beyond a month, the patient is considered to be in a persistent vegetative state.

CONSCIOUSNESS: What this book is all about. At this early point in the scientific exploration of this phenomenon, it is difficult to define it rigorously. Consciousness usually requires some form of selective attention and the short-term storage of information. For strategic reasons, I focus on the brain states sufficient for conscious sensory perception, the NEURONAL CORRELATES OF CONSCIOUSNESS, or NCC. I avoid taking any particular ideological position in the debate concerning the exact relationship between the NCC and conscious experience.

CONSCIOUSNESS-OMETER: A device that would measure the conscious state (or absence of thereof) of humans or animals. No such reliable method exists today. Indeed, many philosophers consider the very idea to be foolish. An alternative is a battery of experiments, including the DELAY TEST, that identify behaviors that require consciousness.

CONTENT OF CONSCIOUSNESS: Specific conscious percept or memory at any one time that forms part of the stream of consciousness (as in seeing a "red apple"). Some specific NCC are sufficient for any one specific content (Section 5.1).

CONTRALATERAL: Common neuroscientific term meaning on the opposite side; as in, "The left primary visual cortex receives input from the right (contralateral) field of view." Ipsilateral means on the same side (Section 4.4).

CORE OF THE THALAMUS: One of two broad classes of thalamic relay cells (see MATRIX). Core neurons convey specific information to the input layers of their cortical target area (Section 7.3).

CORPUS CALLOSUM: About two hundred million fibers that connect the two cortical hemispheres. These are cut in split-brain patients, creating two conscious minds in one skull (Figure 17.1).

CORRELATED FIRING: The extent to which the time at which ACTION POTENTIALS are generated in one neuron is related to the occurrence of action potentials in another neuron. If spikes in one cell are usually followed, a fixed time later, by spikes in the second cell, or if spikes in the first cell are coincident with spikes in the second cell, their firing is highly correlated (Figure 2.7). See also SYNCHRONY.

CORTICAL PROCESSING HIERARCHY: See HIERARCHY.

DEEP LAYERS: Layers 5 and 6 of the neocortex (Section 4.2 and the back endpages). Also called lower layers. Pyramidal neurons whose cell bodies are situated here project outside the cortex, into the thalamus, down to the superior colliculus and to targets beyond (e.g., to the spinal cord).

DELAY TEST: An operational means, by training the subject to enforce a delay between stimulus and motor response, to test for the presence of conscious behaviors in animals, babies, or patients who can't talk (Sections 11.2 and 13.6). See also CONSCIOUSNESS-OMETER.

DEPTH OF COMPUTATION: See LOGICAL DEPTH OF COMPUTATION.

DISPARITY: See BINOCULAR DISPARITY.

DORSAL PATHWAY: Massive anatomical stream that originates in the primary visual cortex and projects through the middle temporal area into regions in the posterior parietal cortex. From there, it sends axons into the dorsolateral prefrontal cortex. Also known as the VISION-FOR-ACTION or WHERE PATHWAY (Figure 7.3).

DREAMING: Vivid and conscious hallucinations that feel as real as life itself. They primarily occur during RAPID-EYE-MOVEMENT SLEEP.

DRIVING CONNECTIONS: see STRONG CONNECTIONS.

EASY PROBLEM: A term used by some philosophers to describe the project at the heart of this book; to discover and characterize the neuronal and, more generally, the material, basis of consciousness. To the extent that consciousness has one or more functions, understanding their mechanistic causes is conceptually and epistemologically straightforward (even if difficult from a scientific and practical perspective). In this view, however, solving the Easy Problem will not explain the mystery of subjective experience. This is the HARD PROBLEM. I suspect that the Hard Problem, like other questions that have occupied philosophers in the past (for example, how it is that humans see the world upright, when the retinal image is inverted) will disappear once we understand the Easy Problem.

ECCENTRICITY: See VISUAL ECCENTRICITY.

ELECTRODE: An electrical conductor, often simply a wire that is insulated everywhere except at its tip, coupled to an amplifier, to record changes in the electrical potential inside or outside nerve cells and/or to directly stimulate neurons. Two types of electrical signals are typically extracted from extracellular recordings: trains of ACTION POTENTIALS from one or more nearby cells, and the LOCAL FIELD POTENTIAL, the collective electrical activity of thousands of cells in the vicinity of the electrode. Arrays of electrodes can eavesdrop on the simultaneous spiking activity of a hundred neurons. Electrode recordings sample the activity of individual neurons with very high temporal (submillisecond) resolution. Their principal limitations are lack of coverage—only a tiny fraction of all neurons in any one area are picked up—and the anonymous nature of the recording.

ELECTROENCEPHALOGRAM (EEG): Noninvasive recordings of the electrical brain potential by attaching numerous electrodes to the top of the head. Oscillatory activity in different frequency bands (theta, alpha, beta, gamma, and so on; Section 2.3) serve as a rough indicator of distinct cognitive states and as a clinical diagnostic tool. The EEG's high temporal (millisecond) but poor spatial (centimeter) resolution severely constrains its ability to identify discrete neuronal populations.

ENABLING FACTORS: The biological mechanisms that need to be in place to be conscious at all (for instance, CHOLINERGIC and GLUTAMERGIC synaptic transmission, and a sufficient blood supply). These are the NCC_e (Section 5.1).

EPHAPTIC INTERACTION: Electrical interaction between neighboring neuronal processes by way of the extracellular potential rather than by specific chemical or electrical synapses. The biophysics of neurons sharply limits the amplitude and specificity of such interactions. The extracellular potential probably plays only a minor role in the processes underlying consciousness (Section 2.3).

ESSENTIAL NODE: A cortical region whose destruction causes the loss of a specific conscious attribute, such as seeing color or motion. Semir Zeki argues that the NCC for this attribute must be located at an essential node (Section 2.2).

EVOKED POTENTIAL: Changes in the electrical potential on the surface of the scalp following presentation of an image (visually evoked potential), sound (auditory evoked potential), or internal cognitive event (e.g., committing an error during some task; event-related potential). The evoked potential is obtained by averaging the EEG over hundreds of trials (Section 2.3).

EXECUTIVE SUMMARY HYPOTHESIS: My proposal that a key function of the neuronal correlates of consciousness is to summarize the present state of affairs in the world and to make this brief summary available to the planning stages of the brain (somewhat similar to the summary demanded by a time-pressed executive who has to make a decision on a complicated topic). This is in contrast to the many SENSORY-MOTOR AGENTS or ZOMBIES who need no such summary, since they deal only with very restricted input and output domains (Section 14.1).

EXPLICIT CODING or EXPLICIT REPRESENTATION: A representation that allows the encoded attribute—orientation, color, or facial identity—to be easily extracted (footnote 9 on page 26). An explicit coding has a larger LOGICAL DEPTH OF COMPUTATION compared to an implicit coding of the same information (Section 2.2). A population of neurons can represent one attribute in an explicit manner and another in an implicit one (for instance, V1 cells encode orientation in an explicit but facial identity in an implicit manner). I argue in Section 2.2 and throughout the book that an explicit representation is a necessary, but not sufficient, condition for the NCC. See also ACTIVITY PRINCIPLE.

EXTINCTION: See NEGLECT.

EXTRASTRIATE CORTEX: A bevy of cortical areas surrounding the PRIMARY VISUAL CORTEX in the occipital lobe, at the back of the brain that subserves vision (Figure 8.1).

FALLACY OF THE HOMUNCULUS: The compelling illusion that at the center of my mind is the conscious I that directs and looks out at the world and initiates all actions. I speculate in Section 18.2 that this illusion is reflected in the neuroanatomy of the connections between the FRONT and the BACK OF THE CORTEX. See also NONCONSCIOUS HOMUNCULUS.

FEEDBACK PATHWAYS: There are higher and lower levels of anatomical organization in the forebrain (see HIERARCHY). Feedback (referred to by Gerald

Edelman as reentrant) pathways are made by axons of pyramidal cells that originate in a higher level and make synaptic connections in one or more lower levels (for instance, from area MT back to V1 or from V1 back to the LGN). I argue that conscious perception would not occur if feedback pathways from the front of the brain to the back were blocked (Section 13.5 and the end of Section 15.3).

FIELD THEORIES OF CONSCIOUSNESS: These postulate the existence of some sort of field that is the physical carrier of conscious sensations. I have little sympathy for such theories, as the electromagnetic field in the brain is too minute and far too unspecific to be able to mediate the specific content of consciousness (see also EPHATIC INTERACTIONS and Section 2.3).

FILLING-IN: A set of processes by which an attribute that is not present is inferred from its immediate context (in space or in time), as at the blind spot (footnote 5 on page 23 and Section 3.3). This can sometimes be misleading.

FIRING RATE CODE: The hypothesis that all of the information carried by a neuron is contained in the (mean) number of spikes triggered within a suitable interval (on the order of 100 msec or more; Section 2.3).

FIRST-PERSON PERSPECTIVE: The unique viewpoint of a conscious being, experiencing and perceiving events in the world. The mystery I address is how a first-person perspective is compatible with, and can be explained in terms of a THIRD-PERSON PERSPECTIVE. While accepting that people *claim* to have experiences, some philosophers deny the reality of subjective states (page 6).

FLEETING MEMORY: See ICONIC MEMORY.

FOREBRAIN: A division of the brain that includes the cortex, the basal ganglia, amygdala, olfactory bulb, and the thalamus (see front endpages). Forebrain neurons mediate the specific CONTENT OF CONSCIOUSNESS. Not to be confused with the FRONT OF THE CORTEX.

FRAMES: See PERCEPTUAL MOMENTS.

FRONT OF THE CORTEX: A shorthand for all cortical regions that lie forward of the central sulcus, including the motor, premotor, prefrontal, and anterior cingulate cortices (the frontal lobe in the front endpages). The front includes cortical regions that receive a significant input, via the thalamus, from the BASAL GANGLIA. Not to be confused with the FOREBRAIN.

FUNCTIONAL MAGNETIC RESONANCE IMAGING or fMRI: A way to record brain signals in conscious subjects in a noninvasive, safe, and convenient manner on the basis of nuclear magnetic resonance. The most commonly used technique is blood-oxygenation level dependent (BOLD) contrast imaging, which measures localized changes in blood volume and blood flow in response to metabolic demand (due to synaptic and spiking activity). fMRI relies on the fact that deoxygenated blood has slightly different magnetic properties than oxygenated blood. fMRI does not directly record the rapid (millisecond) synaptic and spiking events but a proxy, HEMODYNAMIC signals, with a very sluggish time course in the second range and a resolution in the millimeter range (see also footnote 2 on page 135).

FUSIFORM GYRUS: The fusiform gyrus lies on the inferior surface of the cortex, extending from the occipital to the temporal lobe (see INFERIOR TEMPORAL CORTEX, the front endpages, and Section 8.5).

GABA: Principal form of fast synaptic inhibition in the forebrain mediated by the release of the neurotransmitter γ-amino-butyric acid (GABA) from presynaptic terminals.

GAMMA OSCILLATIONS: See OSCILLATIONS.

GIST: Very sparse and high-level description of a visual scene. This makes CHANGE BLINDNESS so compelling: Large changes in the scene are often completely missed since their gist remains the same (Section 9.3).

GLUTAMATE: The principal form of fast, synaptic excitation in the forebrain is based on the neurotransmitter glutamate. Glutamate can act at a variety of postsynaptic receptors. One form acts within a few milliseconds; most of the ordinary synaptic traffic among forebrain neurons uses these glutamate receptors. Another type involves N-methyl-D-aspartate (NMDA) receptors that turn on and off more slowly (50–100 milliseconds). NMDA receptors are important for inducing SYNAPTIC PLASTICITY (Sections 5.1 and 5.3).

HARD PROBLEM: A term popularized by the philosopher David Chalmers to express the grave conceptual difficulty of explaining, in a lawful and reductionist manner, how phenomenal sensations arise out of a physical system (Section 14.4). Why is it that some brain activity goes hand-in-hand with subjective feelings, with QUALIA? In this view, discovering and characterizing the material correlates of consciousness in the brain, the quest to which this book is dedicated, constitutes the EASY PROBLEM.

HEMIANOPIA: Complete blindness or loss of visual perception in half the field of view, caused by a lesion in the pathway from LGN to V1 or upstream from there.

HEMODYNAMIC ACTIVITY: Synaptic release, the generation and propagation of ACTION POTENTIALS, and other neuronal processes use metabolic energy. An increase in metabolic demand, triggered by neural activity, requires the rapid delivery of oxygen via hemoglobin molecules transported in the blood stream. This is accomplished by changes in the blood volume and flow—hemodynamic activity—that are picked up by brain imaging techniques. They include optical (intrinsic) imaging, positron emission tomography (PET), and FUNCTIONAL MAGNETIC RESONANCE IMAGING (fMRI). Their spatio-temporal resolution lies in the sub-millimeter-second range.

HIERARCHY: Based on anatomical criteria, the 30 or more processing areas in the visual brain can be arranged in a hierarchy (front endpages). A particular region receives forward input from an area at a lower level and sends, in turn, a forward projection to an area at a higher level or a sideways connection to a region at the same level of the hierarchy. FEEDBACK PATHWAYS convey information from higher to lower regions. This hierarchy is neither strict nor unique. While similar hierarchical organizations have been reported for somatosensory and auditory regions, it is unclear to what extent regions in the FRONT OF THE CORTEX can be ordered in this manner.

HOMUNCULUS: The little person in the head. See FALLACY OF THE HOMUNCULUS.

ICONIC MEMORY: A form of high-capacity, rapidly decaying (within a second or so) visual memory. It exists in other sensory modalities as well. I call all of these fleeting memory and argue that they are necessary to perceptual consciousness (Secion 11.4).

IMPLICIT CODING or IMPLICIT REPRESENTATION: The opposite of EXPLICIT CODING.

INATTENTIONAL BLINDNESS: Compelling psychophysical demonstrations that unexpected stimuli, even when the subject is looking directly at them, may not be seen (Section 9.1 and footnote 9 on page 155). Inattentional blindness emphasizes the crucial role of expectation in perception.

INFERIOR TEMPORAL or INFEROTEMPORAL CORTEX (IT): In the monkey, the cortical region starting just in front of V4 and continuing almost up to the temporal pole. Includes the dorsal and ventral divisions of PIT, CIT, and AIT (see front endpages and Figure 7.3). Its human homologue is regions anterior to the occipito-temporal cortex, along the ventral surface of the temporal lobe (FUSIFORM GYRUS). This swath of the neocortex is key to conscious, visual perception (Section 8.5).

INTERMEDIATE-LEVEL THEORY OF CONSCIOUSNESS: The hypothesis, put forth by Ray Jackendoff and others, that consciousness only has access to intermediate levels of representations. Neither primitive sensory representations nor the high-level, conceptual representations that underlie many cognitive operations are accessible. One surprising consequence is that thoughts are unconscious. What is conscious about them is their representation in terms of images, silent speech, and other sensory qualities.

INTRALAMINAR NUCLEI OF THE THALAMUS (ILN): A set of small nuclei running through each thalamus. They provide a strong output to the basal ganglia and a more diffuse output to much of the cortex. Their bilateral destruction results in loss of AROUSAL and, if complete enough, in a VEGETATIVE STATE. Part of the NCC_e (Section 5.1).

IPSILATERAL: See CONTRALATERAL.

LAMINAR POSITION: The layer of cortex in which the cell body of a neuron is found. The laminar position is an important determinant of the cell's morphology, input, output, and functional role (Figure 4.1 and the back endpages).

LATERAL GENICULATE NUCLEUS (LGN): Most RETINAL GANGLION CELLS send their axons, making up the optic nerve, into the six-layered lateral geniculate nucleus, one of many thalamic nuclei. Geniculate neurons, in turn, project into the PRIMARY VISUAL CORTEX. Like all thalamic nuclei, the LGN receives massive feedback from the cortex whose function is unknown (Figure 3.6 and the second bottom rung in Figure 7.2).

LGN: See LATERAL GENICULATE NUCLEUS.

LOCAL FIELD POTENTIAL (LFP): The electrical potential recorded in neural tissue from the tip of an electrode. Neuronal processes within a millimeter or so contribute to the LFP (Section 2.3).

LOGICAL DEPTH OF COMPUTATION: A measure of the number of steps necessary for any one computation. The logical depth of a retinal ganglion cell, signaling the occurrence of a spot of light, is far less than that of a cell in the inferior temporal cortex, representing a face. The shallower the logical depth of a neuron's output, the more computations the postsynaptic circuitry has to perform to extract the relevant information (Section 2.2).

LONG-TERM MEMORY: A set of processes that retains information over days, months, and years. Long-term memories includes both implicit, sensory-motor skills as well as declarative memories for autobiographical details and facts (Section 11.2).

LOWER LAYERS: See DEEP LAYERS.

MASKING: When one stimulus eliminates the percept associated with a nearby (in space and/or in time) stimulus, it is said to mask it. Masking visual or auditory stimuli is a sophisticated art (Section 15.3).

MATRIX OF THE THALAMUS: One of two broad classes of thalamic relay cells (see also CORE and THALAMUS). Matrix neurons project widely into the superficial layers of the cortex (Section 7.3).

MEANING: Conscious states mean something, they are about something, they are grounded in the past, in future plans, and in related associations. I argue in Section 14.5 that meaning must be instantiated by myriad synaptic connections among the relevant essential nodes and neurons, the PENUMBRA of any conscious percept.

MEDIAL TEMPORAL LOBE (MTL): Forebrain structure involved in the consolidation of conscious memory and in emotional processing. Includes the hippocampus and surrounding entorhinal (Brodmann's area 28), perirhinal (Brodmann's areas 35 and 36) and parahippocampal cortices (Brodmann's area 37), and the amygdala (see the front endpages, Figure 7.1, and the upper levels of Figure 7.2). Not to be confused with cortical area MT.

MEMORY: A set of distinct psychological processes that operates with different representations, and physiological mechanisms to retain information over time. Important categories include LONG-TERM MEMORY, SHORT-TERM or IMMEDIATE MEMORY, and ICONIC or FLEETING MEMORY (Chapter 11).

MICROCONSCIOUSNESS: Term introduced by Semir Zeki to denote consciousness for individual attributes of any one percept, the associated NCC. Microconsciousness for the motion of an object may be perceived at a slightly different time than microconsciousness for its color. This would make the idea of the unity of consciousness difficult to sustain (Sections 5.4 and 15.2).

MICROELECTRODE: see ELECTRODE.

MICROSTIMULATION: Direct electrical stimulation by an electrode inserted into the relevant brain area. In the cortex, this can evoke elemental or, on occasion, more complex percepts and motor actions (Section 8.3).

MIDDLE TEMPORAL AREA (MT): A small cortical area involved in motion perception. Also referred to as V5 (Figures 7.2 and 8.1). Not to be confused with the MEDIAL TEMPORAL LOBE.

MIND-BODY PROBLEM: A set of problems relating to consciousness. I take the following questions to be the charter for my quest (Section 1.1): To understand how and why the neural basis of a specific conscious sensation is associated with that sensation rather than another, or with a NONCONSCIOUS state; why sensations are structured the way they are, how they acquire MEANING, and why they are PRIVATE; and, finally, how and why so many behaviors occur independent of consciousness (see ZOMBIE AGENTS).

MODULATORY CONNECTIONS: Axons from the thalamus or from a cortical region that terminate in the superficial layers of the cortex or onto the distal dendrites of thalamic neurons. Modulatory connections, by themselves, usually cannot make the target neurons fire strongly, but can modify the firing produced by DRIVING CONNECTIONS. FEEDBACK PATHWAYS are probably modulatory. It is not clear to what extent these distinctions apply to the FRONT OF THE CORTEX.

MONKEYS: They are, like apes and humans, primates (footnote 21 on page 13). Macaque monkeys are not endangered, and can easily be bred and trained in captivity. Although a monkey brain is much smaller than that of a person, its overall organization and processing elements are very similar, making it the most popular model organism to explore the neural basis of perception and cognition (Section 4.1).

MRI: See FUNCTIONAL MAGNETIC RESONANCE IMAGING.

MSEC: Millisecond. One thousandth of a second. Fast, excitatory synaptic inputs and the triggering of an action potential occur within 1 msec.

MT: See MIDDLE TEMPORAL AREA.

μM: Micrometer. One millionth of a meter or one thousandth of a millimeter. A cortical synapse is about 0.5 μm in extent.

NCC: See NEURONAL CORRELATES OF CONSCIOUSNESS.

NCC$_e$: Enabling neuronal conditions for *any* consciousness to occur (Section 5.1).

NEGLECT: A neurological syndrome—often involving damage to the right posterior parietal cortex—in which patients don't respond to information in the affected field of view. Yet their early visual pathways, including the retina and V1, are intact. Known more properly as visuo-spatial hemi-neglect. In the related syndrome of EXTINCTION, the patient can see an isolated object in the affected field, but not if it is presented simultaneously with a stimulus in the opposite, unaffected hemifield (Section 10.3).

NEOCORTEX: See CEREBRAL CORTEX.

NET-WAVE: Wave front of spiking activity, triggered by sensory input, that propagates in a rapid and predictable manner, by leaps and bounds, from the sensory periphery through the various stages of the cortical processing HIERARCHY (Section 7.2).

NEURONAL CORRELATES OF CONSCIOUSNESS or NCC: The minimal set of neuronal mechanisms or events jointly sufficient for a specific conscious percept or experience (Figure 1.1 and Chapter 5). This is what this book is about.

NMDA RECEPTOR: See GLUTAMATE.

NONCLASSICAL RECEPTIVE FIELD: See RECEPTIVE FIELD.

NONCONSCIOUS: Operations or computations that are not directly associated with conscious feelings, sensations, or memories. Subliminal perception is an example of nonconscious processing.

NONCONSCIOUS HOMUNCULUS: A speculation (Section 18.2), according to which networks in part of the front of the cortex look at the back of the cortex, and use this processed sensory information to plan, make decisions and feed these to the relevant motor stages. Much of this neural activity does not contribute to the content of consciousness. These networks act as a nonconscious HOMUNCULUS.

NUCLEUS (plural NUCLEI): A three-dimensional collection of neurons with a prevailing neurochemical and/or neuroanatomical identity (for instance, they all use the same neurotransmitter or they all project to a common destination).

OPTICAL FLOW FIELD: Two-dimensional vector field on the retinae that is induced by changing image intensities. This occurs either during eye or head movement or when an external object moves.

OSCILLATIONS: Semi-regular bouts of periodic activity in the EGG, EVOKED POTENTIAL, or LOCAL FIELD POTENTIAL in a variety of frequency bands (colloquially known as brain waves). Periodic spike discharges can also be picked up with microelectrodes, but with more difficulty. Of particular note are oscillations in the 30 to 70 Hz domain, often referred to as 40 Hz or gamma waves (e.g., Figures 2.6 and 2.7). Their function is probably linked to ATTENTION.

PENUMBRA: A term that I introduce for the neuronal processes that receive synaptic input from the NCC, without being themselves part of them (Section 14.5). The penumbra includes the neural substrate of past associations, the expected consequences, and the cognitive background of the conscious percept. The penumbra provides the meaning, the aboutness of the percept. QUALIA come to symbolize all of this vast, explicit or implicit, information contained in the penumbra.

PERCEPTUAL MOMENTS: The hypothesis that perception occurs in discrete processing episodes, what I call FRAMES or SNAPSHOTS. The stream of consciousness consists of an endless sequence of such frames, not unlike a movie. The attributes *within* a frame, including the perception of motion, are experienced as constant. The NCC need to reflect such quasi-periodic dynamics. The duration of such episodes are quite variable, distributed between 20 and 200 msec.

PERCEPTUAL STIMULI: A sensory input, such as an image, that can be consciously perceived in two or more ways. Examples include bistable illusions, such as the Necker cube (Figure 16.1), BINOCULAR RIVALRY, motion-induced-blindness, and flash suppression. In each case, the same retinal input (the same physical stimulus) can give rise to different percepts. Tracking down the NCC associated with perceptual stimuli offers promising experimental means to identify the neuronal mechanisms underlying consciousness (Chapter 16).

POPULATION CODING: A coding scheme whereby information is distributed across a population of neurons, each of which is relatively broadly tuned. By combining different subsets of them, information can be represented in a robust and efficient manner (Figure 2.3 and Section 2.3). An alternative strategy employs a SPARSE REPRESENTATION.

PRIMARY VISUAL CORTEX: Cortical terminus in the occipital lobe at the very back of the cortex of the visual input from the retina by way of the LATERAL GENICULATE NUCLEUS. Also called V1, striate cortex, or Brodmann's area 17 (Chapter 4 and Figures 7.2 and 8.1).

PRIMATES: The order of primates includes MONKEYS, apes, and humans. See footnote 21 on page 13.

PRIMING: If the processing of one stimulus affects the processing of a much later input, psychologists talk of priming. This is likely to involve changes in synaptic weights. The first input does not even have to be consciously perceived in order for it to increase the detection probability of a later stimulus (Section 11.3).

PRIVACY OF CONSCIOUSNESS: Conscious percepts or memories are private. The CONTENT OF CONSCIOUSNESS cannot be directly communicated, except by way of example or comparison ("this red looks like the red of the Chinese flag"; Section 1.1).

PROSOPAGNOSIA: A specific visual inability to recognize faces. In some patients, an inability to recognize famous or familiar faces (Section 8.5).

QUALIA (singular QUALE): The elemental feelings and sensations making up conscious experience (seeing a face, hearing a tone, and so on). Qualia are at the very heart of the mind-body problem. I argue in Section 14.6 that qualia symbolize, in a compact manner, the vast amount of explicit and implicit information that is contained in the PENUMBRA of the winning coalition. This coalition is sufficient for one particular conscious percept.

RAPID-EYE-MOVEMENT SLEEP: Together with deep sleep, part of the normal sleep cycle. REM sleep is characterized by rapid eye movements, paralysis of other voluntary muscles, and frequent and vivid dream activity.

RATE CODE: See FIRING RATE CODE.

RECEPTIVE FIELD: The classical receptive field of a visual neuron is the location and shape of the visual field from which a stimulus can, by itself, directly excite the cell. While retinal and LGN neurons possess a CENTER-SURROUND ORGANIZATION, cells in the PRIMARY VISUAL CORTEX prefer elongated stimuli of a particular orientation. The much larger region from which the cell's response can be up- or down-regulated is its nonclassical receptive field. For instance, if bars in the nonclassical receptive field have the same orientation at the bar in its center, creating a homogeneous texture, the cell might cease to respond while bars turned at right angle to the central bar evoke a frenzy of spikes (Section 4.4). The nonclassical receptive field places the cell's primary response into a larger context.

REM sleep: See RAPID-EYE-MOVEMENT SLEEP.

RETINAL GANGLION CELLS: Over one million neurons in the retina summarize all of the optic information extracted by photoreceptors, horizontal, bipolar, and amacrine cells and communicate this, in the form of action potentials, to the rest of the brain. Their axons make up the optic nerve. Their activity is insufficient for conscious visual perception (Chapter 3).

RETINOTOPIC ORGANIZATION: An example of a TOPOGRAPHIC ORGANIZATION. Nearby points in visual space are mapped to neighboring neurons, with the representation of the fovea greatly expanded compared to the visual periphery (Figure 4.2).

SACCADE or SACCADIC EYE MOVEMENT: A very rapid, yet directed eye movement. Humans and other primates typically inspect and explore the world by executing a few saccades every second of waking life (Section 3.7).

SEARCHLIGHT: See TOP-DOWN ATTENTION.

SENSORY-MOTOR AGENTS: See ZOMBIE AGENTS.

SHORT-TERM MEMORY: A catch-all term for the temporary storage of information over tens of seconds. WORKING MEMORY is one form of such immediate memory (Section 11.3).

SNAPSHOTS: See PERCEPTUAL MOMENTS.

SPARSE REPRESENTATION: A coding scheme whereby information is expressed by a small number of quite discerning neurons. The advantage over POPULATION CODING is that the information is represented in a explicit manner. In the limit of very sparse coding, a cell may encode only a single, particular individual or category (Figure 2.2 and Section 2.2).

SPARSE TEMPORAL CODING: A code in which information is represented by a handful of spikes, triggered at a particular point in time (like a single note of music) rather than by slower changes in the firing rate over a fraction of a second or longer (Section 2.3). This saves energy and also minimizes interference during learning.

SPIKE: See ACTION POTENTIAL.

SPIKE SYNCHRONY: See SYNCHRONY.

STRIATE CORTEX: Anatomical term for PRIMARY VISUAL CORTEX.

STRONG or DRIVING CONNECTIONS: Axons from the thalamus or from a cortical region that primarily terminate in layer 4 of the cortex or onto the proximal part of thalamic neurons and that can trigger, by themselves, vigorous action potential activity in their target cells. Forward connections that ascend the VISUAL HIERARCHY, from LGN into V1 or from V1 into MT, are driving connections. Francis and I postulate that the thalamo-cortical system avoids loops made up entirely of strong connections (Section 7.4).

SUPERFICIAL LAYERS: Layers 1, 2, and 3 of the neocortex (Section 4.2). Also called upper layers. The forward projection from one cortical region into a region at a higher level in the hierarchy originates from superficial layers. These layers receive massive intracolumnar input from layer 4 neurons, from cortical feedback pathways, and from thalamic matrix neurons. These latter two place the computations carried out here into a more global context.

SYNAPSE: A highly specialized point of contact between a presynaptic and a postsynaptic neuron. A chemical synapse releases neurotransmitter molecules from its presynaptic terminal, a nerve ending. These molecules bind to receptors embedded in the membrane of the postsynaptic neuron to initiate a cascade of rapid electrical (excitatory or inhibitory) and slower biochemical events. In the forebrain, GLUTAMATE and GABA are the dominant excitatory and inhibitory neurotransmitter substances. Several hundred million synapses are packed into one cubic millimeter of cortical tissue. Electrical synapses (so-called gap junctions) are direct, low-resistance connections among cells. In the cortex, they may serve to synchronize the discharge of inhibitory interneurons (footnote 20 on page 36).

SYNAPTIC PLASTICITY: Biophysical and biochemical changes that increase or decrease the effective connection strength of a synapse. These changes can last anywhere from minutes to days or longer. Synaptic plasticity is thought to be key to LONG-TERM MEMORY storage (Section 11.1).

SYNCHRONY or SPIKE SYNCHRONY: The extent to which a spike in one neuron occurs at the same time (or nearly so) as the spike in another neuron (e.g., Figure 2.7). A group of neurons whose firing is tightly synchronized (CORRELATED FIRING) is better at driving its target cells (their synaptic input will carry a stronger punch) than if the spiking activity is disorganized across the group. Spike synchrony is probably an important mechanism to bias the competition among neurons.

TEMPORAL CODE: The hypothesis that the time of occurrence of action potentials within one neuron and among groups of cells contains relevant information. Oscillatory discharges in the 40 Hz range and synchronization are the two most prominent examples of such codes (Section 2.3, Figures 2.6 and 2.7). It is likely that such coding is important as the neuronal expression of selective attention.

THALAMUS: Paired structures situated on top of the midbrain that regulate all inputs into the neocortex. In their absence, no mental life is possible. Each thalamus is divided into many nuclei that don't directly talk to each other.

These receive massive FEEDBACK from the cortex. I consider the thalamus the organ of attention (Figure 5.1 and Section 7.3).

THIRD-PERSON PERSPECTIVE: The standpoint of an external observer, having access to the behavior and brain states (e.g., by observing neurons) of a conscious subject, but not to his or her experiences. Throughout most of history, biology and psychology adopted a purely third-person perspective (as in the Vienna Circle or Behaviorism), totally neglecting the FIRST-PERSON PERSPECTIVE.

TOP-DOWN ATTENTION: A volitional, focal, task-dependent, or endogenous selection mechanism operating in vision and other sensory modalities (Table 9.1). A popular metaphor for top-down visual attention is the SEARCHLIGHT OF ATTENTION that illuminates objects in the field of view, enhancing their processing. At the neuronal level, one important function of attention is to bias the COALITIONS that encode these objects. Attention is a separate process from conscious perception (Section 9.3).

TOPOGRAPHIC ORGANIZATION: The observation that two nearby points in space are represented by neighboring neurons. The LGN, and the early visual cortical, auditory, and somatosensory cortices are topographically organized. Such organization is absent in the higher regions of the ventral pathway.

UPPER LAYERS: See SUPERFICIAL LAYERS.

V1: See PRIMARY VISUAL CORTEX.

VEGETATIVE STATE: See COMA.

VENTRAL PATHWAY: Massive anatomical stream that originates in the primary visual cortex and projects into V4 and the inferior temporal cortex. From there, it sends afferents into the ventrolateral prefrontal cortex. Also known as the VISION-FOR-PERCEPTION or WHAT PATHWAY (Figure 7.3).

VISION-FOR-ACTION PATHWAY: See DORSAL PATHWAY.

VISION-FOR-PERCEPTION PATHWAY: See VENTRAL PATHWAY.

VISUAL ECCENTRICITY: The angle relative to the point of sharpest seeing, the fovea, is referred to as eccentricity. The more eccentric an object, the more difficult it is to see sharply (Figure 3.2).

VISUAL HIERARCHY: The anatomical HIERARCHY found in the visual cortex.

WINNER-TAKE-ALL: A type of operation, easy to implement in neural networks, in which only neurons with the strongest, most vigorous inputs survive. Due to competitive, synaptic interactions, neurons with less active inputs are partially (soft winner-take-all) or completely (hard winner-take-all) suppressed. The coalitions underlying the NCC must have winner-take-all characteristics.

Working memory: One well-studied memory module that stores information needed for ongoing tasks over tens of seconds (such as a phone number; Section 11.3).

Zombie agents: Sensory-motor systems that carry out a specialized behavior in a rapid and effortless manner without, themselves, giving rise to any conscious sensation. This may come later (by feedback), or not at all. Examples include eye movements, walking, running, cycling, dancing, driving, climbing, and other highly trained activities (Chapters 12 and 13).

Bibliography

Abbott, L.F., Rolls, E.T., and Tovee, M.J. "Representational capacity of face coding in monkeys," *Cerebral Cortex* **6**:498–505 (1996).

Abeles, M. *Corticonics: Neural Circuits of the Cerebral Cortex.* Cambridge, UK: Cambridge University Press (1991).

Abeles, M., Bergman, H., Margalit, E., and Vaadia, E. "Spatiotemporal firing patterns in the frontal cortex of behaving monkeys," *J. Neurophysiol.* **70**:1629–1638 (1993).

Aboitiz, F., Scheibel, A.B., Fisher, R.S., and Zaidel, E. "Fiber composition of the human corpus callosum," *Brain Res.* **598**:143–153 (1992).

Abrams, R.A. and Landgraf, J.Z. "Differential use of distance and location information for spatial localization," *Perception & Psychophysics* **47**:349–359 (1990).

Achenbach, J. *Captured by Aliens: The Search for Life and Truth in a Very Large Universe.* New York: Simon & Schuster (1999).

Adolphs, R., Tranel, D., Hamann, S., Young, A.W., Calder, A.J., Phelps, E.A., Anderson, A., Lee G.P., and Damasio, A.R. "Recognition of facial emotion in nine individuals with bilateral amygdala damage," *Neuropsychologia* **37**:1111–1117 (1999).

Aglioto, S., DeSouza, J.F.X., and Goodale, M.A. "Size-contrast illusions deceive the eye but not the hand," *Curr. Biol.* **5**:679–685 (1995).

Ahmed, B., Anderson, J., Douglas, R., Martin, K., and Nelson, C. "Polyneuronal innervation of spiny stellate neurons in cat visual cortex," *J. Comp. Neurol.* **341**:39–49 (1994).

Akelaitis, A.J. "Studies on corpus callosum: Higher visual functions in each homonymous field following complete section of corpus callosum," *Arch. Neurol. Psych. (Chicago)* **45**:788–798 (1941).

Akelaitis, A.J. "A study of gnosis, praxis and language following section of the corpus callosum and anterior commisure," *J. Neurosurg.* **1**:94–102 (1944).

Aksay, E., Gamkrelidze, G., Seung, H.S., Baker, R., and Tank, D.W. "*In vivo* intracellular recording and perturbation of persistent activity in a neural integrator," *Nature Neurosci.* **4**:184–193 (2001).

Alauddin, M.M., Louie, A.Y., Shahinian, A., Meade, T.J., and Conti, P.S. "Receptor mediated uptake of a radiolabeled contrast agent sensitive to beta-galactosidase activity," *Nucl. Med. Biol.* **30**:261–265 (2003).

Albright, T.D. "Cortical processing of visual motion," *Rev. Oculomot. Res.* **51**:77–201 (1993).

Aldrich, M.S., Alessi, A.G., Beck, R.W., and Gilman, S. "Cortical blindness: Etiology, diagnosis and prognosis," *Ann. Neurol.* **21**:149–158 (1987).

Alkire, M.T., Haier, R.J., Shah, N.K., and Anderson, C.T. "Positron emission tomograpy study of regional cerebral metabolism in humans during isoflurane anesthesia," *Anesthesiology* **86**:549–557 (1997).

Alkire, M.T., Pomfrett, C.J.D., Haier, R.J., Gianzero, M.V., Chan, C.M., Jacobsen, B.P., and Fallon, J.H. "Functional brain imaging during anesthesia in humans," *Anesthesiology* **90**:701–709 (1999).

Allen, W. *Getting Even.* New York: Random House (1978).

Allman, J.M. "Stimulus specific responses from beyond the classical receptive field: Neurophysiological mechanisms for local-global comparisons in visual neurons," *Ann. Rev. Neurosci.* **8**:407–430 (1985).

Allman, J.M. *Evolving Brains.* New York: Scientific American Library (1999).

Allman, J.M. and Kaas, J.H. "A representation of the visual field in the caudal third of the middle temporal gyrus of the owl monkey (*Aotus trivirgatus*)," *Brain Res.* **31**:85–105 (1971).

Anderson, M.C. and Green, C. "Suppressing unwanted memories by executive control," *Nature* **410**:366–369 (2001).

Andersen, R.A. "Neural mechanisms of visual motion perception in primates," *Neuron* **18**:865–872 (1997).

Andersen, R.A. "Encoding of intention and spatial location in the posterior parietal cortex," *Cerebral Cortex* **5**:457–469 (1995).

Andersen, R.A., Asanuma, C., Essick, G., and Siegel, R.M. "Cortico-cortical connections of anatomically and physiologically defined subdivisions within the inferior parietal lobule," *J. Comp. Neurol.* **296**:65–113 (1990).

Andersen, R.A, Essick, G., and Siegel, R. "Encoding of spatial location by posterior parietal neurons," *Science* **230**:456–458 (1985).

Andersen, R.A., Snyder L.H., Bradley, D.C., and Xing, J. "Multimodal representation of space in the posterior parietal cortex and its use in planning movements," *Ann. Rev. Neurosci.* **20**:303–330 (1997).

Andrews, T.J., Halpern, S.D., and Purves, D. "Correlated size variations in human visual cortex, lateral geniculate nucleus and optic tract," *J. Neurosci.* **17**:2859–2868 (1997).

Andrews, T.J., and Purves, D. "Similarities in normal and binocularly rivalrous viewing," *Proc. Natl. Acad. Sci. USA* **94**:9905–9908 (1997).

Antkowiak, B. "How do general anesthetics work," *Naturwissenschaften* **88**:201–213 (2001).

Arnold, D.H., Clifford, C.W.G., and Wenderoth, P. "Asynchronous processing in vision: Color leads motion," *Curr. Biol.* **11**:596–600 (2001).

Asenjo, A.B., Rim, J., and Oprian, D.D. "Molecular determinants of human red/green color discrimination," *Neuron* **12**:1131–1138 (1994).

Astafiev, S.V., Shulman, G.L., Stanley, C.M., Snyder, A.Z., Van Essen, D.C., and Corbetta, M. "Functional Organization of Human Intraparietal and Frontal Cortex for Attending, Looking, and Pointing," *J. Neurosci.* **23**:4689–4699 (2003).

Attneave, F. "In defense of homunculi." In: *Sensory Communication*. Rosenblith W.A., ed., pp. 777–782. New York: MIT Press (1961).

Baars, B.J. *A Cognitive Theory of Consciousness*. Cambridge, UK: Cambridge University Press (1988).

Baars, B.J. "Surprisingly small subcortical structures are needed for the *state* of waking consciousness, while cortical projection areas seem to provide perceptual *contents* of consciousness," *Consc. & Cognition* **4**:159–162 (1995).

Baars, B.J. *In the Theater of Consciousness*. New York: Oxford University Press (1997).

Baars, B.J. "The conscious access hypothesis: Origins and recent evidence," *Trends Cogn. Sci.* **6**:47–52 (2002).

Bachmann, T. *Psychophysiology of Visual Masking*. Commack, NY: Nova Science Publishers (1994).

Bachmann T. *Microgenetic Approach to the Conscious Mind*. Amsterdam, Netherlands: Johns Benjamins (2000).

Baddeley, A. *Working Memory*. London, UK: Oxford University Press (1986).

Baddeley, A. *Human Memory: Theory and Practice*. Boston: Allyn & Bacon (1990).

Baddeley, A. "The episodic buffer: A new component of working memory?" *Trends Cogn. Sci.* **4**:417–423 (2000).

Baer, P.E., and Fuhrer, M.J. "Cognitive processes in the differential trace conditioning of electrodermal and vasomotor activity," *J. Exp. Psychology* **84**:176–178 (1970).

Bair, W. "Spike timing in the mammalian visual system," *Curr. Opinion Neurobiol.* **9**:447–453 (1999).

Bair, W. and Koch, C. "Temporal precision of spike trains in extrastriate cortex of the behaving monkey," *Neural Comp.* **8**:1185–1202 (1996).

Baizer, J.A., Ungerleider, L.G., and Desimone, R. "Organization of visual inputs to the inferior temporal and posterior parietal cortex in macaques," *J. Neurosci.* **11**:168–190 (1991).

Bar, M. and Biederman, I. "Subliminal visual priming," *Psychological Science* **9**:464–469 (1998).

Bar, M. and Biederman, I. "Localizing the cortical region mediating visual awareness of object identity," *Proc. Natl. Acad. Sci. USA* **96**:1790–1793 (1999).

Barbas, H. "Pattern in the laminar origin of corticocortical connections," *J. Comp. Neurol.* **252**:415–422 (1986).

Barcelo, F., Suwazono, S., and Knight, R.T. "Prefrontal modulation of visual processing in humans," *Nature Neurosci.* **3**:399–403 (2000).

Bargmann, C.I. "Neurobiology of the *Caenorhabditis elegans* genome," *Science* **282**:2028–2033 (1998).

Barlow, H.B. "Single units and sensation: A neuron doctrine for perceptual psychology," *Perception* **1**:371–394 (1972).

Barlow, H.B. "The neuron doctrine in perception." In: *The Cognitive Neurosciences*. 1st ed., Gazzaniga, M., ed., pp. 415–435. Cambridge, MA: MIT Press (1995).

Barone, P., Batardiere, A., Knoblauch, K., and Kennedy, H. "Laminar distribution of neurons in extrastriate areas projecting to visual areas V1 and V4 correlates with the hierarchical rank and indicates the operation of a distance rule," *J. Neurosci.* **20**:3263–3281 (2000).

Barrow, J.D., and Tipler, F.J. *The Anthropic Cosmological Principle.* Oxford, UK: Oxford University Press (1986).

Bateson, W. "Review of *The Mechanism of Mendelian Heredity* by T.H. Morgan, A.H. Sturtevant, H.J. Muller, and C.B. Bridges," *Science* **44**:536–543 (1916).

Batista, A.P. and Andersen, R.A. "The parietal reach region codes the next planned movement in a sequential reach task," *J. Neurophysiol.* **85**:539–544 (2001).

Bauby, J.-D. *The Diving Bell and the Butterfly: A Memoir of Life in Death.* New York: Alfred A. Knopf (1997).

Bauer, R.M. and Demery, J.A. "Agnosia." In: *Clinical Neuropsychology.* 4th ed., Heilman, K.M., and Valenstein, E., eds., pp. 236–295. New York: Oxford University Press (2003).

Bayne, T. and Chalmers, D.J. "What is the unity of consciousness?" In: *The Unity of Consciousness.* Cleeremans, A., ed., pp. 23–58. Oxford, UK: Oxford University Press (2003).

Beckermann, A., Flohr, H., and Kim, J., eds. *Emergence or Reduction? Essays on the Prospects of Nonreductive Physicalism.* Berlin: Walter de Gruyter (1992).

Beierlein, M., Gibson, J.R., and Connors, B.W. "A network of electrically coupled interneurons drives synchronized inhibition in neocortex," *Nature Neurosci.* **3**:904–910 (2000).

Bennett, C.H. "Logical depth and physical complexity." In: *The Universal Turing Machine. A Half-Century Survey.* Herken, R., ed., pp. 227–258. Oxford, UK: Oxford University Press (1988).

Benton, A. and Tranel, D. "Visuoperceptual, visuospatial, and visuoconstructive disorders." In: *Clinical Neurosychology.* 3rd ed., Heilman, K.M. and Valenstein, E., eds., pp. 165–278. New York: Oxford University Press (1993).

Bergen, J.R. and Julesz, B. "Parallel versus serial processing in rapid pattern discrimination," *Nature* **303**:696–698 (1983).

Berns, G.S., Cohen, J.D., and Mintun, M.A. "Brain regions responsive to novelty in the absence of awareness," *Science* **276**:1272–1275 (1997).

Berti, A. and Rizzolatti, G. "Visual processing without awareness: Evidence from unilateral neglect," *J. Cogn. Neurosci.* **4**:345–351 (1992).

Bhalla, M. and Proffitt, D.R. "Visual-motor recalibration in geographical slant perception," *J. Exp. Psychol.: Human Perception & Performance* **25**:1076–1096 (1999).

Bialek W., Rieke, F., van Steveninck, R.R.D., and Warland, D. "Reading a neural code," *Science* **252**:1854–1857 (1991).

Biederman, I. "Perceiving real-world scenes," *Science* **177**:77–80 (1972).

Billock, V.A. "Very short term visual memory via reverberation: A role for the cortico-thalamic excitatory circuit in temporal filling-in during blinks and saccades?" *Vision Res.* **37**:949–953 (1997).

Bisiach, E. and Luzzatti, C. "Unilateral neglect of representational space," *Cortex* **14**:129–133 (1978).

Bisley, J.W. and Goldberg, M.E. "Neuronal activity in the lateral intraparietal area and spatial attention," *Science* **299**:81–86 (2003).

Blackmore, S.J. *Beyond the Body: An Investigation of Out-Of-The-Body Experiences.* London: Heinemann (1982).

Blackmore, S., Brelstaff, G., Nelson, K., and Tsoscianko, T. "Is the richness of our visual world an illusion? Transsaccadic memory for complex scenes," *Perception* **24**:1075–1081 (1995).

Blake, R. "A neural theory of binocular rivalry," *Psychol. Rev.* **96**:145–167 (1989).

Blake, R. "What can be "perceived" in the absence of visual awareness?" *Curr. Direction Psychol. Sci.* **6**:157–162 (1998).

Blake, R. and Cormack, R.H. "On utrocular discrimination," *Perception & Psychophysics* **26**:53–68 (1979).

Blake, R. and Fox, R. "Adaptation to invisible gratings and the site of binocular rivalry suppression," *Nature* **249**:488–490 (1974).

Blake, R. and Logothetis, N.K. "Visual Competition," *Nature Rev. Neurosci.* **3**:13–21 (2002).

Blanke, O., Ortigue, S., Landis, T., and Seeck, M. "Stimulating illusory own-body perceptions," *Nature* **419**:269–270 (2002).

Blasdel, G.G. "Orientation selectivity, preference, and continuity in monkey striate cortex," *J. Neurosci.* **12**:3139–3161 (1992).

Blasdel, G.G. and Lund, J.S. "Termination of afferent axons in macaque striate cortex," *J. Neurosci.* **3**:1389–1413 (1983).

Blaser, E., Sperling, G., and Lu, Z.-L. "Measuring the amplification of attention," *Proc. Natl. Acad. Sci. USA* **96**:11681–11686 (1999).

Blatow, M., Rozov, A., Katona, I., Hormuzdi, S.G., Meyer, A.H., Whittington, M.A., Caputi, A., and Monyer, H. "A novel network of multipolar bursting interneurons generates theta frequency oscillations in neocortex," *Neuron* **38**:805–817 (2003).

Block, N. "On a confusion about a function of consciousness," *Behav. Brain Sci.* **18**:227–247 (1995).

Block, N. "How can we find the neural correlate of consciousness?" *Trends Neurosci.* **19**:456–459 (1996).

Block, N., Flanagan, O., and Güzeldere, G., eds. *Consciousness: Philosophical Debates.* Cambridge, MA: MIT Press (1997).

Bogen, J.E. "Mental duality in the intact brain," *Bull. Clinical Neurosci.* **51**:3–29 (1986).

Bogen, J.E. "The callosal syndromes." In: *Clinical Neurosychology.* 3rd ed., Heilman, K.M. and Valenstein, E., eds., pp. 337–407. New York: Oxford University Press (1993).

Bogen, J.E. "On the neurophysiology of consciousness: I. An overview," *Consc. & Cognition* **4**:52–62 (1995a).

Bogen, J.E. "On the neurophysiology of consciousness: II. Constraining the semantic problem," *Consc. & Cognition* **4**:137–158 (1995b).

Bogen, J.E. "Some neurophysiologic aspects of consciousness," *Sem. Neurobiol.* **17**:95–103 (1997a).

Bogen, J.E. "The neurosurgeon's interest in the corpus callosum." In: *A History of Neurosurgery in its Scientific and Professional Contexts.* Greenblatt S.H., ed., chapter 24. Park Ridge, IL: American Association of Neurological Surgeons (1997b).

Bogen, J.E. "Does cognition in the disconnected right hemisphere require right hemisphere possession of language?" *Brain & Language* **57**:12–21 (1997c).

Bogen, J.E., Fisher, E.D., and Vogel, P.J. "Cerebral commissurotomy: A second case report," *J. Am. Med. Assoc.* **194**:1328–1329 (1965).

Bogen, J.E. and Gazzaniga, M.S. "Cerebral commissurotomy in man: Minor hemisphere dominance for certain visuospatial functions," *J. Neurosurg.* **23**:394–399 (1965).

Bogen, J.E. and Gordon, H. W. "Musical tests for functional lateralization with intracarotid amobarbital," *Nature* **230**:524–525 (1970).

Bonneh, Y.S., Cooperman, A., and Sagi, D. "Motion-induced blindness in normal observers," *Nature* **411**:798–801 (2001).

Booth, M.C.A. and Rolls, E.T. "View-invariant representations of familiar objects by neurons in the inferior temporal visual cortex," *Cerebral Cortex* **8**:510–523 (1998).

Borrell, V. and Callaway, E.M. "Reorganization of exuberant axonal arbors contributes to the development of laminar specificity in ferret visual cortex," *J. Neurosci.* **22**:6682–6695 (2002).

Bourassa, J. and Deschenes, M. "Corticothalamic projections from the primary visual cortex in rats: A single fiber study using biocytin as an anterograde tracer," *Neurosci.* **66**:253–263 (1995).

Braak, H. "On the striate area of the human isocortex. A Golgi and pigmentarchitectonic study," *J. Comp. Neurol.* **166**:341–364 (1976).

Braak, H. *Architectonics of the Human Telencephalic Cortex.* Berlin: Springer (1980).

Bradley, D.C., Chang, G.C., and Andersen, R.A. "Encoding of three-dimensional structure-from-motion by primate area MT neurons," *Nature* **392**:714–717 (1998).

Braitenberg, V. and Schüz, A. *Anatomy of the Cortex.* Heidelberg: Springer (1991).

Braun, J. "Visual search among items of different salience: Removal of visual attention mimics a lesion in extrastriate area V4," *J. Neurosci.* **14**:554–567 (1994).

Braun, J. "Natural scenes upset the visual applecart," *Trends Cogn. Neurosci.* **7**:7–9 (2003).

Braun, A.R., Balkin, T.J., Wesensten, N.J., Gwadry, F., Carson, R.E., Varga, M., Baldwin, P., Belenky, G., and Herscovitch, P. "Dissociated pattern of activity in visual cortices and their projections during human rapid eye movement sleep," *Science* **279**:91–95 (1998).

Braun, J. and Julesz, B. "Withdrawing attention at little or no cost: Detection and discrimination tasks," *Perception & Psychophysics* **60**:1–23 (1998).

Braun, J., Koch, C., and Davis, J.L., eds. *Visual Attention and Cortical Circuits.* Cambridge, MA: MIT Press (2001).

Braun, J. and Sagi, D. "Vision outside the focus of attention," *Perception & Psychophysics* **48**:277–294 (1990).

Brefczynski, J.A. and DeYoe, E.A. "A physiological correlate of the 'spotlight' of visual attention," *Nature Neurosci.* **2**:370–374 (1999).

Breitmeyer, B.G. *Visual Masking: An Integrative Approach.* Oxford, UK: Oxford University Press (1984).

Breitmeyer, B.G. and Ögmen, H. "Recent models and findings in backward visual masking: A comparison, review and update," *Percept. & Psychophysics* **62**:1572–1595 (2000).

Brewer, A.A., Press, W.A., Logothetis, N.K., and Wandell, B.A. "Visual areas in macaque cortex measured using functional magnetic resonance imaging," *J. Neurosci.* **22**:10416–10426 (2002).

Brickner, R.M. *The Intellectual Functions of the Frontal Lobes.* New York: Macmillan (1936).

Bridgeman, B., Hendry, D., and Stark, L. "Failure to detect displacement of the visual world during saccadic eye movements," *Vision Res.* **15**:719–722 (1975).

Bridgeman, B., Kirch, M., and Sperling, A. "Segregation of cognitive and motor aspects of visual function using induced motion," *Percept. Psychophys.* **29**:336–342 (1981).

Bridgeman, B., Lewis, S., Heit, G., and Nagle, M. "Relation between cognitive and motor-oriented systems of visual position perception," *J. Exp. Psychol. Hum. Percept.* **5**:692–700 (1979).

Bridgeman, B., Peery S., and Anand, S. "Interaction of cognitive and sensorimotor maps of visual space," *Perception & Psychophysics* **59**:456–469 (1997).

Brindley, G.S., Gautier-Smith, P.C., and Lewin, W. "Cortical blindness and the functions of the non-geniculate fibres of the optic tracts," *J. Neurol. Neurosurg. Psychiatry* **32**:259–264 (1969).

Britten, K.H., Newsome, W.T., Shadlen, M.N., Celebrini, S., and Movshon, J.A. "A relationship between behavioral choice and the visual responses of neurons in macaque MT," *Visual Neurosci.* **13**:87–100 (1996).

Britten, K.H., Shadlen, M.N., Newsome, W.T., and Movshon, A. "The analysis of visual motion: A comparison of neuronal and psychophysical performance," *J. Neurosci.* **12**:4745–4765 (1992).

Broca, A. and Sulzer, D. "La sensation lumineuse fonction du temps," *J. de Physiol. Taphol. Generale* **4**:632–640 (1902).

Brodmann, K. "Physiologie des Gehirns," *Neue Deutsche Chirurgie* **11**:85–426 (1914).

Brooke, R.N., Downes, J., and Powell, T.P. "Centrifugal fibres to the retina in the monkey and cat," *Nature* **207**:1365–1367 (1965).

Broughton, R., Billings, R., Cartwright, R., Doucette, D., Edmeads, J., Edwardh, M., Ervin, F., Orchard, B., Hill, R., and Turrell, G. "Homicidal somnambulism: A case report," *Sleep* **17**:253–264 (1994).

Brown, E.N., Frank, L.M., Tang, D., Quirk, M.C., and Wilson, M.A. "A statistical paradigm for neural spike train decoding applied to position prediction from ensemble firing patterns of rat hippocampal place cells," *J. Neurosci.* **18**:7411–7425 (1998).

Brown, W.S., Murphy, N., and Malony, H.N., eds. *Whatever Happened to the Soul? Scientific and Theological Portraits of Human Nature*. Minneapolis, MN: Fortress Press (1998).

Bruce, C.J., Desimone, R., and Gross, C.G. "Both striate cortex and superior colliculus contribute to visual properties of neurons in superior temporal polysensory area of the macaque monkey," *J. Neurophysiol.* **55**:1057–1075 (1986).

Budd, J.M. "Extrastriate feedback to primary visual cortex in primates: A quantitative analysis of connectivity," *Proc. R. Soc. Lond. B* **265**:1037–1044 (1998).

Bullier, J. "Feedback connections and conscious vision," *Trends Cogn. Sci.* **5**:369–370 (2001).

Bullier, J., Girard, P., and Salin, P.-A. "The role of area 17 in the transfer of information to extrastriate visual cortex." In: *Cerebral Cortex Vol. 10*. Peters, A. and Rockland, K.S., eds., pp. 301–330. New York: Plenum Press (1994).

Burkhalter, A. and Van Essen, D.C. "Processing of color, form and disparity information in visual areas VP and V2 of ventral extrastiriate cortex in the macaque monkey," *J. Neurosci.* **6**:2327–2351 (1986).

Burle, B. and Bonnet, M. "Further argument for the existence of a pacemaker in the human information processing system," *Acta Psychol.* **97**:129–143 (1997).

Burle, B. and Bonnet, M. "What's an internal clock for? From temporal information processing to temporal processing of information," *Behavioural Processes* **45**:59–72 (1999).

Burr, D.C., Morrone, M.C., and Ross, R. "Selective suppression of the magnocellular visual pathway during saccadic eye movements," *Nature* **371**:511–513 (1994).

Buxhoeveden, D.P. and Casanova, M.F. "The minicolumn hypothesis in neuroscience," *Brain* **125**:935–951 (2002).

Buzsáki, G. "Theta oscillations in the hippocampus," *Neuron* **33**:325–340 (2002).

Byrne, A. and Hilbert, D.R., eds. *Readings on Color: The Science of Color*. Vol. 2. Cambridge, MA: MIT Press (1997).

Calkins, D.J. "Representation of cone signals in the primate retina," *J. Optical Soc. Am. A* **17**:597–606 (2000).

Callaway, E.M. and Wiser, A.K. "Contributions of individual layer 2–5 spiny neurons to local circuits in macaque primary visual cortex," *Vis. Neurosci.* **13**:907–922 (1996).

Calvin, W.H. "Competing for consciousness: A Darwinian mechanism of an appropriate level of explanation." *J. Consc. Studies* **5**:389–404 (1998).

Calvin, W.H. and Ojemann, G.A. *Conversations with Neil's Brain*. Reading, MA: Addison-Wesley (1994).

Campbell, K.K. *Body and Mind*. New York: Doubleday (1970).

Carey, D.P. "Do action systems resist visual illusions?" *Trends Cogn. Sci.* **5**:109–113 (2001).

Carmichael, S.T. and Price, J.L. "Architectonic subdivision of the orbital and medial prefrontal cortex in the macaque monkey," *J. Comp. Neurol.* **346**:366–402 (1994).

Carrillo, M.C., Gabrieli, J.D.E., and Disterhoft, J.F. "Selective effects of division of attention on discrimination conditioning," *PsychoBiol.* **28**:293–302 (2000).

Carter, R.M., Hofstötter, C., Tsuchiya, N., and Koch, C. "Working memory and fear conditoning," *Proc. Natl. Acad. Sci. USA* **100**:1399–1404 (2003).

Castet, E. and Masson, G.S. "Motion perception during saccadic eye movements," *Nature Neurosci.* **3**:177–183 (2000).

Castiello, U., Paulignan, Y., and Jeannerod, M. "Temporal dissociation of motor responses and subjective awareness," *Brain* **114**:2639–2655 (1991).

Cauller, L.J. and Kulics, A.T. "The neural basis of the behaviorally relevant N1 component of the somatosensory-evoked potential in SI cortex of awake monkeys: Evidence that backward cortical projections signal conscious touch sensation," *Exp. Brain Res.* **84**:607–619 (1991).

Cave, K.R. and Bichot, N.P. "Visuospatial attention: Beyond a spotlight model," *Psychonomic Bull. Rev.* **6**:204–223 (1999).

Celesia, G.G. "Persistent vegetative state: Clinical and ethical issues," *Theor. Medicine* **18**:221–236 (1997).

Celesia, G.G., Bushnell, D., Cone-Toleikis, S., and Brigell, M.G. "Cortical blindness and residual vision: Is the second visual system in humans capable of more than rudimentary visual perception?" *Neurol.* **41**:862–869 (1991).

Chalmers, D.J. *The Conscious Mind: In Search of a Fundamental Theory.* New York: Oxford University Press (1996).

Chalmers, D.J. "What is a neural correlate of consciousness?" In: *Neural Correlates of Consciousness: Empirical and Conceptual Questions.* Metzinger, T., ed., pp. 17–40. Cambridge, MA: MIT Press (2000).

Chalmers, D.J., ed. *Philosophy of Mind: Classical and Contemporary Readings.* Oxford, UK: Oxford University Press (2002).

Changeux, J.P. *L'homme neuronal.* Paris: Fayard (1983).

Chatterjee, S. and Callaway, E.M. "S cone contributions to the magnocellular visual pathway in macaque monkey," *Neuron* **35**:1135–1146 (2002).

Cheesman J. and Merikle, P.M. "Distinguishing conscious from unconscious perceptual processes," *Can. J. Psychol.* **40**:3433–367 (1986).

Chelazzi, L., Miller, E.K., Duncan, J., and Desimone, R. "A neural basis for visual search in inferior temporal cortex," *Nature* **363**:345–347 (1993).

Cherniak, C. "Neural component placement," *Trends Neurosci.* **18**:522–527 (1995).

Chun, M. M. and Wolfe, J. M. "Just say no: How are visual searches terminated when there is no target present?" *Cogn. Psychology* **30**:39–78 (1996).

Churchland, P.S. *Neurophilosophy.* Cambridge, MA: MIT Press (1986).

Churchland, P.S. *Brain-Wise: Studies in Neurophilosophy.* Cambridge, MA: MIT Press (2002).

Churchland, P.S. and Ramachandran, V.S. "Filling in: Why Dennett is wrong." In: *Dennett and His Critics: Demystifying Mind*. Dahlbom, B., ed., pp. 28–52. Oxford, UK: Blackwell Scientific (1993).

Clark, R.E. and Squire, L.R. "Classical conditioning and brain systems: The role of awareness," *Science* **280**:77–81 (1998).

Clark, R.E. and Squire, L.R. "Human eyeblink classical conditioning: Effects of manipulating awareness of the stimulus contingencies," *Psychological Sci.* **10**:14–18 (1999).

Cleeremans, A., et al. "Implicit learning: News from the front," *Trends Cogn. Sci.* **2**:406–416 (1998).

Cleeremans, A., ed. *The Unity of Consciousness*. Oxford, UK: Oxford University Press (2003).

Clifford, C.W.G., Arnold, D.H., and Pearson, J. "A paradox of temporal perception revealed by a stimulus oscillating in colour and orientation," *Vision Res.* **43**:2245–2253 (2003).

Colby, C.L. and Goldberg, M.E. "Space and attention in parietal cortex," *Ann. Rev. Neurosci.* **22**:319–349 (1999).

Cole, J. *Pride and a Daily Marathon*. Cambridge, MA: MIT Press (1995).

Coltheart, M. "Iconic memory," *Phil. Trans. R. Soc. Lond. B* **302**:283–294 (1983).

Coltheart, V., ed. *Fleeting Memories: Cognition of Brief Visual Stimuli*. Cambridge, MA: MIT Press (1999).

Colvin, M.K., Dunbar, K., and Grafman, J. "The effects of frontal lobe lesions on goal achievement in the water jug task," *J. Cogn. Neurosci.* **13**:1139–1147 (2001).

Compte, A., Brunel, N., Goldman-Rakic, P.S., and Wang, X.J. "Synaptic mechanisms and network dynamics underlying spatial working memory in a cortical network model," *Cerebral Cortex* **10**:10–123 (2000).

Conway, B.R., Hubel, D.H., and Livingstone, M.S. "Color contrast in macaque V1," *Cerebral Cortex* **12**:915–925 (2002).

Cook, E.P. and Maunsell, J.H.R. "Dynamics of neuronal responses in macaque MT and VIP during motion detection," *Nature Neurosci.* **5**:985–994 (2002).

Coppola, D. and Purves, D. "The extraordinary rapid disappearance of entoptic images," *Proc. Natl. Acad. Sci. USA* **93**:8001–8004 (1996).

Corbetta, M. "Frontoparietal cortical networks for directing attention and the eye to visual locations: Identical, independent, or overlapping neural systems?" *Proc. Natl. Acad. Sci. USA* **95**:831–838 (1998).

Corkin, S., Amaral, D.G., Gonzalez, R.G., Johnson, K.A., and Hyman, B.T. "H. M.'s medial temporal lobe lesion: Findings from magnetic resonance imaging," *J. Neurosci.* **17**:3964–3979 (1997).

Cornell-Bell, A.H., Finkbeiner, S.M., Cooper, M.S., and Smith, S.J. "Glutamate induces calcium waves in cultured astrocytes: Long-range glial signaling," *Science* **247**:470–473 (1990).

Cotterill, R. *Enchanted Looms: Conscious Networks in Brains and Computers*. Cambridge, UK: Cambridge University Press (1998).

Courtney, S.M., Petit, L., Maisog, J.M., Ungerleider, L.G., and Haxby, J.V. "An area specialized for spatial working memory in human frontal cortex," *Science* **279**:1347–1351 (1998).

Cowan, N. "The magical number 4 in short-term memory: A reconsideration of mental storage capacity," *Behav. Brain Sci.* **24**:87–185 (2001).

Cowey, A. and Heywood, C.A. "Cerebral achromatopsia: Color blindness despite wavelength processing," *Trends Cogn. Sci.* **1**:133–139 (1997).

Cowey, A. and Stoerig, P. "The neurobiology of blindsight," *Trends Neurosci.* **14**:140–145 (1991).

Cowey, A. and Stoerig, P. "Blindsight in monkeys," *Nature* **373**:247–249 (1995).

Cowey, A. and Walsh, V. "Tickling the brain: Studying visual sensation, perception and cognition by transcranial magnetic stimulation," *Prog Brain Research* **134**:411–425 (2001).

Creutzfeldt, O.D. *Cortex Cerebri: Performance, Structural and Functional Organization of the Cortex.* Oxford, UK: Oxford University Press (1995).

Creutzfeldt, O.D. and Houchin, J. "Neuronal basis of EEG waves." In: *Handbook of Electroencephalography and Clinical Neurophysiology.* Vol. 2., Remond, A., ed., pp. 3–55. Amsterdam, Netherlands: Elsevier (1984).

Crick, F.C. "Thinking about the brain," *Scientific American* **241**:219–232 (1979).

Crick, F.C. "Function of the thalamic reticular complex: The searchlight hypothesis," *Proc. Natl. Acad. Sci. USA* **81**:4586–4590 (1984).

Crick, F.C. *The Astonishing Hypothesis.* New York: Charles Scribner's Sons (1994).

Crick, F.C. and Jones, E.G. "Backwardness of human neuroanatomy," *Nature* **361**:109–110 (1993).

Crick, F.C. and Koch, C. "Towards a neurobiological theory of consciousness," *Sem. Neurosci.* **2**:263–275 (1990a).

Crick, F.C. and Koch, C. "Some reflections on visual awareness," *Cold Spring Harbor Symp. Quant. Biol.* **55**:953–962 (1990b).

Crick, F.C. and Koch, C. "The problem of consciousness," *Sci. Am.* **267**:153–159 (1992).

Crick, F.C. and Koch, C. "Are we aware of neural activity in primary visual cortex?" *Nature* **375**:121–123 (1995a).

Crick, F.C. and Koch, C. "Why neuroscience may be able to explain consciousness," *Sci. Am.* **273**:84–85 (1995b).

Crick, F.C. and Koch, C. "Constraints on cortical and thalamic projections: The no-strong-loops hypothesis," *Nature* **391**:245–250 (1998a).

Crick, F.C. and Koch, C. "Consciousness and neuroscience," *Cerebral Cortex* **8**:97–107 (1998b).

Crick, F.C. and Koch, C. "The Unconscious Homunculus. With commentaries by multiple authors," *Neuro-Psychoanalysis* **2**:3–59 (2000).

Crick, F.C. and Koch, C. "A framework for consciousness," *Nature Neurosci.* **6**:119–126 (2003).

Crunelli, V. and Leresche, N. "Childhood absence epilepsy: Genes, channels, neurons and networks," *Nature Rev. Neurosci.* **3**:371–382 (2002).

Culham, J.C., Brandt, S.A., Cavanagh, P., Kanwisher, N.G., Dale, A.M., and Tootell, R.B. "Cortical fMRI activation produced by attentive tracking of moving targets," *J. Neurophysiol.* **80**:2657–2670 (1998).

Cumming, B.G. and DeAngelis, G.C. "The physiology of stereopsis," *Ann. Rev. Neurosci.* **24**:203–238 (2001).

Cumming, B.G. and Parker, A.J. "Responses of primary visual cortical neurons to binocular disparity without depth perception," *Nature* **389**:280–283 (1997).

Cumming, B.G. and Parker, A.J. "Binocular neurons in V1 of awake monkeys are selective for absolute, not relative, disparity," *J. Neurosci.* **19**:5602–5618 (1999).

Cumming, B.G. and Parker, A.J. "Local disparity not perceived depth is signalled by binocular neurons in cortical area V1 of the macaque," *J. Neurosci.* **20**:4758–4767 (2000).

Curcio, C.A., Allen, K.A., Sloan, K.R., Lerea, C.L. Hurley, J.B., Klock, I.B., and Milam, A.H. "Distribution and morphology of human cone photoreceptors stained with anti-blue opsin," *J. Comp. Neurol.* **312**:610–624 (1991).

Curran, T. "Implicit learning revealed by the method of opposition," *Trends Cogn. Sci.* **5**:503–504 (2001).

Cytowic, R.E. *The Man Who Tasted Shapes.* Cambridge, MA: MIT Press (1993).

Dacey, D.M. "Circuitry for color coding in the primate retina," *Proc. Natl. Acad. Sci. USA* **93**:582–588 (1996).

Dacey, D.M., Peterson, B.B., Robinson, F.R., and Gamlin, P.D. "Fireworks in the primate retina: In vitro photodynamics reveals diverse LGN-projecting ganglion cell types," *Neuron* **37**:15–27 (2003).

Damasio, A.R. *The Feeling of What Happens: Body and Emotion in the Making of Consciousness.* New York: Harcourt Brace (1999).

Damasio, A.R. "A neurobiology for consciousness." In: *Neural Correlates of Consciousness: Empirical and Conceptual Questions.* Metzinger, T., ed., pp. 111–120. Cambridge, MA: MIT Press (2000).

Damasio, A.R. and Anderson, S.W. "The frontal lobes." In: *Clinical Neuropsychology.* 4th ed., Heilman, K.M. and Valenstein, E. eds., pp. 404–446. New York: Oxford University Press (2003).

Damasio, A.R., Eslinger, P., Damasio, H., Van Hoesen, G.W., and Cornell, S. "Multimodal amnesic syndrome following bilateral temporal and basal forebrain damage," *Arch. Neurol.* **42**:252–259 (1985).

Damasio, A.R., Tranel, D., and Rizzo, M. "Disorders of complex visual processing." In: *Principles of Behavioral and Cognitive Neurology.* Mesulam, M.M., ed., pp. 332–372. Oxford, UK: Oxford University Press (2000).

Damasio, A.R., Yamada, T., Damasio, H., Corbet, J., and McKee, J. "Central achromatopsia: Behavioral, anatomic and physiologic aspects," *Neurol.* **30**:1064–1071 (1980).

Dantzker, J.L. and Callaway, E.M. "Laminar sources of synaptic input to cortical inhibitory interneurons and pyramidal neurons," *Nature Neurosci.* **7**:701–707 (2000).

Das, A. and Gilbert, C.D. "Distortions of visuotopic map match orientation singularities in primary visual cortex," *Nature* **387**:594–598 (1997).

Davis, W. *Passage of Darkness: The Ethnobiology of the Haitian Zombie.* Chapel Hill, NC: University of North Carolina Press (1988).

Dawson M.E. and Furedy, J.J. "The role of awareness in human differential autonomic classical conditioning: The necessary gate hypothesis," *Psychophysiology* **13**:50–53 (1976).

Dayan P. and Abbott, L. *Theoretical Neuroscience.* Cambridge, MA: MIT Press (2001).

DeAngelis, G.C., Cumming, B.G., and Newsome, W.T. "Cortical area MT and the perception of stereoscopic depth," *Nature* **394**:677–680 (1998).

DeAngelis, G.C. and Newsome, W.T. "Organization of disparity-selective neurons in macaque area MT," *J. Neurosci.* **19**:1398–1415 (1999).

de Fockert, J.W., Rees, G., Frith, C.D., and Lavie, N. "The role of working memory in visual selective attention," *Science* **291**:1803–1806 (2001).

Dehaene, S. "Temporal oscillations in human perception," *Psychol. Sci.* **4**:264–270 (1993).

Dehaene, S. and Changeux, J.-P. "Neural mechanisms for access to consciousness." In: *The Cognitive Neurosciences.* 3rd ed., Gazzaniga, M., ed., in press. Cambridge, MA: MIT Press (2004).

Dehaene, S. and Naccache, L. "Towards a cognitive neuroscience of consciousness: Basic evidence and a workspace framework," *Cognition* **79**:1–37 (2001).

Dehaene, S., Naccache, L., Cohen, L., Le Bihan, D., Mangin J.-F., Poline J.-B., and Rivère, D. "Cerebral mechanisms of word masking and unconscious repetition priming," *Nature Neurosci.* **4**:752–758 (2001).

Dehaene, S., Sergent, C., and Changeux, J.P. "A neuronal model linking subjective report and objective neurophysiological data during conscious perception," *Proc. Natl. Acad. Sci. USA* **100**:8520–8525 (2003).

de Lima, A.D., Voigt, T., and Morrison, J.H. "Morphology of the cells within the inferior temporal gyrus that project to the prefrontal cortex in the macaque monkey," *J. Comp. Neurol.* **296**:159–172 (1990).

Dennett, D. *Content and Consciousness.* Cambridge, MA: MIT Press (1969).

Dennett, D. *Brainstorms.* Cambridge, MA: MIT Press (1978).

Dennett, D. *Consciousness Explained.* Boston: Little & Brown (1991).

Dennett, D. "Are we explaining consciousness yet?" *Cognition* **79**:221–237 (2001).

Dennett, D. "The gift horse of philosophical instruction," *Trends Cogn. Sci.*, in press (2004).

Dennett, D. and Kinsbourne, M. "Time and the observer," *Behavioral & Brain Sci.* **15**:183–247 (1992).

Desimone, R. and Duncan, J. "Neural mechanisms of selective visual attention," *Ann. Rev. Neurosci.* **18**:193–222 (1995).

Desimone, R., Wessinger M., Thomas, L., and Schneider, W. "Attentional control of visual perception: Cortical and subcortical mechanisms," *Cold Spring Harbor Symp. Quant. Biol.* **55**:963–971 (1990).

Destrebecqz, A. and Cleeremans, A. "Can sequence learning be implicit? New evidence with the process dissociation procedure," *Psychonomic Bull. Rev.* **8**:343–350 (2001).

DeVries, S.H. and Baylor, D.A. "Mosaic arrangement of ganglion cell receptive fields in rabbit retina," *J. Neurophysiol.* **78**:2048–2060 (1997).

DeWeerd, P., Gattass, R., Desimone, R., and Ungerleider, L.G. "Responses of cells in monkey visual cortex during perceptual filling-in of an artificial scotoma," *Nature* **377**:731–734 (1995).

DeWeerd, P., Peralta, III M.R., Desimone, R., and Ungerleider, L.G. "Loss of attentional stimulus selection after extrastriate cortical lesions in macaques," *Nature Neurosci.* **2**:753–758 (1999).

DeYoe, E.A., Carman, G.J., Bandettini, P., Glickman, S., Wieser, J., Cox, R., Miller, D., and Neitz, J. "Mapping striate and extrastriate visual areas in human cerebral cortex," *Proc. Natl. Acad. Sci. USA* **93**:2382–2386 (1996).

DiCarlo, J.J. and Maunsell, J.H.R. "Form representation in monkey inferotemporal cortex is virtually unaltered by free viewing," *Nature Neurosci.* **3**:814–821 (2000).

DiLollo, V., Enns, J.T., and Rensink, R.A. "Competition for consciousness among visual events: The psychophysics of reentrant visual processes," *J. Exp. Psychol. Gen.* **129**:481–507 (2000).

Ditterich, J., Mazurek, M.E., and Shadlen, M.N. "Microstimulation of visual cortex affects the speed of perceptual decisions," *Nature Neurosci.* **6**:891–898 (2003).

Di Virgilio, G. and Clarke, S. "Direct interhemisphere visual input to human speech areas," *Human Brain Map.* **5**:347–354 (1997).

Dmytryk, E. *On Film Editing: An Introduction to the Art of Film Construction*. Boston: Focal Press (1984).

Dobelle, W.H. "Artificial vision for the blind by connecting a television camera to the visual cortex," *Am. Soc. Artificial Internal Organs J.* **46**:3–9 (2000).

Dolan, R.J. "Emotion, cognition, and behavior," *Science* **298**:1191–1194 (2002).

Dosher, B. A. and Sperling, G. "A century of human information processing theory: Vision, attention, memory." In: *Perception and Cognition at Century's End.* Hochberg J., ed., pp. 201–254. New York: Academic Press (1998).

Douglas, R., Koch, C., Mahowald, M., Martin, K., and Suarez, H. "Recurrent excitation in neocortical circuits," *Science* **269**:981–985 (1995).

Dow, B.M. "Orientation and color columns in monkey visual cortex," *Cerebral Cortex* **12**:1005–1015 (2002).

Dowling, J.E. *The Retina: An Approachable Part of the Brain.* Cambridge, MA: Harvard University Press (1987).

Doyle, D.A., Cabral, J.M., Pfuetzner, R.A., Kuo, A., Gulbis, J.M., Cohen, S.L., Chait, B.T., and MacKinnon, R. "The structure of the potassium channel: Molecular basis of K^+ conduction and selectivity," *Science* **280**:69–77 (1998).

Dragoi, V., Sharma, J., and Sur, M. "Adaptation-induced plasticity of orientation tuning in adult visual cortex," *Neuron* **28**:287–298 (2000).

Dragunow, M. and Faull, R. "The use of c-fos as a metabolic marker in neuronal pathway tracing," *J. Neurosci. Methods*, **29**:261–265 (1989).

Driver, J. and Baylis, G.C. "Attention and visual object segmentation." In: *The Attentive Brain*. Parasurama R., ed., pp. 299–325. Cambridge, MA: MIT Press (1998).

Driver, J. and Mattingley, J.B. "Parietal neglect and visual awareness," *Nature Neurosci.* **1**:17–22 (1998).

Drummond, J.C. "Monitoring depth of anesthesia: With emphasis on the application of the bispectral index and the middle latency auditory evoked response to the prevention of recall," *Anesthesiology* **93**:876–882 (2000).

Dudai, Y. *The Neurobiology of Memory: Concepts, Findings, Trends*. New York: Oxford University Press (1989).

Duncan, J. "Selective attention and the organization of visual information," *J. Exp. Psychology: General* **113**:501–517 (1984).

Duncan, J. "Converging levels of analysis in the cognitive neuroscience of visual attention," *Phil. Trans. R. Soc. Lond. B* **353**:1307–1317 (1998).

Duncan, J. "An adaptive coding model of neural function in prefrontal cortex," *Nature Rev. Neurosci.* **2**:820–829 (2001).

Eagleman, D.M. and Sejnowski, T.J. "Motion integration and postdiction in visual awareness," *Science* **287**:2036–2038 (2000).

Ebner, A., Dinner, D.S., Noachtar, S., and Lüders, H. "Automatisms with preserved responsiveness: A lateralizing sign in psychomotor seizures," *Neurology* **45**:61–64 (1995).

Eccles, J.C. "Do mental events cause neural events analogously to the probability fields of quantum mechanics?" *Proc. Roy. Soc. Lond. B* **227**:411–428 (1986).

Eccles, J.C. *Evolution of the Brain: Creation of the Self*. London: Routledge (1988).

Eckhorn, R., Bauer, R., Jordan, W., Brosch, M., Kruse, W., Munk, M., and Reitböck, H.J. "Coherent oscillations: a mechanism of feature linking in the visual cortex?" *Biol. Cybern.* **60**:121–130 (1988).

Eckhorn, R., Frien, A., Bauer, R., Woelbern, T., and Kehr, H. "High frequency (60–90 Hz) oscillations in primary visual cortex of awake monkey," *Neuroreport* **4**:243–246 (1993).

Edelman, G.M. *The Remembered Present: A Biological Theory of Consciousness*. New York: Basic Books (1989).

Edelman, G.M. "Naturalizing consciousness: A theoretical framework," *Proc. Natl. Acad. Sci. USA* **100**:5520–5524 (2003).

Edelman, G.M. and Tononi, G. *A Universe of Consciousness*. New York: Basic Books (2000).

Efron, R. "The duration of the present," *Annals New York Acad. Sci.* **138**:713–729 (1967).

Efron, R. "The minimum duration of a perception," *Neuropsychologia* **8**:57–63 (1970a).

Efron, R. "The relationship between the duration of a stimulus and the duration of a perception," *Neuropsychologia* **8**:37–55 (1970b).

Efron, R. "An invariant characteristic of perceptual systems in the time domain," *Attention and Performance* **4**:713–736 (1973a).

Efron, R. "Conservation of temporal information by perceptual systems," *Perception & Psychophysics* **14**:518–530 (1973b).

Egeth, H.E. and Yantis, S. "Visual attention: Control, representation, and time course," *Ann. Rev. Psychol.* **48**:269–297 (1997).

Eichenbaum, H. *The Cognitive Neuroscience of Memory.* New York: Oxford University Press (2002).

Ekstrom, A.D., Kahana, M.J., Caplan, J.B., Fields, T.A., Isham, E.A., Newman, E.L., and Fried, I. "Cellular networks underlying human spatial navigation," *Nature* **425**:184–188 (2003).

Elger, C.E. "Semeiology of temporal lobe seizures." In: *Intractable Focal Epilepsy.* Oxbury, J., Polkey, C.E., and Duchowny, M., eds., pp. 63–68. Philadelphia: Saunders (2000).

Eliasmith, C. *How Neurons Mean: A Neurocomputational Theory of Representational Content.* Ph.D. Dissertation, Dept. of Philosophy, Washington University, St. Louis, MO (2000).

Ellenberger, H.F. *The Discovery of the Unconscious.* New York: Basic Books (1970).

Elston, G.N. "Pyramidal cells of the frontal lobe: All the more spinous to think with," *J. Neurosci.* **20**:RC95 (1–4) (2000).

Elston, G.N. and Rosa, M.G.P. "The occipitoparietal pathway of the macaque monkey: Comparison of pyramidal cell morphology in layer III of functionally related cortical visual areas," *Cerebral Cortex* **7**:432–452 (1997).

Elston, G.N. and Rosa, M.G.P. "Morphological variation of layer III pyramidal neurones in the occipitotemporal pathway of the macaque monkey visual cortex," *Cerebral Cortex* **8**:278–294 (1998).

Elston, G.N., Tweedale, R., and Rosa, M.G.P. "Cortical integration in the visual system of the macaque monkey: Large-scale morphological differences in the pyramidal neurons in the occipital, parietal and temporal lobes," *Proc. R. Soc. Lond. B* **266**:1367–1374 (1999).

Engel, A.K., Fries, P., König, P., Brecht, M., and Singer, W. "Temporal binding, binocular rivalry, and consciousness," *Consc. & Cognition* **8**:128–151 (1999).

Engel, S.A., Glover, G.H., and Wandell, B.A. "Retinotopic organization in human visual cortex and the spatial precision of functional MRI," *Cerebral Cortex* **7**:181–192 (1997).

Engel, A.K., König, P., Gray, C.M., and Singer, W. "Stimulus-dependent neuronal oscillations in cat visual cortex: Inter-columnar interaction as determined by cross-correlation analysis," *Eur. J. Neurosci.* **2**:588–606 (1990).

Engel, A.K., König, P., Kreiter, A.K., and Singer, W. "Interhemispheric synchronization of oscillatory neuronal responses in cat visual cortex," *Science* **252**:1177–1179 (1991).

Engel, A.K. and Singer, W. "Temporal binding and the neural correlates of sensory awareness," *Trends Cogn. Sci.* **5**:16–25 (2001).

Engel, S.A., Zhang, X., and Wandell, B.A. "Colour tuning in human visual cortex measured with functional magnetic resonance imaging," *Nature* **388**:68–71 (1997).

Enns, J.T. and DiLollo, V. "What's new in visual masking," *Trends Cogn. Sci.* **4**:345–352 (2000).

Enroth-Cugell, C. and Robson, J.G. "Functional characteristics and diversity of cat retinal ganglion cells," *Inv. Ophthalmol. Vis. Sci.* **25**:250–267 (1984).

Epstein, R. and Kanwisher, N. "A cortical representation of the local visual environment," *Nature* **392**:598–601 (1998).

Ermentrout, B.G. and Kleinfeld, D. "Traveling electrical waves in cortex: Insights form phase dynamics and speculation on a computational role," *Neuron* **29**:33–44 (2001).

Fahle, M. "Figure-ground discrimination from temporal information," *Proc. R. Soc. Lond. B* **254**:199–203 (1993).

Farah, M.J. *Visual Agnosia.* Cambridge, MA: MIT Press (1990).

Farber, I. and Churchland, P.S. "Consciousness and the neurosciences: Philosophical and theoretical issues." In: *The Cognitive Neurosciences.* 1st ed., Gazzaniga, M.S., ed., pp. 1295–1306. Cambridge, MA: MIT Press (1995).

Fearing, F. *Reflex Action.* Cambridge, MA: MIT Press (1970).

Feldman, M.H. "Physiological observations in a chronic case of locked-in syndrome," *Neurol.* **21**:459–478 (1971).

Felleman, D.J. and Van Essen, D.C. "Distributed hierarchical processing in the primate cerebral cortex," *Cerebral Cortex* **1**:1–47 (1991).

Fendt, M. and Fanselow, M.S. "The neuroanatomical and neurochemical basis of conditioned fear," *Neurosci. & Biobehavioral Rev.* **23**:743–760 (1999).

Ffytche, D.H., Guy, C.N., and Zeki, S. "Motion specific responses from a blind hemifield," *Brain* **119**:1971–1982 (1996).

Ffytche, D.H., Howard, R.J., Brammer, M.J., David, A., Woodruff, P., and Williams, S. "The anatomy of conscious vision: An fMRI study of visual hallucinations," *Nature Neurosci.* **1**:738–742 (1998).

Finger, S. *Origins of Neuroscience.* New York: Oxford University Press (1994).

Fiorani, M. Jr., Rosa, M.G.P., Gattass, R., and Rocha-Miranda, C.E. "Dynamic surrounds of receptive fields in primate striate cortex: A physiological basis for perceptual completion?" *Proc. Natl. Acad. Sci. USA* **89**:8547–8551 (1992).

Flaherty, M.G. *A Watched Pot: How We Experience Time.* New York: University Press (1999).

Flanagan, O. *Consciousness Reconsidered.* Cambridge, MA: MIT Press (1992).

Flanagan, O. *Dreaming Souls.* New York: Oxford University Press (2000).

Flanagan, O. *The Problem of the Soul.* New York: Basic Books (2002).

Flohr, H. "NMDA receptor-mediated computational processes and phenomenal consciousness." In: *Neural Correlates of Consciousness: Empirical and Conceptual Questions.* Metzinger, T., ed., pp. 245–258. Cambridge, MA: MIT Press (2000).

Flohr, H., Glade, U., and Motzko, D. "The role of the NMDA synapse in general anesthesia," *Toxicology Lett.* **100**:23–29 (1998).

Foote, S.L., Aston-Jones, G., and Bloom, F.E. "Impulse activity of locus coeruleus neurons in awake rats and monkeys is a function of sensory stimulation and arousal," *Proc. Natl. Acad. Sci. USA* **77**:3033–3037 (1980).

Foote, S.L. and Morrison, J.H. "Extrathalamic modulation of cortical function," *Ann. Rev. Neurosci.* **10**:67–95 (1987).

Forster, E.M. and Whinnery, J.E. "Recovery from G_z-induced loss of consciousness: Psychophysiologic considerations," *Aviation, Space, Env. Med.* **59**:517–522 (1988).

Frank, L.M., Brown, E.N., and Wilson, M. "Trajectory encoding in the hippocampus and entorhinal cortex," *Neuron* **27**:169–178 (2000).

Franks, N.P. and Lieb, W.R. "Molecular and cellular mkechanisms of general anesthesia," *Nature* **367**:607–614 (1994).

Franks, N.P. and Lieb, W.R. "The molecular basis of general anesthesia: Current ideas." In: *Toward a Science of Consciousness II.* Hameroff, S.R., Kaszniak, A.W., and Scott, A.C., eds., pp.443–457. Cambridge, MA: MIT Press (1998).

Franks, N.P. and Lieb, W.R. "The role of NMDA receptors in consciounsess: What can we learn from anesthetic mechanisms?" In: *Neural Correlates of Consciousness: Empirical and Conceptual Questions.* Metzinger, T., ed., pp. 265–269. Cambridge, MA: MIT Press (2000).

Franz, V.H., Gegenfurtner, K.R., Bülthoff, H.H., and Fahle, M. "Grasping visual illusions: No evidence for a dissociation between perception and action," *Psychol. Sci.* **11**:20–25 (2000).

Freedman, D.J., Riesenhuber, M., Poggio, T., and Miller, E.K. "Categorical representation of visual stimuli in the primate prefrontal cortex," *Science* **291**:312–316 (2001).

Freedman, D.J., Riesenhuber, M., Poggio, T., and Miller, E.K. "Visual categorization and the primate prefrontal cortex: Neurophysiology and behavior," *J. Neurophysiol.* **88**:929–941 (2002).

Freeman, W.J. *Mass Action in the Nervous System.* New York: Academic Press (1975).

Freud, S. "Das Unbewusste," *Int. Zeitschrift Psychoanal.* **3**(4):189–203 and **3**(5):257–269 (1915).

Freud, S. *The Standard Edition of the Complete Psychological Works of Sigmund Freund,* Vol. 1: 1886–1899. Strachey, J., ed., London: The Hogart Press (1966).

Freund, T.F. and Buzsáki, G. "Interneurons in the hippocampus," *Hippocampus* **6**:347–470 (1996).

Fried, I. "Auras and experiental responses arising in the temporal lobe." In: *The Neuropsychiatry of Limbic and Subcortical Disorders.* Salloway S., Malloy P., and Cummings J.L., eds., pp. 113–122. Washington, DC: American Psychiatric Press (1997).

Fried, I., Wilson, C.L., MacDonald, K.A., and Behnke, E.J. "Electric current stimulates laughter," *Nature* **391**:650 (1998).

Friedman-Hill, S., Maldonado, P.E., and Gray, C.M. "Dynamics of striate cortical activity in the alert macaque: I. Incidence and stimulus-dependence of gamma-band neuronal oscillations," *Cerebral Cortex* **10**:1105–1116 (2000).

Fries, P., Neuenschwander, S., Engel, A.K., Goebel, R., and Singer, W. "Rapid feature selective neuronal synchronization through correlated latency shifting," *Nature Neurosci.* **4**:194–200 (2001a).

Fries, P., Reynolds, J.H., Rorie, A.E., and Desimone, R. "Modulation of oscillatory neuronal synchronization by selective visual attention," *Science* **291**:1560–1563 (2001b).

Fries, P., Schröder, J.-H., Singer, W., and Engel, A.K. "Conditions of perceptual selection and suppression during interocular rivalry in strabismic and normal cats," *Vision Res.* **41**:771–783 (2001c).

Fries, W. "Pontine projection from striate and prestriate visual cortex in the macaque monkey: An anterograde study," *Vis. Neurosci.* **4**:205–216 (1990).

Fries, P., Roelfsema, P.R., Engel, A.K., König, P., and Singer, W. "Synchronization of oscillatory responses in visual cortex correlates with perception in interocular rivalry," *Proc. Natl. Acad. Sci. USA* **94**:12699–12704 (1997).

Frith, C.D. "The role of prefrontal cortex in self-consciousness: The case of auditory hallucinations," *Phil. Trans. Roy. Soc. Lond. B* **351**:1505–1512 (1996).

Fuster, J.M. "Unit activity in prefrontal cortex during delayed-response performance: Neuronal correlates of transient memory," *J. Neurophysiol.* **36**:61–78 (1973).

Fuster, J.M. *Memory in the Cerebral Cortex*. Cambridge, MA: MIT Press (1995).

Fuster, J.M. *The Prefrontal Cortex: Anatomy, Physiology, and Neuropsychology of the Frontal Lobe*. 3rd ed. Philadelphia: Lippincott-Raven (1997).

Fuster, J.M. "Executive frontal functions," *Exp. Brain Res.* **133**:66–70 (2000).

Gail, A., Brinksmeyer, H.J., and Eckhorn, R. "Perception-related modulations of local field potential power and coherence in primary visual cortex of awake monkey during binocular rivalry," *Cerebral Cortex*, in press (2004).

Galambos, R., Makeig, S., and Talmachoff, P.J. "A 40-Hz auditory potential recorded from the human scalp," *Proc. Natl. Acad. Sci.* **78**:2643–2647 (1981).

Galin, D. "The structure of awareness: Contemporary applications of William James' forgotten concept of 'the fringe'," *J. Mind & Behavior* **15**:375–402 (1997).

Gallant, J.L., Connor, C.E., and Van Essen, D.C. "Neural activity in areas V1, V2 and V4 during free viewing of natural scenes compared to controlled viewing," *Neuroreport* **9**:2153–2158 (1997).

Gallant, J.L., Shoup, R.E., and Mazer, J.A. "A human extrastriate area functionally homologous to macaque V4," *Neuron* **27**:227–235 (2000).

Gallistel, C.R. *The Organization of Learning*. Cambridge, MA: MIT Press (1990).

Gandhi, S.P., Heeger, D.J., and Boynton, G.M. "Spatial attention affects brain activity in human primary visual cortex," *Proc. Natl. Acad. Sci. USA* **96**:3314–3319 (1999).

Gangestad, S.W., Thornhill, R., and Garver, C.E. "Changes in women's sexual interests and their partners' mate-retention tactics across the menstrual cycle: Evidence for shifting conflicts of interest," *Proc. Roy. Soc. Lond. B* **269**:975–982 (2002).

Gawne, T.J. and Martin, J.M. "Activity of primate V1 cortical neurons during blinks," *J. Neurophysiol.* **84**:2691–2694 (2000).

Gazzaniga, M.S. "Principles of human brain organization derived from split-brain studies," *Neuron* **14**:217–228 (1995).

Gegenfurtner, K. R. and Sperling, G. "Information transfer in iconic memory experiments," *J. Exp. Psychol.* **19**:845–866 (1993).

Geissler, H.G., Schebera, F.U., and Kompass, R. "Ultra-precise quantal timing: evidence from simultaneity thresholds in long-range apparent movement," *Percept. Psychophys.* **61**:707–726 (1999).

Gershon, M.D. *The Second Brain: The Scientific Basis of Gut Instinct.* New York: Harper Collins (1998).

Geschwind, N. and Galaburda, A.M. *Cerebral Laterization.* Cambridge, MA: MIT Press (1987).

Gho, M. and Varela, F.J. "A quantitative assessment of the dependency of the visual temporal frame upon the cortical rhythm," *J. Physiol. Paris* **83**:95–101 (1988).

Ghose, G.M. and Maunsell, J.H.R. "Attentional modulation in visual cortex depends on task timing," *Nature* **419**:616–620 (2002).

Giacino, J.T. "Disorders of consciousness: Differential diagnosis and neuropathologic features," *Seminars Neurol.* **17**:105–111 (1997).

Gibson, J.J. *The Senses Considered as a Perceptual System.* Boston: Houghton Mifflin (1966).

Gibson, J.R., Beierlein, M., and Connors, B.W. "Two networks of electrically coupled inhibitory neurons in neocortex," *Nature* **402**:75–79 (1999).

Gladwell, M. "Wrong turn," *The New Yorker*, June 11, 50–61 (2001).

Glickstein, M. "How are visual areas of the brain connected to motor areas for the sensory guidance of movement?" *Trends Neurosci.* **23**:613–617 (2000).

Gloor, P. "Consciousness as a neurological concept in epileptology: A critical review," *Epilepsia* **27** (**Suppl 2**):S14–S26 (1986).

Gloor, P., Olivier A., and Ives J. "Loss of consciousness in temporal lobe seizures: Observations obained with stereotaxic depth electrode recordings and stimulations." In: *Adv. in Epileptology: 11th Epilepsy Intl. Symposium.* Canger, R., Angeleri, F., and Penry, J.K., eds., pp. 349–353. New York: Raven Press (1980).

Goebel, R., Khorram-Sefat, D., Muckli, L., Hacker, H., and Singer, W. "The constructive nature of vision: Direct evidence from functional magnetic resonance imaging studies of apparent motion and motion imagery," *Eur. J. Neurosci.* **10**:1563–1573 (1998).

Gold, J.L. and Shadlen, M.N. "Banburismus and the brain: Decoding the relationship between sensory stimuli, decisions, and reward," *Neuron* **36**:299–308 (2002).

Goldberg, E. *The Executive Brain: Frontal Lobes and the Civilized Mind.* New York: Oxford University Press (2001).

Goldman-Rakic, P.S. "Architecture of the prefrontal cortex and the central executive," *Annals New York Acad. Sci.* **769**:71–83 (1995).

Goldman-Rakic, P.S., Scalaidhe, S.P.O., and Chafee, M.W. "Domain specificity in cognitive systems." In: *The New Cognitive Neurosciences*. 2nd ed., Gazzaniga, M.S., ed., pp. 733–742. Cambridge, MA: MIT Press (2000).

Goldstein, K. and Gelb, A. "Psychologische Analysen hirnpathologischer Fälle auf Grund von Untersuchungen Hirnverletzter. I Zur Psychologie des optische Wahrnehmungs-und Erkennungsvorganges," *Z. Neurologie & Psychiatrie* **41**:1–142 (1918).

Goodale, M.A. "Perception and action in the human visual system." In: *The New Cognitive Neurosciences*. 2nd ed., Gazzaniga, M.S., ed., pp. 365–377. Cambridge, MA: MIT Press (2000).

Goodale, M.A., Jakobson, L.S., and Keillor, J.M. "Differences in the visual control of pantomimed and natural grasping movements," *Neuropsychologia* **32**:1159–1178 (1994).

Goodale, M.A. and Milner, A.D. *Sight Unseen*. Oxford, UK: Oxford University Press (2004).

Goodale, M.A., Pélisson, D., and Prablanc, C. "Large adjustments in visually guided reaching do not depend on vision of the hand or perception of target displacement," *Nature* **320**:748–750 (1986).

Gordon, H. W. and Bogen, J.E. "Hemispheric lateralization of singing after intracarotid sodium amylobarbitone," *J. Neurol. Neurosurg. Psychiat.* **37**:727–738 (1974).

Gottlieb, J.P., Kusunoki, M., and Goldberg, M.E. "The representation of visual salience in monkey parietal cortex," *Nature* **391**:481–484 (1998).

Gowdy, P.D., Stromeyer, C.F. III, and Kronauer, R.E. "Detection of flickering edges: Absence of a red-green edge detector," *Vision Res.* **39**:4186–4191 (1999).

Grafman, J., Holyoak, K.J., and Boller, F., eds. *Structure and Function of the Human Prefrontal Cortex. Annals New York Acad. Sci.* **769** (1995).

Granon, S., Faure, P., and Changeux, J.P. "Executive and social behaviors under nicotinic receptor regulation," *Proc. Natl. Acad. Sci. USA* **100**:9596–9601 (2003).

Gray, C.M. "The temporal correlation hypothesis of visual feature integration: Still alive and well," *Neuron* **24**:31–47 (1999).

Gray, C.M., König, P., Engel, A.K., and Singer, W. "Oscillatory responses in cat visual cortex exhibit inter-columnar synchronization which reflects global stimulus properties," *Nature* **338**:334–337 (1989).

Gray, C.M. and Singer, W. "Stimulus-specific neuronal oscillations in orientation columns of cat visual cortex," *Proc. Natl. Acad. Sci. USA* **86**:1698–1702 (1989).

Graziano, M.S.A., Taylor, C.R.S., and Moore, T. "Complex movements evoked by microstimulation of precentral cortex," *Neuron* **34**:841–851 (2002).

Greenfield, S.A. *Journeys to the Centers of the Mind. Toward a Science of Consciousness*. New York: W.H. Freeman (1995).

Gregory, R.L. "Cognitive contours," *Nature* **238**:51–52 (1972).

Gregory, R.L. *Eye and Brain: The Psychology of Seeing*. 5th ed. Princeton, NJ: Princeton University Press (1997).

Grieve, K.L., Acuna, C., and Cudeiro, J. "The primate pulvinar nuclei: Vision and action," *Trends Neurosci.* **23**:35–38 (2000).

Griffin, D.R. *Animal Minds: Beyond Cognition to Consciousness.* Chicago, IL: University of Chicago Press (2001).

Griffin, D.R. and Speck, G.B. "New evidence of animal consciousness," *Animal Cognition,* in press (2004).

Grimes, J. "On the failure to detect changes in scenes across saccades." In: *Perception (Vancouver Studies in Cognitive Science, Vol. 2).* Akins, K., ed., pp. 89–110. Oxford, UK: Oxford University Press (1996).

Gross, C.G. *Brain, Vision, Memory: Tales in the History of Neuroscience.* Cambridge, MA: MIT Press (1998).

Gross, C.G. "Genealogy of the 'Grandmother cell'," *Neuroscientist* **8**:512–518 (2002).

Gross, C.G., Bender, D.B., and Rocha-Miranda, C.E. "Visual receptive fields of neurons in inferotemporal cortex of the monkey," *Science* **166**:1303–1306 (1969).

Gross, C.G. and Graziano, M.S.A. "Multiple representations of space in the brain," *Neuroscientist* **1**:43–50 (1995).

Gross, C.G., Rocha-Miranda C.E., and Bender D.B. "Visual properties of neurons in inferotemporal cortex of the macaque," *J. Neurophysiol.* **35**:96–111 (1972).

Grossberg, S. "The link between brain learning, attention, and consciousness," *Conscious. Cogn.* **8**:1–44 (1999).

Grossenbacher, P.G. and Lovelace, C.T. "Mechanisms of synaesthesia: Cognitive and physiological constraints," *Trends Cogn. Sci.* **5**:36–41 (2001).

Grossmann, R.G. "Are current concepts and methods in neuroscience inadequate for studying the neural basis of consciosuness and mental activity?" In: *Information Processing in the Nervous System,* Pinsker, H.M. and Willis, W.D. Jr., eds. New York: Raven Press (1980).

Grunewald, A., Bradley, D.C., and Andersen, R.A. "Neural correlates of structure-from-motion perception in macaque V1 and MT," *J. Neurosci.* **22**:6195–6207 (2002).

Grush, R. and Churchland, P.S. "Gaps in Penrose's toiling," *J. Consc. Studies* **2**:10–29 (1995).

Grüsser, O.J. and Landis, T. *Visual Agnosias and Other Disturbances of Visual Perception and Cognition.* Houndmills, UK: MacMillan Press (1991).

Guilleminault, C. "Cataplexy." In: *Narcolepsy.* Guilleminault, C., Dennet, W.C., and Passouant, P. eds., pp. 125–143. New York: Spectrum (1976).

Gur, M. and Snodderly, D.M. "A dissociation between brain activity and perception: Chromatically opponent cortical neurons signal chromatic flicker that is not perceived," *Vision Res.* **37**:377–382 (1997).

Haarmeier, T., Thier, P., Repnow, M., and Petersen, D. "False perception of motion in a patient who cannot compensate for eye movements," *Nature* **389**:849–852 (1997).

Hadamard, J. *The Mathematician's Mind.* Princeton, NJ: Princeton University Press (1945).

Hadjikhani, N., Liu, A.K., Dale, A.M., Cavanagh, P., and Tootell, R.B. "Retinotopy and color sensitivity in human visual cortical area V8," *Nature Neurosci.* **1**:235–241 (1998).

Hahnloser, R.H.R., Kozhevnikov, A.A., and Fee, M.S. "An ultra-sparse code underlies the generation of neural sequences in a songbird," *Nature* **419**:65–70 (2002).

Haines, R.F. "A breakdown in simultaneous information processing." In: *Presbyopia Research: From Molecular Biology to Visual Adaptation.* Obrecht, G. and Stark, L., eds., pp. 171–175. New York: Plenum Press (1991).

Hameroff, S.R. and Penrose, R. "Orchestrated reduction of quantum coherence in brain microtubules: A model for consciousness." In: *Toward a Science of Consciousness.* Hameroff, S.R., Kaszniak, A.W., and Scott, A.C., eds., pp. 507–540. Cambridge, MA: MIT Press (1996).

Hamker, F.H. "A dynamic model of how feature cues guide spatial attention," *Vision Res.*, in press (2004).

Hamker, F.H. and Worcester, J. "Object detection in natural scenes by feedback." In: *Biologically Motivated Computer Vision. Lecture Notes in Computer Science.* Büelthoff, H.H., ed., pp. 398–407. Berlin: Springer (2002).

Han, C.J., O'Tuathaigh, C.M., van Trigt, L., Quinn, J.J., Fanselow, M.S., Mongeau, R., Koch, C., and Anderson, D.J. "Trace but not delay fear conditioning requires attention and the anterior cingulate cortex," *Proc. Natl. Acad. Sci. USA*, **100**:13087–13092 (2003).

Hardcastle, V.G. "Attention versus consciousness." In: *Neural Basis of Consciousness.* Osaka N., ed., pp. 105–121. Amsterdam, Netherlands: John Benjamins (2003).

Hardin, C.L. *Color for Philosophers: Unweaving the Rainbow.* Indianapolis, IN: Hackett Publishing Company (1988).

Harris, K.D., Csicsvar, J., Hirase, H., Dragoi, G., and Buzsáki, G. "Organization of cell assembles in the hippocampus," *Nature* **424**:552–556 (2003).

Harrison, R.V., Harel, N., Panesar, J., and Mount, R.J. "Blood capillary distribution correlates with hemodynamic-based functional imaging in cerebral cortex," *Cerebral Cortex* **12**:225–233 (2002).

Harter, M.R., "Excitability cycles and cortical scanning: A review of two hypotheses of central intermittency in perception," *Psychol. Bull.* **68**:47–58 (1967).

Haxby, J.V., Gobbini, M.I., Furey, M.L., Ishai, A., Schouten, J.L., and Pietrini, P. "Distributed and overlapping representations of faces and objects in ventral temporal cortex," *Science* **293**:2425–2430 (2001).

Haxby, J.V., Hoffman, E.A., and Gobbini, M.I. "The distributed human neural system for face perception," *Trends Cogn. Sci.* **4**:223–233 (2000).

He, S., Cavanagh, P., and Intrilligator, J. "Attentional resolution and the locus of visual awareness," *Nature* **383**:334–337 (1996).

He, S., Cohen, E.R., and Hu, X. "Close correlation between activity in brain area MT/V5 and the perception of a visual motion aftereffect," *Curr. Biol.* **8**:1215–1218 (1998).

He, S. and MacLeod, D.I.A. "Orientation-selective adaptation and tilt aftereffect from invisible patterns," *Nature* **411**:473–476 (2001).

Hebb, D.O. *The Organization of Behavior: A Neuropsychological Theory.* New York: Wiley (1949).

Heeger, D.J., Boynton, G.M., Demb, J.B., Seideman, E., and Newsome, W.T. "Motion opponency in visual cortex," *J. Neurosci.* **19**:7162–7174 (1999).

Heeger, D.J., Huk, A.C., Geisler, W.S., and Albrecht, D.G. "Spikes versus BOLD: What does neuroimaging tell us about neuronal activity," *Nature Neurosci.* **3**:631–633 (2000).

Heilman, K.M., Watson, R.T., and Valenstein, E. "Neglect and related disorders." In: *Clinical Neuropsychology.* 4th ed., Heilman, K.M. and Valenstein, E., eds., pp. 296–346. New York: Oxford University Press (2003).

Heinemann, S.H., Terlau, H., Stühmer, W., Imoto, K., and Numa, S. "Calcium-channel characteristics conferred on the sodium-channel by single mutations," *Nature* **356**:441–443 (1992).

Heisenberg, M. and Wolf, R. *Vision in Drosophila: Genetics of Microbehavior. Studies in Brain Function, Vol. 12.* Heidelberg, Germany: Springer (1984).

Herrigel, E. *Zen in the Art of Archery.* New York: Pantheon Books (1953).

Herzog, M. and Koch, C. "Seeing properties of an invisible object: Feature inheritance and shine-through," *Proc. Natl. Acad. Sci. USA* **98**:4271–4275 (2001).

Herzog, M., Parish, L., Koch, C., and Fahle, M. "Fusion of competing features is not serial," *Vision Res.* **43**:1951–1960 (2003).

Hess, R.H., Baker, C.L., and Zihl, J. "The motion-blind patient: Low-level spatial and temporal filters," *J. Neurosci.* **9**:1628–1640 (1989).

Heywood, C.A. and Zihl, J. "Motion blindness." In: *Case Studies in the Neuropsychology of Vision.* Humphreys, G.W., ed., pp. 1–16. Psychology Press (1999).

Hilgetag, C.-C., O'Neill, M.A., and Young, M.P. "Indeterminate organization of the visual system," *Science* 271: 776–777 (1996).

Hille, B. *Ionic Channels of Excitable Membranes.* 3rd ed. Sunderland, MA: Sinauer Associates: (2001).

Hirsh, I.J. and Sherrick, C.E. "Perceived order in different sense modalities," *J. Exp. Psychol.* **62**:423–432 (1961).

Hobson, J.A. *Sleep.* New York: Scientific American Library, Freeman (1989).

Hobson, J.A. *Consciousness.* New York: Scientific American Library, Freeman (1999).

Hobson, J.A., Stickgold, R., and Pace-Schott, E.F. "The neurophysiology of REM sleep dreaming," *Neuroreport* **9**:R1–R14 (1998).

Hochstein, S. and Ahissar, M. "View from the top: Hierarchies and reverse hierarchies in the visual system," *Neuron* **36**:791–804 (2002).

Hofstötter, C., Koch, C., and Kiper, D.C. "Absence of high-level contributions to the formation of afterimages," *Soc. Neurosci. Abstr.*, **819**:24 (2003).

Holender, D. "Semantic activation without conscious identification in dichotic listening, parafoveal vision, and visual masking: A survey and appraisal," *Behav. Brain Sci.* **9**:1–23 (1986).

Holt, G.R. and Koch, C. "Electrical interactions via the extracellular potential near cell bodies," *J. Computat. Neurosci.* **6**:169–184 (1999).

Holy, T.E., Dulac, C., and Meister, M. "Responses of vomeronasal neurons to natural stimuli," *Science* **289**:1569–1572 (2000).

Horgan, J. *The End of Science.* Reading, MA: Addison-Wesley (1996).

Horton, J.C. and Hedley-Whyte, E.T. "Mapping of cytochrome oxidase patches and ocular dominance columns in human visual cortex," *Phil. Trans. Roy. Soc. Lond. B* **304**:255–272 (1984).

Horton, J.C. and Hoyt, W.F. "The representation of the visual field in human striate cortex," *Arch. Opthalmology* **109**:816–824 (1991a).

Horton, J.C. and Hoyt, W.F. "Quadratic visual field defects: A hallmark of lesions in extrastriate (V2/V3) cortex," *Brain* **114**:1703–1718 (1991b).

Hu, Y. and Goodale, M.A. "Grasping after a delay shifts size-scaling from absolute to relative metrics," *J. Cogn. Neurosci.* **12**:856–868 (2000).

Hubel, D.H. *Eye, Brain, and Vision.* New York: Scientific American Library (1988).

Hubel, D.H. and Wiesel, T.N. "Receptive fields of single neurons in the cat's striate cortex," *J. Physiol.* **148**:574–591 (1959).

Hubel, D.H. and Wiesel, T.N. "Receptive fields, binocular interaction and functional architecture in the cat's visual cortex," *J. Physiol.* **160**:106–154 (1962).

Hubel, D.H. and Wiesel, T.N. "Receptive fields and functional architecture of monkey striate cortex," *J. Physiol.* **195**:215–243 (1968).

Hübener M., Shoham, D., Grinvald, A., and Bonhoeffer, T. "Spatial relationships among three columnar systems in cat area 17," *J. Neurosci.* **17**:9270–9284 (1997).

Huerta, M.F., Krubitzer, L.A., and Kaas, J.H. "Frontal eye field as defined by intracortical microstimulation in squirrel monkeys, owl monkeys and macaque monkeys: I. Subcortical connections," *J. Comp. Neurol.* **253**:415–439 (1986).

Huk, A.C., Ress, D., and Heeger, D.J. "Neuronal basis of the motion aftereffect reconsidered," *Neuron* **32**:161–172 (2001).

Hunter, J. and Jasper, H.H. "Effects of thalamic stimulation in unanesthetized cats," *EEG Clin. Neurophysiol.* **1**:305–315 (1949).

Hupe, J.M., James, A.C., Payne, B.R., Lomber, S.G., Girard, P., and Bullier, J. "Cortical feedback improves discrimination between figure and background by V1, V2, and V3 neurons," *Nature* **394**:784–787 (1998).

Husain, M. and Rorden, C. "Non-spatially lateralized mechanisms in hemispatial neglect," *Nature Rev. Neurosci.* **4**:26–36 (2003).

Huxley, T.H. *Animal Automatism, and Other Essays.* Humboldt Library of Popular Science Literature. New York: J. Fitzgerald (1884).

Ilg, U.J. and Thier, P. "Inability of rhesus monkey area V1 to discriminate between self-induced and externally induced retinal image slip," *Eur. J. Neurosci.* **8**:1156–1166 (1996).

Inoue, Y. and Mihara, T. "Awareness and responsiveness during partial seizures," *Epilepsia* **39**:7–10 (1998).

Ishai, A., Ungerleider, L.G., Martin, A., and Haxby, J.V. "The representation of objects in the human occipital and temporal cortex," *J. Cogn. Neurosci.* **12 (Suppl. 2)**:35–51 (2000).

Ito, M. and Gilbert, C.D. "Attention modulates contextual influences in the primary visual cortex of alert monkeys," *Neuron* **22**:593–604 (1999).

Ito, M., Tamura, H., Fujita, I., and Tanaka, K. "Size and position invariance of neuronal responses in monkey inferotemporal cortex," *J. Neurophysiol.* **73**:218–226 (1995).

Itti, L. and Koch, C. "A saliency-based search mechanism for overt and covert shifts of visual attention," *Vision Res.* **40**:1489–1506 (2000).

Itti, L. and Koch, C. "Computational modeling of visual attention," *Nature Rev. Neurosci.* **2**:194–204 (2001).

Itti, L., Koch, C., and Niebur, E. "A model of saliency-based visual attention for rapid scene analysis," *IEEE Trans. Pattern Analysis & Machine Intell. (PAMI)* **20**:1254–1259 (1998).

Jackendoff, R. *Consciousness and the Computational Mind.* Cambridge, MA: MIT Press (1987).

Jackendoff, R. "How language helps us think," *Pragmatics & Cognition* **4**:1–34 (1996).

Jacobson, A., Kales, A., Lehmann, D., and Zweizig, J.R. "Somnambulism: All-night electroencephalographic studies," *Science* **148**:975–977 (1965).

Jacoby, L.L. "A process dissociation framework: Separating automatic from intentional uses of memory," *J. Memory Lang.* **30**:513–541 (1991).

James, W. *The Principles of Psychology.* New York: Dover Publications (1890).

James, W. *Psychology: Briefer Course.* New York: Collier Books (1962).

Jameson, K.A., Highnote, S.M., and Wasserman, L.M. "Richer color experience in observers with multiple photopigment opsin genes," *Psychonomic Bulletin & Rev.* **8**:244–261 (2001).

Järvilehto, T. "The theory of the organism-environment system: IV. The problem of mental activity and consciousness," *Int. Physiol. Behav. Sci.* **35**:35–57 (2000).

Jasper, H.H. "Sensory information and conscious experience," *Adv. Neurol.* **77**:33–48 (1998).

Jaynes, J. *The Origin of Consciousness in the Breakdown of the Bicameral Mind.* Boston: Houghton Mifflin (1976).

Jeannerod, M. *The Cognitive Neuroscience of Action.* Oxford, UK: Blackwell (1997).

Johnson, R.R. and Burkhalter, A. "A polysynaptic feedback circuit in rat visual cortex," *J. Neurosci.* **17**:129–140 (1997).

Johnson-Laird, P.N. "A computational analysis of consciousness," *Cognition & Brain Theory* **6**:499–508 (1983).

Johnston, R.W. "Pheromones, the vomeronasal system, and communication." In: *Olfaction and Taste XII: An International Symposium*. Murphy, C., ed., pp. 333–348. *Annals New York Acad. Sci.* **855** (1998).

Jolicoeur, P., Ullman, S., and MacKay, M. "Curve tracing: A possible basic operation in the perception of spatial relations," *Mem. Cognition* **14**:129–140 (1986).

Jones, E.G. *The Thalamus*. New York: Plenum Press (1985).

Jones, E.G. "Thalamic organization and function after Cajal," *Progress Brain Res.* **136**:333–357 (2002).

Jordan, G. and Mollon, J.D. "A study of women heterozygous for color deficiencies," *Vision Res.* **33**:1495–1508 (1993).

Jovicich, J., Peters, R.J., Koch, C., Braun, J., Chang, L., and Ernst, T. "Brain areas specific for attentional load in a motion tracking task," *J. Cogn. Neurosci.* **13**:1048–1058 (2001).

Judson, H.J. *The Eighth Day of Creation*. London: Penguin Books (1979).

Julesz, B. *Foundations of Cyclopean Perception*. Chicago, IL: University of Chicago Press (1971).

Julesz, B. "Textons, the elements of texture perception, and their interactions," *Nature* **290**:91–97 (1981).

Kahana, M.K., Sekuler, R., Caplan, J.B., Kirschen, M., and Madsen, J.R. "Human theta oscillations exhibit task dependence during virtual maze navigation," *Nature* **399**:781–784 (1999).

Kamitani, Y. and Shimojo, S. "Manifestation of scotomas created by transcranial magnetic stimulation of human visual cortex," *Nature Neurosci.* **2**:767–771 (1999).

Kandel, E.R. "A new intellectual framework for psychiatry," *Am. J. Psychiatry* **155**:457–469 (1998).

Kandel, E.R. "The molecular biology of memory storage: A dialogue between genes and synapses," *Science* **294**:1030–1038 (2001).

Kanizsa, G. *Organization in Vision: Essays in Gestalt Perception*. New York: Praeger (1979).

Kanwisher, N. and Driver, J. "Objects, attributes, and visual attention: Which, what and where," *Curr. Direct. Psychol. Sci.* **1**:26–31 (1997).

Kanwisher, N., McDermott, J., and Chun, M.M. "The fusiform face area: A module in human extrastriate cortex specialized for face perception," *J. Neurosci.* **17**:4302–4311 (1997).

Kaplan, E. "The receptive field structure of retinal ganglion cells in cat and monkey." In: *The Neural Basis of Visual Function*. Leventhal, A.G., ed., pp. 10–40. Boca Raton, FL: CRC Press (1991).

Kaplan-Solms, K. and Solms M. *Clinical Studies in Neuro-Psychoanalysis*. London: Karnac Books (2000).

Karnath, H.-O. "New insights into the functions of the superior temporal cortex," *Nature Rev. Neurosci.* **2**:568–576 (2001).

Karnath, H.-O., Ferber, S., and Himmelbach, M. "Spatial awareness is a function of the temporal, not the posterior parietal lobe," *Nature* **411**:950–954 (2001).

Kastner, S., De Weerd, P., Desimone, R., and Ungerleider, L.G. "Mechanisms of directed attention in the human extrastriate cortex as revealed by functional MRI," *Science* **282**:108–111 (1998).

Kastner, S. and Ungerleider, L.G. "Mechanisms of visual attention in the human cortex," *Ann. Rev. Neurosci.* **23**:315–341 (2000).

Kavey, N.B., Whyte, J., Resor, S.R. Jr., and Gidro-Frank, S. "Somnambulism in adults," *Neurol.* **40**:749–752 (1990).

Keil, A., Müller, M.M., Ray, W.J., Gruber, T., and Elbert, T. "Human gamma band activity and perception of a gestalt," *J. Neurosci.* **19**:7152–7161 (1999).

Keller, E.F. *The Century of the Gene.* Cambridge, MA: Harvard University Press (2000).

Kennedy, H. and Bullier, J. "A double-labelling investigation of the afferent connectivity to cortical areas V1 and V2," *J. Neurosci.* **5**:2815–2830 (1985).

Kentridge, R.W., Heywood, C.A., and Weiskrantz, L. "Residual vision in multiple retinal locations within a scotoma: Implications for blindsight," *J. Cogn. Neurosci.* **9**:191–202 (1997).

Kentridge, R.W., Heywood, C.A., and Weiskrantz, L. "Attention without awareness in blindsight," *Proc. Roy. Soc. Lond. B* **266**:1805–1811 (1999).

Kessel, R.G. and Kardon, R.H. *Tissues and Organs: A Text-Atlas of Scanning Electron Microscopy.* San Francisco, CA: Freeman (1979).

Keverne, E.B. "The vomeronasal organ," *Science* **286**:716–720 (1999).

Keysers, C. and Perrett, D.I. "Visual masking and RSVP reveal neural competition," *Trends Cogn. Sci.* **6**:120–125 (2002).

Keysers, C., Xiao, D.-K., Földiák, P., and Perrett, D.I. "The speed of sight," *J. Cogn. Neurosci.* **13**:1–12 (2001).

Kinney, H.C., Korein, J., Panigrahy, A., Dikkes, P., and Goode, R. "Neuropathological findings in the brain of Karen Ann Quinlan," *New England J. Med.* **330**:1469–1475 (1994).

Kinomura, S., Larsson, J., Gulyás, B., and Roland, P.E. "Activation by attention of the human reticular formation and thalamic intralaminar nuclei," *Science* **271**:512–515 (1996).

Kirk, R. "Zombies versus materialists," *Aristotelian Society* **48 (suppl.)**:135–152 (1974).

Kitcher, P. *Freud's Dream: A Complete Interdisciplinary Science of Mind.* Cambridge, MA: MIT Press (1992).

Kleinschmidt, A., Buchel, C., Zeki, S., and Frackowiak, R.S.J. "Human brain activity during spontaneously reversing perception of ambiguous figures," *Proc. R. Soc. Lond. B* **265**:2427–2433 (1998).

Klemm, W.R., Li, T.H., and Hernandez, J.L. "Coherent EEG indicators of cognitive binding during ambigious figure tasks," *Consc. & Cognition* **9**:66–85 (2000).

Klimesch, W. "EEG alpha and theta oscillations reflect cognitive and memory performance: A review and analysis," *Brain Res. Rev.* **29**:169–195 (1999).

Knuttinen, M.-G., Power, J.M., Preston, A.R., and Disterhoft, J.F. "Awareness in classical differential eyeblink conditioning in young and aging humans," *Behav. Neurosci.* **115**:747–757 (2001).

Kobatake, E., Wang, G., and Tanaka, K. "Effects of shape-discrimination training on the selectivity of inferotemporal cells in adult monkeys," *J. Neurophysiol.* **80**:324–330 (1998).

Koch, C. "The action of the corticofugal pathway on sensory thalamic nuclei: A hypothesis," *Neurosci.* **23**:399–406 (1987).

Koch, C. "Visual awareness and the thalamic intralaminar nuclei," *Consc. & Cognition* **4**:163–165 (1995).

Koch, C. *Biophysics of Computation.* New York: Oxford University Press (1999).

Koch, C. and Crick, F.C. "Some further ideas regarding the neuronal basis of awareness." In: *Large-Scale Neuronal Theories of the Brain.* Koch, C. and Davis, J., eds., pp. 93–110, Cambridge, MA: MIT Press (1994).

Koch, C. and Laurent, G. "Complexity and the nervous system," *Science* **284**:96–98 (1999).

Koch, C. and Tootell, R.B. "Stimulating brain but not mind," *Nature* **383**:301–303 (1996).

Koch, C. and Ullman, S. "Shifts in selective visual attention: Towards the underlying neural circuitry," *Human NeuroBiol.* **4**:219–227 (1985).

Koffka, K. *Principles of Gestalt Psychology.* New York: Hartcourt (1935).

Kohler, C.G., Ances, B.M., Coleman, A.R., Ragland, J.D., Lazarev, M., and Gur, R.C. "Marchiafava-Bignami disease: Literature review and case report," *Neuropsychiatry, Neuropsychol. Behav. Neurol.* **13**:67–76 (2000).

Köhler, W. *The Task of Gestalt Psychology.* Princeton, NJ: Princeton University Press (1969).

Kolb, F.C. and Braun, J. "Blindsight in normal observers," *Nature* **377**:336–338 (1995).

Komatsu, H., Kinoshita, M., and Murakami, I. "Neural responses in the retinotopic representation of the blind spot in the macaque V1 to stimuli for perceptual filling-in," *J. Neurosci.* **20**:9310–9319 (2000).

Komatsu, H. and Murakami, I. "Behavioral evidence of filling-in at the blind spot of the monkey," *Vis. Neurosci.* **11**:1103–1113 (1994).

Konorski, J. *Integrative Activity of the Brain.* Chicago, IL: University of Chicago Press (1967).

Kosslyn, S.M. "Visual Consciousness." In: *Finding Consciousness in the Brain.* Grossenbacher P.G., ed., pp. 79–103. Amsterdam, Netherlands: John Benjamins (2001).

Kosslyn, S.M., Ganis, G., and Thompson, W.L. "Neural foundations of imagery," *Nature Rev. Neurosci.* **2**:635–642 (2001).

Kosslyn, S.M., Thompson, W.L., and Alpert, N.M. "Neural systems shared by visual imagery and visual perception: A PET study," *Neuroimage* **6**:320–334 (1997).

Koulakov, A.A. and Chklovskii, D.B. "Orientation preference patterns in mammalian visual cortex: A wire length minimization approach," *Neuron* **29**:519–527 (2001).

Krakauer, J. *Eiger Dreams*. New York: Lyons & Burford (1990).

Kreiman, G. *On the neuronal activity in the human brain during visual recognition, imagery and binocular rivalry*. Ph.D. Thesis. Pasadena: California Institute of Technology (2001).

Kreiman G., Fried, I., and Koch, C. "Single-neuron correlates of subjective vision in the human medial temporal lobe," *Proc. Natl. Acad. Sci. USA* **99**:8378–8383 (2002).

Kreiman, G., Koch, C., and Fried, I. "Category-specific visual responses of single neurons in the human medial temporal lobe," *Nature Neurosci.* **3**:946–953 (2000a).

Kreiman, G., Koch, C., and Fried, I. "Imagery neurons in the human brain," *Nature* **408**:357–361 (2000b).

Kreiter, A.K. and Singer, W. "Oscillatory neuronal responses in the visual cortex of the awake macaque monkey," *Eur. J. Neurosci.* **4**:369–375 (1992).

Kreiter, A.K. and Singer, W. "Stimulus-dependent synchronization of neuronal responses in the visual cortex of the awake macaque monkey," *J. Neurosci.* **16**:2381–2396 (1996).

Krekelberg, B. and Lappe, M. "Neuronal latencies and the position of moving objects," *Trends Neurosci.* **24**:335–339 (2001).

Kretschmann, H.-J. and Weinrich, W. *Cranial Neuroimaging and Clinical Neuroanatomy*. Stuttgart, Germany: Georg Thieme (1992).

Kristofferson, A.B. "Successiveness discrimination as a two-state, quantal process," *Science* **158**:1337–1339 (1967).

Kuffler, S.W. "Neurons in the retina: Organization, inhibition and excitatory problems," *Cold Spring Harbor Symp. Quant. Biol.* **17**:281–292 (1952).

Kulli, J. and Koch, C. "Does anesthesia cause loss of consciousness?" *Trends Neurosci.* **14**:6–10 (1991).

Kunimoto, C., Miller, J., and Pashler, H. "Confidence and accuracy of near-threshold discrimination responses," *Cons. & Cogn.* **10**:294–340 (2001).

Kustov, A.A. and Robinson, D.L. "Shared neural control of attentional shifts and eye movements," *Nature* **384**:74–77 (1996).

LaBerge, D. and Buchsbaum, M.S. "Positron emission tomographic measurements of pulvinar activity during an attention task. *J. Neurosci.* **10**:613–619 (1990).

Laming, P.R., Syková, E., Reichenbach, A., Hatton, G.I., and Bauer, H., *Glia Cells: Their Role in Behavior*. Cambridge, UK: Cambridge University Press (1998).

Lamme, V.A.F. "Why visual attention and awareness are different," *Trends Cogn. Sci.* **7**:12–18 (2003).

Lamme, V.A.F. and Roelfsema, P.R. "The distinct modes of vision offered by feedforward and recurrent processing," *Trends Neurosci.* **23**:571–579 (2000).

Lamme, V.A.F. and Spekreijse, H. "Contextual modulation in primary visual cortex and scene perception." In: *The New Cognitive Neurosciences*. 2nd ed., Gazzaniga, M.S., ed., pp. 279–290. Cambridge, MA: MIT Press (2000).

Lamme, V.A.F., Zipser, K., and Spekreijse, H. "Figure-ground activity in primary visual cortex is suppressed by anesthesia," *Proc. Natl. Acad. Sci. USA* **95**:3263–3268 (1998).

Langston, J.W. and Palfreman, J. *The Case of the Frozen Addicts.* New York: Vintage Books (1995).

Lashley, K.S. "Cerebral organization and behavior." In: *The Brain and Human Behavior. Proc. Ass. Nervous & Mental Disease*, pp. 1–18. New York: Hafner (1956).

Laurent, G. "A systems perspective on early olfactory coding," *Science* **286**:723–728 (1999).

Laurent, G., Stopfer, M., Friedrich, R.W., Rabinovich, M.I., Volkovskii, A., and Abarbanel, H.D. "Odor encoding as an active, dynamical process: Experiments, computation, and theory," *Ann. Rev. Neurosci.* **24**:263–297 (2001).

Laureys, S., Faymonville, M.E., Degueldre, C., Fiore, G.D., Damas, P, Lambermont, B., Janssens, N., Aerts, J., Franck, G., Luxen, A., Moonen, G., Lamy, M., and Maquet, P. "Auditory processing in the vegetative state," *Brain* **123**:1589–1601 (2000).

Laureys, S., Faymonville, M.E., Peigneux, P., Damas, P., Lambermont, B., Del Fiore, G., Degueldre, C., Aerts, J., Luxen, A., Franck, G., Lamy, M., Moonen, G., and Maquet, P. "Cortical processing of noxious somatosensory stimuli in the persistent vegetative state," *Neuroimage* **17**:732–741 (2002).

Le Bihan, D., Mangin, J.F., Poupon, C., Clark, C.A., Pappata, S., Molko, N., and Chabriat, H. "Diffusion tensor imaging: Concepts and applications," *J. Magnetic Resonance Imaging* **13**:534–546 (2001).

Lechner, H.A.E., Lein, E.S., and Callaway, E.M. "A genetic method for selective and quickly reversible silencing of mammalian neurons," *J. Neurosci.* **22**:5287–5290 (2002).

LeDoux, J. *The Emotional Brain.* New York: Simon and Schuster (1996).

Lee, D.K., Itti, L., Koch, C., and Braun, J. "Attention activates winner-take-all competition amongst visual filters," *Nature Neurosci.* **2**:375–381 (1999).

Lee, D.N. and Lishman, J.R. "Visual proprioceptive control of stance," *J. Human Movement Studies* **1**:87–95 (1975).

Lee, S.-H. and Blake, R. "Rival ideas about binocular rivalry," *Vision Res.* **39**:1447–1454 (1999).

Lehky, S.R. and Maunsell, J.H.R. "No binocular rivalry in the LGN of alert macaque monkeys," *Vision Res.* **36**:1225–1234 (1996).

Lehky, S.R. and Sejnowski, T. J. "Network model of shape-from-shading: Neural function arises from both receptive and projective fields", *Nature* **333**:452–454 (1988).

Lennie, P. "Color vision." In: *Principles of Neural Science.* 4th ed., Kandel, E.R., Schwartz, J.H., and Jessel, T.M. eds., pp. 583–599. New York: McGraw Hill (2000).

Lennie, P. "The cost of cortical computation," *Current Biol.* **13**:493–497 (2003).

Leopold, D.A. and Logothetis, N.K. "Activity changes in early visual cortex reflects monkeys' percepts during binocular rivalry," *Nature* **379**:549–553 (1996).

Leopold, D.A. and Logothetis, N.K. "Multistable phenomena: Changing views in perception," *Trends Cogn. Sci.* **3**:254–264 (1999).

Leopold, D.A., Wilke, M., Maier, A., and Logothetis, N.K. "Stable perception of visually ambiguous patterns," *Nature Neurosci.* **5**:605–609 (2002).

LeVay, S., Connolly, M., Houde, J., and Van Essen, D.C. "The complete pattern of ocular dominance stripes in the striate cortex and visual field of the macaque monkey," *J. Neurosci.* **5**:486–501 (1985).

LeVay, S. and Gilbert, C.D. "Laminar patterns of geniculocortical projection in the cat," *Brain Res.* **113**:1–19 (1976).

LeVay, S. and Nelson, S.B. "Columnar organization of the visual cortex." In: *The Neural Basis of Visual Function.* Leventhal, A.G., ed., pp. 266–314. Boca Raton, FL: CRC Press (1991).

Levelt, W. *On Binocular Rivalry.* Soesterberg, Netherlands: Institute for Perception RVO-TNO (1965).

Levick, W.R. and Zacks, J.L. "Responses of cat retinal ganglion cells to brief flashes of light," *J. Physiol.* **206**:677–700 (1970).

Levine, J. "Materialism and qualia: The explanatory gap." *Pacific Philos. Quart.* **64**:354–361 (1983).

Levitt, J.B., Kiper, D.C., and Movshon, J.A. "Receptive fields and functional architecture of macaque V2," *J. Neurophysiol.* **71**:2517–2542 (1994).

Lewis, J.W. and Van Essen, D.C. "Mapping of architectonic subdivisions in the macaque monkey, with emphasis on parieto-occipital cortex," *J. Comp. Neurol.* **428**:79–111 (2000).

Li, F.F., VanRullen, R., Koch, C., and Perona, P. "Rapid natural scene categorization in the near absence of attention," *Proc. Natl. Acad. Sci. USA* **99**:9596–9601 (2002).

Li, W.H., Parigi, G., Fragai, M., Luchinat, C., and Meade, T.J. "Mechanistic studies of a calcium-dependent MRI contrast agent," *Inorg. Chem.* **41**:4018–4024 (2002).

Liang, J., Williams, D.R., and Miller, D.T. "Supernormal vision and high-resolution retinal imaging through adaptive optics," *J. Opt. Soc. Am. A* **14**:2884–2892 (1997).

Libet, B. "Brain stimulation and the threshold of conscious experience." In: *Brain and Conscious Experience.* Eccles, J.C., ed., pp. 165–181. Berlin: Springer (1966).

Libet, B. "Electrical stimulation of cortex in human subjects and conscious sensory aspects." In: *Handbook of Sensory Physiology, Vol II: Somatosensory Systems.* Iggo, A. ed., pp. 743–790. Berlin: Springer (1973).

Libet, B. *Neurophysiology of Consciousness: Selected Papers and New Essays by Benjamin Libet.* Boston: Birkhäuser (1993).

Lichtenstein, M. "Phenomenal simultaneity with irregular timing of components of the visual stimulus," *Percept. Mot. Skills* **12**:47–60 (1961).

Lisman, J.E. "Bursts as a unit of neural information: Making unreliable synapses reliable," *Trends Neurosci.* **20**:38–43 (1997).

Lisman, J.E. and Idiart, M. A. "Storage of 7 ± 2 short-term memories in oscillatory subcycles," *Science* **267**:1512–1515 (1995).

Livingstone, M.S. "Mechanisms of direction selectivity in macaque V1," *Neuron* **20**:509–526 (1998).

Livingstone, M.S. and Hubel, D.H. "Effects of sleep and rousal on the processing of visual information in the cat," *Science* **291**:554–561 (1981).

Livingstone, M.S. and Hubel, D.H. "Anatomy and physiology of a color system in the primate visual system," *J. Neurosci.* **4**:309–356 (1984).

Livingstone, M.S. and Hubel, D.H. "Connections between layer 4B of area 17 and thick cytochrome oxidase stripes of area 18 in the squirrel monkey," *J. Neurosci.* **7**:3371–3377 (1987).

Llinás, R.R. and Paré, D. "Of dreaming and wakefulness," *Neurosci.* **44**:521–535 (1991).

Llinás, R.R., Ribary, U., Contreras, D., and Pedroarena, C. "The neuronal basis for consciousness," *Phil. Trans. R. Soc. Lond. B. Biol. Sci.* **353**:1841–1849 (1998).

Loftus, G.R., Duncan, J., and Gehrig, P. "On the time course of perceptual information that results from a brief visual presentation," *J. Exp. Psychol. Human Percept. & Perform.* **18**:530–549 (1992).

Logothetis, N.K. "Single units and conscious vision," *Phil. Trans. R. Soc. Lond. B* **353**:1801–1818 (1998).

Logothetis, N.K. "The neural basis of the blood-oxygen-level-dependent functional magnetic resonance imaging signal," *Phil. Trans. R. Soc. Lond. B* **357**:1003–1037 (2002).

Logothetis, N.K. "MR imaging in the non-human primate: Studies of function and dynamic connectivity," *Curr. Opinion Neurobiol.* in press (2004).

Logothetis, N.K., Guggenberger, H., Peled, S., and Pauls, J. "Functional imaging of the monkey brain," *Nature Neurosci.* **2**:555–562 (1999).

Logothetis, N.K., Leopold, D.A., and Sheinberg, D.L. "What is rivalling during binocular rivalry," *Nature* **380**:621–624 (1996).

Logothetis, N.K. and Pauls, J. "Psychophysical and physiological evidence for viewer-centered object representations in the primate," *Cerebral Cortex* **5**:270–288 (1995).

Logothetis, N.K., Pauls, J., Augath, M., Trinath, T., and Oeltermann, A. "Neurophysiological investigation of the basis of the fMRI signal," *Nature* **412**:150–157 (2001).

Logothetis, N.K., Pauls, J., Bülthoff, H.H., and Poggio, T. "View-dependent object recognition by monkeys," *Curr. Biol.* **4**:401–414 (1994).

Logothetis, N.K. and Schall, J.D. "Neuronal correlates of subjective visual perception," *Science* **245**:761–763 (1989).

Logothetis, N.K. and Sheinberg, D.L. "Visual object recognition," *Ann. Rev. Neurosci.* **19**:577–621 (1996).

Louie, K. and Wilson, M.A. "Temporally structured replay of awake hippocampal ensemble activity during rapid eye movement sleep," *Neuron* **29**:145–156 (2001).

Lovibond, P.F. and Shanks, D.R. "The role of awareness in Pavlovian conditioning: Empirical evidence and theoretical implications," *J. Exp. Psychology: Animal Behavior Processes* **28**:3–26 (2002).

Lucas, J.R. "Minds, machines and Gödel," *Philosophy* **36**:112–127 (1961).

Luce, R.D. *Response Times.* Oxford, UK: Oxford University Press (1986).

Luck, S.J., Chelazzi, L., Hillyard, S.A., and Desimone, R. "Neural mechanisms of spatial attention in areas V1, V2, and V4 of macaque visual cortex," *J. Neurophysiol.* **77**:24–42 (1997).

Luck, S.J., Hillyard, S.A., Mangun, G.R., and Gazzaniga, M.S. "Independent hemispheric attentional systems mediate visual search in split-brain patients," *Nature* **342**:543–545 (1989).

Luck, S.J., Hillyard, S.A., Mangun, G.R., and Gazzaniga, M.S. "Independent attentional scanning in the separated hemispheres of split-brain patients," *J. Cogn. Neurosci.* **6**:84–91 (1994).

Lumer, E.D., Friston, K.J., and Rees, G. "Neural correlates of perceptual rivalry in the human brain," *Science* **280**:1930–1934 (1998).

Lumer, E.D. and Rees, G. "Covariation of activity in visual and prefrontal cortex associated with subjective visual perception," *Proc. Natl. Acad. Sci. USA* **96**:1669–1673 (1999).

Lux, S., Kurthen, M., Helmstaedter C., Hartje, W., Reuber, M., and Elger, C.E. "The localizing value of ictal consciousness and its constituent functions," *Brain* **125**:2691–2698 (2002).

Lyon, D.C. and Kaas, J.H. "Evidence for a modified V3 with dorsal and ventral halves in macaque monkeys," *Neuron* **33**:453–461 (2002).

Lytton, W.W. and Sejnowski, T.J. "Simulations of cortical pyramidal neurons synchronized by inhibitory interneurons," *J. Neurophysiol.* **66**:1059–1079 (1991).

Mack, A. and Rock, I. *Inattentional Blindness.* Cambridge, MA: MIT Press (1998).

Mackintosh, N.J. *Conditioning and Associative Learning.* Oxford, UK: Clarendon Press (1983).

Macknik, S.L. and Livingstone, M.S. "Neuronal correlates of visibility and invisibility in the primate visual system," *Nat Neurosci.* **1**:144–149 (1998).

Macknik, S.L. and Martinez-Conde, S. "Dichoptic visual masking in the geniculocortical system of awake primates," *J. Cogn. Neurosci.* in press (2004).

Macknik, S.L., Martinez-Conde, S., and Haglund, M.M. "The role of spatiotemporal edges in visibility and visual masking," *Proc. Natl. Acad. Sci. USA.* **97**:7556–7560 (2000).

MacLeod, K., Backer, A., and Laurent, G. "Who reads temporal information contained across synchronized and oscillatory spike trains?" *Nature* **395**:693–698 (1998).

MacNeil, M.A. and Masland, R.H. "Extreme diversity among amacrine cells: Implication for function," *Neuron* **20**:971–982 (1998).

Macphail, E.M. *The Evolution of Consciousness.* Oxford, UK: Oxford University Press (1998).

Madler, C. and Pöppel, E. "Auditory evoked potentials indicate the loss of neuronal oscillations during general anaesthesia," *Naturwissenschaften* **74**:42–43 (1987).

Magoun, H.W. "An ascending reticular activating system in the brain stem," *Arch. Neurol. Psychiatry* **67**:145–154 (1952).

Makeig, S., Westerfield, M., Jung, T.P., Enghoff, S., Townsend, J., Courchesne, E., and Sejnowski, T.J. "Dynamic brain sources of visual evoked responses," *Science* **295**:690–694 (2002).

Mandler, G. *Consciousness Recovered: Psychological Functions and Origins of Conscious Thought*. Amsterdam, Netherlands: John Benjamins (2002).

Manford, M. and Andermann, F. "Complex visual hallucinations: Clinical and neurobiological insights," *Brain* **121**:1819–1840 (1998).

Mark, V. "Conflicting communicative behavior in a split-brain patient: Support for dual consciousness." In: *Toward a Science of Consciousness: The First Tucson Discussions and Debates*. Hameroff, S.R., Kaszniak, A.W., and Scott, A.C., eds., pp. 189–196. Cambridge, MA: MIT Press (1996).

Marr, D. *Vision*. San Francisco, CA: Freeman (1982).

Marsálek, P., Koch, C., and Maunsell, J.H.R. "On the Relationship between Synaptic Input and Spike Output Jitter in Individual Neurons," *Proc. Natl. Acad. Sci. USA* **94**:735–740 (1997).

Martinez, J.L. and Kesner, R.P., eds. *Neurobiology of Learning and Memory*. New York: Academic Press (1998).

Masand P., Popli, A.P., and Weilburg, J.B. "Sleepwalking," *Am. Fam. Physician* **51**:649–654 (1995).

Masland, R.H. "Neuronal diversity in the retina," *Curr. Opinion Neurobiol.* **11**:431–436 (2001).

Mather, G., Verstraten, F., and Anstis, S. *The Motion Aftereffect: A Modern Perspective*. Cambridge, MA: MIT Press (1998).

Mathiesen, C., Caesar, K., Ören, N.A., and Lauritzen, M. "Modification of activity-dependent increases of cerebral blood flow by excitatory synaptic activity and spikes in rat cerebellar cortex," *J. Physiology* **512**:555–566 (1998).

Mattingley, J.B., Husain, M., Rorden, C., Kennard, C., and Driver, J. "Motor role of human inferior parietal lobe revealed in unilateral neglect patients," *Nature* **392**:179–182 (1998).

Maunsell, J.H.R. and Van Essen, D.C. "Functional properties of neurons in middle temporal visual area of the macaque monkey. II. Binocular interactions and sensitivity to binocular disparity," *J. Neurophysiol.* **49**:1148–1167 (1983).

McAdams, C.J. and Maunsell, J.H.R. "Effects of attention on orientation-tuning functions of single neurons in macaque cortical area V4," *J. Neurosci.* **19**:431–441 (1999).

McAdams, C.J. and Maunsell, J.H.R. "Attention to both space and feature modulates neuronal responses in macaque area V4," *J. Neurophysiol.* **83**:1751–1755 (2000).

McBain, C.J. and Fisahn, A. "Interneurons unbound," *Nature Rev. Neurosci.* **2**:11–23 (2001).

McClintock, M.K. "Whither menstrual synchrony?" *Ann. Rev. Sex Res.* **9**:77–95 (1998).

McComas, A.J. and Cupido, C.M. "The RULER model. Is this how somatosensory cortex works?" *Clinical Neurophysiol.* **110**:1987–1994 (1999).

McConkie, G.W. and Currie, C.B. "Visual stability across saccades while viewing complex pictures," *J. Exp. Psych.: Human Perception & Performance* **22**:563–581 (1996).

McCullough, J.N., Zhang, N., Reich, D.L., Juvonen, T.S., Klein, J.J., Spielvogel, D., Ergin, M.A., and Griepp, R.B. "Cerebral metabolic suppression during hypothermic circulatory arrest in humans," *Ann. Thorac. Surg.* **67**:1895–1899 (1999).

McGinn, C. *The Problem of Consciousness.* Oxford, UK: Blackwell (1991).

McMullin, E. "Biology and the theology of the human." In: *Controlling Our Destinies.* Sloan, P.R., ed., pp. 367–400. Notre Dame, IN: University of Notre Dame Press (2000).

Meador, K.J., Ray, P.G., Day, L.J., and Loring, D.W. "Train duration effects on perception: Sensory deficit, neglect and cerebral lateralization," *J. Clinical Neurophysiol.* **17**:406–413 (2000).

Meadows, J.C. "Disturbed perception of colours associated with localized cerebral lesions," *Brain* **97**:615–632 (1974).

Medina, J.F., Repa, J.C., Mauk, M.D., and LeDoux, J.E. "Parallels between cerebellum- and amygdala-dependent conditioning," *Nature Rev. Neurosci.* **3**:122–131 (2002).

Meenan, J.P. and Miller, L.A. "Perceptual flexibility after frontal or temporal lobectomy," *Neuropsychologia* **32**:1145–1149 (1994).

Meister, M. "Multineuronal codes in retinal signaling," *Proc. Natl. Acad. Sci. USA* **93**:609–614 (1996).

Merigan, W.H. and Maunsell, J.H.R. "How parallel are the primate visual pathways?" *Ann. Rev. Neurosci.* **16**:369–402 (1993).

Merigan, W.H., Nealey, T.A., and Maunsell, J.H.R. "Visual effects of lesions of cortical area V2 in macaques," *J. Neurosci.* **13**:3180–3191 (1993).

Merikle, P.M. "Perception without awareness. Critical issues," *Am. Psychol.* **47**:792–795 (1992).

Merikle, P.M. and Daneman, M. "Psychological investigations of unconscious perception," *J. Consc. Studies* **5**:5–18 (1998).

Merikle, P.M., Smilek, D., and Eastwood, J.D. "Perception without awareness: Perspectives from cognitive psychology," *Cognition* **79**:115–134 (2001).

Merleau-Ponty, M. *The Phenomenology of Perception.* C. Smith, transl., London: Routledge & Kegan Paul (1962).

Metzinger, T., ed. *Conscious Experience.* Exeter, UK: Imprint Academic (1995).

Metzinger, T., ed. *Neural Correlates of Consciousness: Empirical and Conceptual Questions.* Cambridge, MA: MIT Press (2000).

Michael, C.R. "Color vision mechanisms in monkey striate cortex: Dual-opponent cells with concentric receptive fields," *J. Neurophysiol.* **41**:572–588 (1978).

Michael, C.R. "Columnar organization of color cells in monkey's striate cortex," *J. Neurophysiol.* **46**:587–604 (1981).

Miller, E.K. "The prefrontal cortex: Complex neural properties for complex behavior," *Neuron* **22**:15–17 (1999).

Miller, E.K. and Cohen, J.D. "An integrative theory of prefrontal cortex function," *Ann. Rev. Neurosci.* **24**:167–202 (2001).

Miller, E.K., Gochin, P.M., and Gross, C.G. "Suppression of visual responses of neurons in inferior temporal cortex of the awake macaque by addition of a second stimulus," *Brain Res.* **616**:25–29 (1993).

Miller, E.K., Erickson, C.A., and Desimone, R. "Neural mechanisms of visual working memory in prefrontal cortex of the macaque," *J. Neurosci.* **16**:5154–5167 (1996).

Miller, G.A. "The magical number seven, plus or minus two: Some limits on our capacity for processing information," *Psychol. Rev.* **63**:81–97 (1956).

Miller, K.D., Chapman, B., and Stryker, M.P. "Visual responses in adult cat visual cortex depend on *N*-methyl-D-aspartate receptors," *Proc. Natl. Acad. Sci. USA* **86**:5183–5187 (1989).

Miller, S.M., Liu, G.B., Ngo, T.T., Hooper, G., Riek, S., Carson, R.G., and Pettigrew, J.D. "Interhemispheric switching mediates perceptual rivalry," *Curr. Biol.* **10**:383–392 (2000).

Millican, P. and Clark, A., eds. *Machines and Thought: The Legacy of Alan Turing.* Oxford, UK: Oxford University Press (1999).

Milner, A.D. and Dyde, R. "Why do some perceptual illusions affect visually guided action, when others don't?" *Trends Cogn. Sci.* **7**:10–11 (2003).

Milner, A.D. and Goodale, M.A. *The Visual Brain in Action.* Oxford, UK: Oxford University Press (1995).

Milner, A.D., Perrett, D.I., Johnston, R.S., Benson, P.J., Jordan, T.R., Heeley, D.W., Bettucci, D., Mortara, F., Mutani, R., Terazzi, E., and Davidson, D.L.W. "Perception and action in form agnosia," *Brain* **114**:405–428 (1991).

Milner, B. "Disorders of learning and memory after temporal lobe lesions in man," *Clin. Neurosurg.* **19**:421–446 (1972).

Milner, B., Squire, L.R., and Kandel, E.R. "Cognitive neuroscience and the study of memory," *Neuron* **20**:445–468 (1998).

Milner, P. "A model for visual shape recognition," *Psychol. Rev.* **81**:521–535 (1974).

Minamimoto, T. and Kimura, M. "Participation of the thalamic CM-Pf complex in attentional orienting," *J. Neurophysiol.* **87**:3090–3101 (2002).

Minsky, M. *The Society of Mind.* New York: Simon and Schuster (1985).

Mitchell, J.P., Macrae, C.N., and Gilchrist, I.D. "Working memory and the suppression of reflexive saccades," *J. Cogn. Neurosci.* **14**:95–103 (2002).

Miyashita, Y., Okuno, H., Tokuyama, W., Ihara, T., and Nakajima, K. "Feedback signal from medial temporal lobe mediates visual associative mnemonic codes of inferotemporal neurons," *Brain Res. Cogn. Brain Res.* **5**:81–86 (1996).

Moldofsky, H., Gilbert, R., Lue, F.A., and MacLean, A.W. "Sleep-related violence," *Sleep* **18**:731–739 (1995).

Montaser-Kouhsari, L., Moradi, F., Zand-Vakili, A., and Esteky, H. "Orientation selective adaptation during motion-induced blindness," *Perception*, in press (2004).

Moore, G.E. *Philosophical Studies*. London: Routledge & Kegan Paul (1922).

Moran, J. and Desimone, R. "Selective attention gates visual processing in extrastriate cortex," *Science* **229**:782–784 (1985).

Morris, J.S., Ohman, A., and Dolan, R.J. "A subcortical pathway to the right amygdala mediating 'unseen' fear," *Proc. Natl. Acad. Sci. USA* **96**:1680–1685 (1999).

Moruzzi, G. and Magoun, H.W. "Brain stem reticular formation and activation of the EEG," *EEG Clin. Neurophysiol.* **1**:455–473 (1949).

Motter, B.C. "Focal attention produces spatially selective processing in visual cortical areas V1, V2, and V4 in the presence of competing stimuli," *J. Neurophysiol.* **70**:909–919 (1993).

Mountcastle, V.B. "Modality and topographic properties of single neurons of cat's somatic sensory cortex," *J. Neurophysiol.* **20**:408–434 (1957).

Mountcastle, V.B. *Perceptual Neuroscience*. Cambridge, MA: Harvard University Press (1998).

Mountcastle, V.B., Andersen, R.A., and Motter, B.C. "The influence of attentive fixation upon the excitability of light-sensitive neurons of the posterior parietal cortex," *J. Neurosci.* **1**:1218–1235 (1981).

Moutoussis, K. and Zeki, S. "Functional segregation and temporal hierarchy of the visual perceptive systems," *Proc. R. Soc. Lond. B* **264**:1407–1415 (1997a).

Moutoussis, K. and Zeki, S. "A direct demonstration of perceptual asynchrony in vision," *Proc. R. Soc. Lond. B* **264**:393–399 (1997b).

Mumford, D. "On the computational architecture of the neocortex. I. The role of the thalamo-cortical loop," *Biol. Cybernetics* **65**:135–145 (1991).

Mumford, D. "Neuronal architectures for pattern-theoretic problems." In: *Large Scale Neuronal Theories of the Brain*. Koch, C., and Davis, J.L., eds, pp. 125–152. Cambridge, MA: MIT Press (1994).

Murakami, I., Komatsu, H., and Kinoshita, M. "Perceptual filling-in at the scotoma following a monocular retinal lesion in the monkey," *Visual Neurosci.* **14**:89–101 (1997).

Murayama, Y., Leopold, D.A., and Logothetis, N.K. "Neural activity during binocular rivalry in the anesthetized monkey," *Soc. Neurosci. Abstr.* 448.11 (2000).

Murphy, N. "Human nature: Historical, scientific, and religious issues." In: *Whatever Happened to the Soul? Scientific and Theological Portraits of Human Nature*. Brown, W.S., Murphy, N., and Malony H.N., eds., pp. 1–30. Minneapolis, MN: Fortress Press (1998).

Myerson, J., Miezin, F., and Allman, J.M. "Binocular rivalry in macaque monkeys and humans: A comparative study in perception," *Behav. Anal. Lett.* **1**:149–159 (1981).

Naccache, L., Blandin, E., and Dehaene, S. "Unconscious masked priming depends on temporal attention," *Psychol. Sci.* **13**:416–424 (2002).

Nadel, L. and Eichenbaum, H. "Introduction to the special issue on place cells," *Hippocampus* **9**:341–345 (1999).

Nagarajan, S., Mahncke, H., Salz, T., Tallal, P., Roberts, T., and Merzenich, M.M. "Cortical auditory signal processing in poor readers," *Proc. Natl. Acad. Sci. USA* **96**:6483–6488 (1999).

Nagel, T. "What is it like to be a bat?" *Philosophical Rev.* **83**:435–450 (1974).

Nagel, T. "Panpsychism." In: *Mortal Questions*. Nagel, T., ed., pp. 181–195. Cambridge, UK: Cambridge University Press (1988).

Nakamura, R.K. and Mishkin, M. "Blindness in monkeys following non-visual cortical lesions," *Brain Res.* **188**:572–577 (1980).

Nakamura, R.K. and Mishkin, M. "Chronic 'blindness' following lesions of nonvisual cortex in the monkey," *Exp. Brain Res.* **63**:173–184 (1986).

Nakayama, K. and Mackeben, M. "Sustained and transient components of focal visual attention," *Vision Res.* **29**:1631–1647 (1989).

Nathans, J. "The evolution and physiology of human color vision: Insights from molecular genetic studies of visual pigments," *Neuron* **24**:299–312 (1999).

Naya, Y., Yoshida, M., and Miyashita, Y. "Backward spreading of memory-retrieval signal in the primate temporal cortex," *Science* **291**:661–664 (2001).

Newman, J.B. "Putting the puzzle together: Toward a general theory of the neural correlates of consciousness," *J. Consc. Studies* **4**:47–66 (1997).

Newsome, W.T., Britten, K.H. and Movshon, J.A. "Neuronal correlates of a perceptual decision," *Nature* **341**:52–54 (1989).

Newsome, W.T., Maunsell, J.H.R., and Van Essen, D.C. "Ventral posterior visual area of the macaque: Visual topography and areal boundaries," *J. Comp. Neurol.* **252**:139–153 (1986).

Newsome, W.T. and Pare, E.B. "A selective impairment of motion perception following lesions of the Middle Temporal visual area (MT)," *J. Neurosci.* **8**:2201–2211 (1988).

Niebur, E. and Erdős, P. "Theory of the locomotion of nematodes: Control of the somatic motor neurons by interneurons," *Math. Biosci.* **118**:51–82 (1993).

Niebur, E., Hsiao, S.S., and Johnson, K.O. "Synchrony: A neuronal mechanism for attentional selection?" *Curr. Opinion Neurobiol.* **12**:190–194 (2002).

Niebur, E. and Koch, C. "A model for the neuronal implementation of selective visual attention based on temporal correlation among neurons," *J. Computational Neurosci.* **1**:141–158 (1994).

Niebur, E., Koch, C., and Rosin, C. "An oscillation-based model for the neuronal basis of attention," *Vision Research* **33**:2789–2802 (1993).

Nijhawan, R. "Motion extrapolation in catching," *Nature* **370**:256–257 (1994).

Nijhawan, R. "Visual decomposition of colour through motion extrapolation," *Nature* **386**:66–69 (1997).

Nimchinsky, E.A., Gilissen, E., Allman, J.M., Perl, D.P., Erwin J.M., and Hof, P.R. "A neuronal morphologic type unique to humans and great apes," *Proc. Natl. Acad. Sci. USA* **96**:5268–5273 (1999).

Nirenberg, S., Carcieri, S.M., Jacobs, A.L., and Latham, P.E. "Retinal ganglion cells act largely as independent encoders," *Nature* **411**:698–701 (2001).

Nishida, S. and Johnston, A. "Marker correspondence, not processing latency, determines temporal binding of visual attributes," *Curr. Biol.* **12**:359–368 (2002).

Noë, A. *Action in Perception.* Cambridge, MA: MIT Press (2004).

Noesselt, T., Hillyard, S.A., Woldorff, M.G., Schoenfeld, A., Hagner, T., Jancke, L., Tempelmann, C., Hinrichs, H., and Heinze, H.J. "Delayed striate cortical activation during spatial attention," *Neuron* **35**:575–587 (2002).

Nordby, K. "Vision in a complete achromat: A personal account." In: *Night Vision: Basic, Clinical and Applied Aspects.* Hess, R.F., Sharpe, L.T., and Nordby, K., eds., pp. 290–315. Cambridge, UK: Cambridge University Press (1990).

Norman, R.A., Maynard, E.M., Guillory, K.S., and Warren, D.J. "Cortical implants for the blind," *IEEE Spectrum* **33**:54–59 (1996).

Norretranders, T. *The User Illusion.* New York: Penguin (1998).

Nowak, L.G. and Bullier, J. "The timing of information transfer in the visual system." In: *Extrastriate Cortex in Primates, Vol. 12.* Rockland, K.S., Kaas, J.H., and Peters, A., eds., pp. 205–241. New York: Plenum (1997).

Nunn, J.A., Gregory, L.J., Brammer, M., Williams, S.C.R., Parslow, D.M., Morgan, M.J., Morris, R.G., Bullmore, E.T., Baron-Cohen, S., and Gray, J.A. "Functional magnetic resonance imaging of synesthesia: Activation of V4/V8 by spoken words," *Nature Neurosci.* **5**:371–375 (2002).

O'Connor, D.H., Fukui, M.M., Pinsk, M.A., and Kastner, S. "Attention modulates responses in the human lateral geniculate nucleus," *Nature Neurosci.* **5**:1203–1209 (2002).

O'Craven, K. and Kanwisher, N. "Mental imagery of faces and places activates corresponding stimulus-specific brain regions," *J. Cogn. Neursci.* **12**:1013–1023 (2000).

Öhman, A. and Soares, J.J. "Emotional conditioning to masked stimuli: Expectancies for aversive outcomes following nonrecognized fear-relevant stimuli," *J. Exp. Psychol. Gen.* **127**:69–82 (1998).

Ojemann, G.A., Ojemann, S.G., and Fried, I. "Lessons from the human brain: Neuronal activity related to cognition," *Neuroscientist* **4**:285–300 (1998).

Ojima, H. "Terminal morphology and distribution of corticothalamic fibers originating from layers 5 and 6 of cat primary auditory cortex," *Cerebral Cortex* **4**:646–663 (1994).

O'Keefe, J. and Nadel, L. *The Hippocampus as a Cognitive Map.* Oxford, UK: Clarendon (1978).

O'Keefe, J. and Recce, M.L. "Phase relationship bteween hippocampal place units and the EEG theta rhythm," *Hippocampus* **3**:317–330 (1993).

Ono, H. and Barbeito, R. "Ultocular discrimination is not sufficient for utrocular identification," *Vision Res.* **25**:289–299 (1985).

O'Regan, J.K. "Solving the 'real' mysteries of visual perception: The world as an outside memory," *Canadian J. Psychol.* **46**:461–488 (1992).

O'Regan, J.K. and Noë, A. "A sensorimotor account of vision and visual consciousness," *Behav. Brain Sci.* **24**:939–1001 (2001).

O'Regan, J.K., Rensink, R.A., and Clark, J.J. "Change-blindness as a result of mud-splashes," *Nature* **398**:34 (1999).

O'Shea, R.P. and Corballis, P.M. "Binocular rivalry between complex stimuli in split-brain observers," *Brain & Mind* **2**:151–160 (2001).

Oxbury, J., Polkey, C.E., and Duchowny, M., eds. *Intractable Focal Epilepsy.* Philadelphia: Saunders (2000).

Pagels, H. *The Dreams of Reason.* New York: Simon and Schuster (1988).

Palm, G. *Neural Assemblies: An Alternative Approach to Artificial Intelligence.* Berlin: Springer (1982).

Palm, G. "Cell assemblies as a guideline for brain research," *Concepts Neurosci.* **1**:133–147 (1990).

Palmer, L.A., Jones, J.P., and Stepnoski, R.A. "Striate receptive fields as linear filters: Characterization in two dimensions of space." In: *The Neural Basis of Visual Function.* Leventhal, A.G., ed., pp. 246–265. Boca Raton, FL: CRC Press (1991).

Palmer, S. *Vision Science: Photons to Phenomenology.* Cambridge, MA: MIT Press (1999).

Pantages, E. and Dulac, C. "A novel family of candidate pheromone receptors in mammals," *Neuron* **28**:835–845 (2000).

Parasuraman, R., ed. *The Attentive Brain.* Cambridge, MA: MIT Press (1998).

Parker, A.J. and Krug, K. "Neuronal mechanisms for the perception of ambiguous stimuli," *Curr. Opinion Neurobiol.* **13**:433–439 (2003).

Parker, A.J. and Newsome, W.T. "Sense and the single neuron: Probing the physiology of perception," *Ann. Rev. Neurosci.* **21**:227–277 (1998).

Parra, G., Gulyas, A.I., and Miles, R. "How many subtypes of inhibitory cells in the hippocampus?" *Neuron* **20**:983–993 (1998).

Parvizi, J. and Damasio, A.R. "Consciousness and the brainstem," *Cognition* **79**:135–159 (2001).

Pashler, H.E. *The Psychology of Attention.* Cambridge, MA: MIT Press (1998).

Passingham, R. *The Frontal Lobes and Voluntary Action.* Oxford, UK: Oxford University Press (1993).

Pastor, M.A. and Artieda, J., eds. *Time, Internal Clocks, and Movement.* Amsterdam, Netherlands: Elsevier (1996).

Paulesu, E., Harrison, J., Baron-Cohen, S., Watson, J.D., Goldstein, L., Heather, J., Frackowiak, R.S.J., and Frith, C.D. "The physiology of coloured hearing. A PET activation study of colour-word synaesthesia," *Brain* **118**:661–676 (1995).

Payne, B.R., Lomber, S.G., Villa, A.E., and Bullier, J. "Reversible deactivation of cerebral network components," *Trends Neurosci.* **19**:535–542 (1996).

Pedley, T.A. and Guilleminault, C. "Episodic nocturnal wanderings responsive to anti-convulsant drug therapy," *Ann. Neurol.* **2**:30–35 (1977).

Penfield, W. *The Mystery of the Mind.* Princeton, NJ: Princeton University Press (1975).

Penfield, W. and Jasper, H. *Epilepsy and the Functional Anatomy of the Human Brain.* Boston: Little & Brown (1954).

Penfield, W. and Perot, P. "The brain's record of auditory and visual experience: A final summary and discussion," *Brain* **86**:595–696 (1963).

Penrose, R. *The Emperor's New Mind*. Oxford, UK: Oxford University Press (1989).

Penrose, R. *Shadows of the Mind*. Oxford, UK: Oxford University Press (1994).

Perenin, M.T. and Rossetti, Y. "Grasping without form discrimination in a hemianopic field," *Neuroreport* **7**:793–797 (1996).

Perez-Orive, J., Mazor, O., Turner, G.C., Cassenaer, S., Wilson, R.I., and Laurent, G. "Oscillations and sparsening of odor representation in the mushroom body," *Science* **297**:359–365 (2002).

Perrett, D.I., Hietanen, J.K., Oram, M.W., and Benson, P.J. "Organization and functions of cells responsive to faces in the temporal cortex," *Phil. Trans. Roy. Soc. Lond. B* **335**:23–30 (1992).

Perry, E., Ashton, H., and Young, A., eds. *Neurochemistry of Consciousness*. Amsterdam, Netherlands: John Benjamins (2002).

Perry, E., Walker, M., Grace, J., and Perry, R. "Acetylcholine in mind: A neurotransmitter correlate of consciousness," *Trends Neurosci.* **22**:273–280 (1999).

Perry, E. and Young, A. "Neurotransmitter networks." In: *Neurochemistry of Consciousness*. Perry, E., Ashton, H., and Young, A., eds., pp. 3–23. Amsterdam, Netherlands: John Benjamins (2002).

Pessoa, L. and DeWeerd, P., eds. *Filling-In: From Perceptual Completion to Cortical Reorganization*. New York: Oxford University Press (2003).

Pessoa, L., Thompson, E., and Noë, A. "Finding out about filling in: A guide to perceptual completion for visual science and the philosophy of perception," *Behavioral and Brain Sci.* **21**:723–802 (1998).

Peterhans, E. "Functional organization of area V2 in the awake monkey." In: *Cerebral Cortex, Vol 12*. Rockland, K.S., Kaas, J.H., and Peters, A., eds., pp. 335–358. New York: Plenum Press (1997).

Peterhans, E. and von der Heydt, R. "Subjective contours: Bridging the gap between psychophysics and physiology," *Trends Neurosci.* **14**:112–119 (1991).

Peters, A. and Rockland, K.S., eds. *Cerebral Cortex. Vol. 10*. New York: Plenum Press (1994).

Pettigrew, J.D. and Miller, S.M. "A 'sticky' interhemishperic switch in bipolar disorder?" *Proc. R. Soc. Lond. B Biol. Sci.* **265**:2141–2148 (1998).

Philbeck, J.W. and Loomis, J.M. "Comparisons of two indicators of perceived egocentric distance under full-cue and reduced-cue conditions," *J. Exp. Psychology: Human Perception & Performance* **23**:72–85 (1997).

Pickersgill, M.J. "On knowing with which eye one is seeing," *Quart. J. Exp. Psychol.* **13**:168–172 (1961).

Pitts, W. and McCulloch, W.S. "How we know universals: The perception of auditory and visual forms," *Bull. Math. Biophysics* **9**:127–147 (1947).

Plum, F. and Posner, J.B. *The Diagnosis of Stupor and Coma*. 3rd ed. Philadelphia: FA Davis (1983).

Pochon, J.-B., Levy, R., Poline, J.-B., Crozier, S., Lehéricy, S., Pillon, B., Deweer, B., Le Bihan, D., and Dubois, B. "The role of dorsolateral prefrontal cortex in the preparation of forthcoming actions: An fMRI study," *Cerebral Cortex* **11**:260–266 (2001).

Poggio, G.F. and Poggio, T. "The analysis of stereopsis," *Ann. Rev. Neurosci.* **7**:379–412 (1984).

Poggio, T. "A theory of how the brain might work," *Cold Spring Harbor Symp. Quant. Biol.* **55**:899–910 (1990).

Poggio, T., Torre, V., and Koch, C. "Computational vision and regularization theory," *Nature* **317**:314–319 (1985).

Poincaré, H. "Mathematical discovery." In: *Science and Method.* pp. 46–63. New York: Dover Books (1952).

Pollen, D.A. "Cortical areas in visual awareness," *Nature* **377**:293–294 (1995).

Pollen, D.A. "On the neural correlates of visual perception," *Cerebral Cortex* **9**:4–19 (1999).

Pollen, D.A. "Explicit neural representations, recursive neural networks and conscious visual perception," *Cerebral Cortex* **13**:807–814 (2003).

Polonsky, A., Blake, R., Braun, J., and Heeger, D. "Neuronal activity in human primary visual cortex correlates with perception during binocular rivalry," *Nature Neurosci.* **3**:1153–1159 (2000).

Polyak, S.L. *The Retina.* Chicago, IL: University of Chicago Press (1941).

Pöppel, E. "Time perception." In: *Handbook of Sensory Physiology. Vol. 8: Perception.* Held, R., Leibowitz, H.W., and Teuber, H.-L. eds., pp. 713–729. Berlin: Springer (1978).

Pöppel, E. "A hierarchical model of temporal perception," *Trends Cogn. Sci.* **1**:56–61 (1997).

Pöppel, E., Held, R., and Frost, D. "Residual visual function after brain wounds involving the central visual pathways in man," *Nature* **243**:295–296 (1973).

Pöppel, E. and Logothetis, N.K. "Neural oscillations in the brain. Discontinuous initiations of pursuit eye movements indicate a 30-Hz temporal framework for visual information processing," *Naturwissenschaften* **73**:267–268 (1986).

Popper, K.R. and Eccles, J.C. *The Self and its Brain.* Berlin: Springer (1977).

Porac, C. and Coren, S. "Sighting dominance and utrocular discrimination," *Percept. Psychophys.* **39**:449–41 (1986).

Posner, M.I. and Gilbert, C.D. "Attention and primary visual cortex," *Proc. Natl. Acad. Sci. USA* **16**:2585–2587 (1999).

Posner, M.I., Snyder, C.R.R. and Davidson, B.J. "Attention and the detection of signals," *J. exp. Psychol.: General* **109**:160–174 (1980).

Potter, M.C. "Very short-term conceptual memory," *Memory & Cognition* **21**:156–161 (1993).

Potter, M.C. and Levy, E.I. "Recognition memory for a rapid sequence of pictures," *J. Exp. Psychol.* **81**:10–15 (1969).

Pouget, A. and Sejnowski, T.J. "Spatial transformations in the parietal cortex using basis functions," *J. Cogn. Neurosci.* **9**:222–237 (1997).

Preuss, T.M. "What's human about the human brain?" In: *The New Cognitive Neurosciences.* 2nd ed., Gazzaniga, M.S., ed., pp. 1219–1234. Cambridge, MA: MIT Press (2000).

Preuss, T.M., Qi, H., and Kaas, J.H. "Distinctive compartmental organization of human primary visual cortex," *Proc. Natl. Acad. Sci. USA* **96**:11601–11606 (1999).

Pritchard, R.M., Heron, W., and Hebb, D.O. "Visual perception approached by the method of stabilized images," *Canad. J. Psychol.* **14**:67–77 (1960).

Proffitt, D.R., Bhalla, M., Gossweiler, R., and Midgett, J. "Perceiving geographical slant," *Psychonomic Bulletin & Rev.* **2**:409–428 (1995).

Przybyszewski, A.W., Gaska, J.P., Foote, W., and Pollen, D.A. "Striate cortex increases contrast gain of macaque LGN neurons," *Visual Neurosci.* **17**:485–494 (2000).

Puccetti, R. *The Trial of John and Henry Norton.* London: Hutchinson (1973).

Purpura, K.P. and Schiff, N.D. "The thalamic intralaminar nuclei: Role in visual awareness," *Neuroscientist* **3**:8–14 (1997).

Purves, D., Paydarfar, J.A., and Andrews, T.J. "The wagon wheel illusion in movies and reality," *Proc. Natl. Acad. Sci. USA* **93**:3693–3697 (1996).

Quinn, J.J., Oommen, S.S., Morrison, G.E., and Fanselow, M.S. "Post-training excitotoxic lesions of the dorsal hippocampus attenuate forward trace, backward trace, and delay fear conditioning in a temporally-specific manner," *Hippocampus* **12**:495–504 (2002).

Rafal, R.D. "Hemispatial neglect: Cognitive neuropsychological aspects." In: *Behavioral Neurology and Neuropsychology.* Feinberg, T.E. and Farah, M.J., eds., pp. 319–336. New York: McGraw-Hill (1997a).

Rafal, R.D. "Balint syndrome." In: *Behavioral Neurology and Neuropsychology.* Feinberg, T.E. and Farah, M.J., eds., pp. 337–356. New York: McGraw-Hill (1997b).

Rafal, R.D. and Posner, M. "Deficits in human visual spatial attention following thalamic lesions," *Proc. Natl. Acad. Sci. USA* **84**:7349–7353 (1987).

Rakic, P. "A small step for the cell, a giant leap for mankind: A hypothesis of neocortical expansion during evolution," *Trends Neurosci.* **18**:383–388 (1995).

Ramachandran, V.S. "Blind spots," *Sci. Am.* **266**:86–91 (1992).

Ramachandran, V.S. and Gregory, R.L. "Perceptual filling in of artificially induced scotomas in human vision," *Nature* **350**:699–702 (1991).

Ramachandram, V.S. and Hubbard, E.M. "Psychophysical investigations into the neural basis of synaesthesia," *Proc. R. Soc. Lond. B* **268**:979–983 (2001).

Ramòn y Cajal, S. "New ideas on the structure of the nervous system of man and vertebrates." Translated by Swanson, N. and Swanson, L.M. from *Les nouvelles idées sur la structure du système nerveux chez l'homme et chez les vertébrés.* Cambridge, MA: MIT Press (1991).

Rao, R.P.N. and Ballard, D.H. "Predictive coding in the visual cortex: A functional interpretation of some extra-classical receptive-field effects," *Nature Neurosci.* **2**:79–87 (1999).

Rao, R.P.N, Olshausen, B.A., and Lewicki, M.S., eds. *Probabilistic Models of the Brain.* Cambridge, MA: MIT Press (2002).

Rao, S.C., Rainer, G., and Miller, E.K. "Integration of what and where in the primate prefrontal cortex," *Science* **276**:821–824 (1997).

Ratliff, F. and Hartline, H.K. "The responses of Limulus optic nerve fibers to patterns of illumination on the receptor mosaic," *J. Gen. Physiol.* **42**:1241–1255 (1959).

Ray, P.G., Meador, K.J., Smith, J.R., Wheless, J.W., Sittenfeld, M., and Clifton, G.L. "Cortical stimulation and recording in humans," *Neurology* **52**:1044–1049 (1999).

Reddy, L., Wilken, P., and Koch, C. "Face-gender discrimination in the near-absence of attention," *J. Vision*, in press (2004).

Rees, G., Friston, K., and Koch, C. "A direct quantitative relationship between the functional properties of human and macaque V5," *Nature Neurosci.* **3**:716–723 (2000).

Rees, G., Wojciulik, E., Clarke, K., Husain, M., Frith, C., and Driver, J. "Unconscious activation of visual cortex in the damaged right hemisphere of a parietal patient with extinction," *Brain* **123**:1624–1633 (2000).

Reeves, A.G., ed. *Epilepsy and the Corpus Callosum.* New York: Plenum Press (1985).

Reingold, E.M. and Merikle, P.M. "On the inter-relatedness of theory and measurement in the study of unconscious processes," *Mind Lang.* **5**:9–28 (1990).

Rempel-Clower, N.L. and Barbas, H. "The laminar pattern of connections between prefrontal and anterior temporal cortices in the rhesus monkey is related to cortical structure and function," *Cerebral Cortex* **10**:851–865 (2000).

Rensink, R.A. "Seeing, sensing, and scrutinizing," *Vision Res.* **40**:1469–1487 (2000a).

Rensink, R.A. "The dynamic representation of scenes," *Visual Cognition* **7**:17–42 (2000b).

Rensink, R.A., O'Regan, J.K., and Clark, J.J. "To see or not to see: The need for attention to perceive changes in scenes," *Psychological Sci.* **8**:368–373 (1997).

Revonsuo, A. "The reinterpretation of dreams: An evolutionary hypothesis of the function of dreaming," *Behav. Brain Sci.* **23**:877–901 (2000).

Revonsuo, A., Johanson, M., Wedlund, J.-E., and Chaplin, J. "The zombie among us." In: *Beyond Dissociation.* Rossetti, Y. and Revonsuo, A., eds., pp. 331–351. Amsterdam, Netherlands: John Benjamins (2000).

Revonsuo, A., Wilenius-Emet, M., Kuusela, J., and Lehto, M. "The neural generation of a unified illusion in human vision," *Neuroreport* **8**:3867–3870 (1997).

Reynolds, J.H., Chelazzi, L., and Desimone, R. "Competitive mechanisms subserve attention in macaque areas V2 and V4," *J. Neurosci.* **19**:1736–1753 (1999).

Reynolds, J.H. and Desimone, R. "The role of neural mechanisms of attention in solving the binding problem," *Neuron* **24**:19–29 (1999).

Rhodes P.A. and Llinás, R.R. "Apical tuft input efficacy in layer 5 pyramidal cells from rat visual cortex," *J. Physiol.* **536**:167–187 (2001).

Ricci, C. and Blundo, C. "Perception of ambiguous figures after focal brain lesions," *Neuropsychologia* **28**:1163–73 (1990).

Riddoch, M.J. and Humphreys, G.W. "17 + 14 = 41? Three cases of working memory impairment." In: *Broken Memories: Case Studies in Memory Impairment*. Campbell, R. and Conway, M.A., eds., pp. 253–266. Oxford, UK: Blackwell (1995).

Ridley, M. *Nature Via Nurture*. New York: Harper Collins (2003).

Rieke, F., Warland, D., van Steveninck, R.R.D., and Bialek, W. *Spikes: Exploring the Neural Code*. Cambridge, MA: MIT Press (1996).

Ritz, R. and Sejnowski, T.J. "Synchronous oscillatory activity in sensory systems: New vistas on mechanisms," *Curr. Opinion Neurobiol.* **7**:536–546 (1997).

Rizzuto, D.S., Madsen, J.R., Bromfield, E.B., Schulze-Bonhage, A., Seelig, D., Aschenbrenner-Scheibe, R., and Kahana, M.J. "Reset of human neocortical oscillations during a working memory task," *Proc. Natl. Acad. Sci. USA* **100**:7931–7936 (2003).

Robertson, L. "Binding, spatial attention, and perceptual awareness," *Nature Rev. Neurosci.* **4**:93–102 (2003).

Robertson, I.H. and Marshall, J.C., eds. *Unilateral Neglect: Clinical and Experimental Studies*. Hove, UK: Lawrence Erlbaum (1993).

Robertson, L., Treisman, A., Friedman-Hill, S., and Grabowecky, M. "The interaction of spatial and object pathways: Evidence from Balint's syndrome," *J. Cogn. Neurosci.* **9**:295–317 (1997).

Robinson, D.L. and Cowie, R.J. "The primate pulvinar: Stuctural, functional, and behavioral components of visual salience." In: *The Thalamus*. Jones, E.G., Steriade, M., and McCormick, D.A., eds., pp. 53–92. Amsterdam: Elsevier (1997).

Robinson, D.L. and Petersen, S.E. "The pulvinar and visual salience," *Trends Neurosci.* **15**:127–132 (1992).

Rock, I. and Gutman, D. "The effect of inattention on form perception," *J. Exp. Psychol. Hum. Perception & Performance* **7**:275–285 (1981).

Rockel, A.J., Hiorns, R.W., and Powell, T.P.S. "The basic uniformity in structure of the neocortex," *Brain* **103**:221–244 (1980).

Rockland, K.S. "Further evidence for two types of corticopulvinar neurons," *Neuroreport* **5**:1865–1868 (1994).

Rockland, K.S. "Two types of corticopulvinar terminations: Round (type 2) and elongate (type 1)," *J. Comp. Neurol.* **368**:57–87 (1996).

Rockland, K.S. "Elements of cortical architecture: Hierarchy revisited." In: *Cerebral Cortex, Vol. 12*. Rockland, K.S., Kaas, J.H., and Peters, A., eds., pp. 243–293. New York: Plenum Press (1997).

Rockland, K.S. and Pandya, D.N. "Laminar origins and terminations of cortical connections of the occipital lobe in the rhesus monkey," *Brain Res.* **179**:3–20 (1979).

Rockland, K.S. and Van Hoesen, G.W. "Direct temporal-occipital feedback connections to striate cortex (V1) in the macaque monkey," *Cerebral Cortex* **4**:300–313 (1994).

Rodieck, R.W. *The First Steps in Seeing*. Sunderland, MA: Sinauer Associates (1998).

Rodieck, R.W., Binmoeller, K.F., and Dineen, J.T. "Parasol and midget ganglion cells of the human retina," *J. Comp. Neurol.* **233**:115–132 (1985).

Rodriguez, E., George, N., Lachaux, J.-P., Martinerie, J., Renault, B., and Varela, F.J. "Perception's shadow: Long-distance synchronziation of human brain activity," *Nature* **397**:430–433 (1999).

Roe, A.W. and Ts'o, D.Y. "The functional architecture of area V2 in the macaque monkey: Physiology, topography, and connectivity." In *Cerebral Cortex, Vol 12: Extrastriate Cortex in Primates*, Rockland, K.S., Kaas, J.H., and Peters, A., eds., pp. 295–334. New York: Plenum Press (1997).

Roelfsema, P.R., Lamme, V.A.F., and Spekreijse, H. "Oject-based attention in the primary visual cortex of the macaque monkey," *Nature* **395**:376–381 (1998).

Rolls, E.T. "Spatial view cells and the representation of place in the primate hippocampus," *Hippocampus* **9**:467–480 (1999).

Rolls, E.T., Aggelopoulos, N.C., and Zheng, F. "The receptive fields of inferior temporal cortex neurons in natural scenes," *J. Neurosci.* **23**:339–348 (2003).

Rolls, E.T. and Deco, G. *Computational Neuroscience of Vision*. Oxford, UK: Oxford University Press (2002).

Rolls, E.T. and Tovee, M.J. "Processing speed in the cerebral cortex and the neurophysiology of visual masking," *Proc. R. Soc. Lond. B* **257**:9–15 (1994).

Rolls, E.T. and Tovee, M.J. "The responses of single neurons in the temporal visual cortical areas of the macaque when more than one stimulus is present in the receptive field," *Exp. Brain Res.* **103**:409–420 (1995).

Romo, R., Brody, C.D., Hernández, A., and Lemus, L. "Neuronal correlates of parametric working memory in the prefrontal cortex," *Nature* **399**:470–473 (1999).

Roorda, A. and Williams, D.R. "The arrangement of the three cone classes in the living human eye," *Nature* **397**:520–522 (1999).

Rosen, M. and Lunn, J.N., eds. *Consciousness, Awareness, and Pain in General Anaesthesia*. London: Butterworths (1987).

Rossen, R., Kabat, H., and Anderson, J.P. "Acute arrest of cerebral circulation in man," *Arch. Neurol. Psychiatry* **50**:510–528 (1943).

Rossetti, Y. "Implicit short-lived motor representations of space in brain damaged and healthy subjects," *Consc. & Cognition* **7**:520–558 (1998).

Rousselet, G., Fabre-Thorpe, M., and Thorpe, S. "Parallel processing in high-level visual scene categorization," *Nature Neurosci.* **5**:629–630 (2002).

Ryle, G. *The Concept of the Mind* London: Hutchinson (1949).

Sacks, O. *Migraine*. Rev. ed. Berkeley, CA: University of California Press (1970).

Sacks, O. *Awakenings*. New York: E.P. Dutton (1973).

Sacks, O. *A Leg to Stand On*. New York: Summit Books (1984).

Sacks, O. *The Man Who Mistook His Wife for a Hat*. New York: Harper & Row (1985).

Sacks, O. "The mind's eye: What the blind see." *The New Yorker*, July 28, pp. 48–59 (2003).

Saenz, M., Buracas, G.T., and Boynton, G.M. "Global effects of feature-based attention in human visual cortex," *Nature Neurosci.* **5**:631–632 (2002).

Saint-Cyr, J.A., Ungerleider, L.G., and Desimone, R. "Organization of visual cortical inputs to the striatum and subsequent outputs to the pallido-nigral complex in the monkey," *J. Compa. Neurol.* **298**:129–156 (1990).

Sakai, K., Watanabe, E., Onodera, Y., Uchida, I., Kato, H., Yamamoto, E., Koizumi, H., and Miyashita, Y. "Functional mapping of the human colour centre with echo-planar magnetic resonance imaging," *Proc. R. Soc. Lond. B* **261**:89–98 (1995).

Saleem, K.S., Suzuki, W., Tanaka, K., and Hashikawa, T. "Connections between anterior inferotemporal cortex and superior temporal sulcus regions in the macaque monkey," *J. Neurosci.* **20**:5083–5101 (2000).

Salin, P.-A. and Bullier, J. "Corticocortical connections in the visual system: Structure and Function," *Physiol. Rev.* **75**:107–154 (1995).

Salinas, E. and Abbott, L.F. "Transfer of coded information from sensory to motor networks," *J. Neurosci.* **15**:6461–6474 (1995).

Salinas, E. and Sejnowski, T.J. "Correlated neuronal activity and the flow of neural information," *Nature Rev. Neurosci.* **2**:539–550 (2001).

Salzman, C.D., Murasugi, C.M., Britten, K.H., and Newsome, W.T. "Microstimulation in visual area MT: Effects on direction discrimination performance," *J. Neurosci.* **12**:2331–2355 (1992).

Salzman, C.D. and Newsome, W.T. "Neural mechanisms for forming a perceptual decision," *Science* **264**:231–237 (1994).

Sammon, P.M. *Future Noir: The Making of Blade Runner*. New York, HarperPrims (1996).

Sanderson, M.J. "Intercellular waves of communication," *New Physiol. Sci.* **11**:262–269 (1996).

Sanford, A.J. "A periodic basis for perception and action." In: *Biological Rhythms and Human Performance*. Colquhuon, W., ed., pp. 179–209. New York: Academic Press (1971).

Savic, I. "Imaging of brain activation by odorants in humans," *Curr. Opinion Neurobiol.* **12**:455–461 (2002).

Savic, I., Berglund, H., Gulyas, B., and Roland, P. "Smelling of odorous sex hormone-like compounds causes sex-differentiated hypothalamic activations in humans," *Neuron* **31**:661–668 (2001).

Sawatari, A. and Callaway, E.M. "Diversity and cell type specificity of local excitatory connections to neurons in layer 3B of monkey primary visual cortex," *Neuron* **25**:459–471 (2000).

Scalaidhe, S.P., Wilson, F.A., and Goldman-Rakic, P.S. "Areal segregation of face-processing neurons in prefrontal cortex," *Science* **278**:1135–1138 (1997).

Schall, J.D. "Neural basis of saccadic eye movements in primates." In: *The Neural Basis of Visual Function*. Leventhal, A.G., ed., pp. 388–441. Boca Raton, FL: CRC Press (1991).

Schall, J.D. "Visuomotor areas of the frontal lobe. In: *Cerebral Cortex. Vol. 12*. Rockland, K.S., Kaas, J.H., and Peters, A., eds., pp. 527–638. New York: Plenum Press (1997).

Schall, J.D. "Neural basis of deciding, choosing and acting," *Nature Rev. Neurosci.* **2**:33–42 (2001).

Schank, J.C. "Menstrual-cycle synchrony: Problems and new directions for research," *J. Comp. Psychology* **115**:3–15 (2001).

Schenck, C.H. and Mahowald, M.W. "An analysis of a recent criminal trial involving sexual misconduct with a child, alcohol abuse and a successful sleepwalking defence: Arguments supporting two proposed new forensic categories," *Med. Sci. Law* **38**:147–152 (1998).

Schiff, N.D. "The neurology of impaired consciousness: Challenges for cognitive neuroscience." In: *The New Cognitive Neurosciences.* Gazzaniga, M., ed. Cambridge, MA: MIT Press (2004).

Schiff, N.D. and Plum, F. "The role of arousal and 'gating' systems in the neurology of impaired consciousness," *J. Clinical Neurophysiol.* **17**:438–452 (2000).

Schiffer, F. "Can the different cerebral hemispheres have distinct personalities? Evidence and its implications for theory and treatment of PTSD and other disorders?" *J. Traum. Dissoc.* **1**:83–104 (2000).

Schiller, P.H. and Chou, I.H. "The effects of frontal eye field and dorsomedial frontal-cortex lesions on visually guided eye-movements," *Nature Neurosci.* **1**:248–253 (1998).

Schiller, P.H. and Logothetis, N.K. "The color-opponent and broad-based channels of the primate visual system," *Trends Neurosci.* **13**:392–398 (1990).

Schiller, P.H., True, S.D., and Conway, J.L. "Effects of frontal eye field and superior colliculus ablations on eye movements," *Science* **206**:590–592 (1979).

Schlag, J. and Schlag-Rey, M. "Visuomotor functions of central thalamus in monkey. II. Unit activity related to visual events, targeting, and fixation," *J. Neurophysiol.* **51**:1175–1195 (1984).

Schlag, J. and Schlag-Rey, M. "Through the eye, slowly: Delays and localization errors in the visual system," *Nature Rev. Neurosci.* **3**:191–215 (2002).

Schmidt, E.M., Bak, M.J., Hambrecht, F.T., Kufta, C.V., O'Rourke, D.K., and Vallabhanath, P. "Feasibility of a visual prosthesis for the blind based on intracortical microstimulation of the visual cortex," *Brain* **119**:507–522 (1996).

Schmolesky, M.T., Wang, Y., Hanes, D.P., Leutgeb, S., Schall, J.B., and Leventhal, A.G. "Signal timing across the macaque visual system," *J. Neurophysiol.* **79**:3272–3280 (1998).

Schooler, J.W. and Melcher, J. "The ineffability of insight." In: *The Creative Cognition Approach.* Smith, S.M., Ward, T.B., and Finke, R.A., eds., pp. 97–133. Cambridge, MA: MIT Press (1995).

Schooler, J.W., Ohlsson, S., and Brooks, K. "Thoughts beyond words: When language overshadows insight," *J. Exp. Psychol. Gen.* **122**:166–183 (1993).

Schrödinger, E. *What Is Life?* Cambridge, UK: Cambridge University Press (1944).

Scoville, W.B. and Milner, B. "Loss of recent memory after bilateral hippocampal lesions," *J. Neurochem.* **20**:11–21 (1957).

Searle, J.R. *The Mystery of Consciousness*. New York: The New York Review of Books (1997).

Searle, J.R. "Consciousness," *Ann. Rev. Neurosci.* **23**:557–578 (2000).

Seckel, A. *The Art of Optical Illusions*. Carlton Books (2000).

Seckel, A. *More Optical Illusions*. Carlton Books (2002).

Sennholz, G. "Bispectral analysis technology and equipment," *Minerva Anestesiol.* **66**:386–388 (2000).

Shadlen, M.N., Britten, K.H., Newsome, W.T., and Movshon, J.A. "A computational analysis of the relationship between neuronal and behavioral responses to visual motion," *J. Neurosci.* **16**:1486–1510 (1996).

Shadlen, M.N. and Movshon, J.A. "Synchrony unbound: A critical evaluation of the temporal binding hypothesis," *Neuron* **24**:67–77 (1999).

Shallice, T. *From Neuropsychology to Mental Structure*. Cambridge, UK: Cambridge University Press (1988).

Shapley, R. and Ringach, D. "Dynamics of responses in visual cortex." In: *The New Cognitive Neurosciences*. 2nd ed., Gazzaniga, M.S., ed., pp. 253–261. Cambridge, MA: MIT Press (2000).

Shear, J., ed. *Explaining Consciousness: The Hard Problem*. Cambridge, MA: MIT Press (1997).

Sheinberg, D.L. and Logothetis, N.K. "The role of temporal cortical areas in perceptual organization," *Proc. Natl. Acad. Sci. USA* **94**:3408–3413 (1997).

Sheinberg, D.L. and Logothetis, N.K. "Noticing familiar objects in real world scenes: The role of temporal cortical neurons in natural vision," *J. Neurosci.* **15**:1340–1350 (2001).

Sheliga, B.M., Riggio, L., and Rizzolatti, G. "Orienting of attention and eye movements," *Exp. Brain Res.* **98**:507–522 (1994).

Shepherd, G.M. *Foundations of the Neuron Doctrine*. New York: Oxford University Press (1991).

Shepherd, M., Findlay, J.M., and Hockey, R.J. "The relationship between eye movements and spatial attention," *Quart. J. Exp. Psychol.* **38**:475–491 (1986).

Sherk, H. "The claustrum." In: *Cerebral Cortex Vol. 5*. Jones, E.G. and Peters, A., eds., pp. 467–499. New York: Plenum (1986).

Sherman, S.M. and Guillery, R. *Exploring the Thalamus*. San Diego, CA: Academic Press (2001).

Sherman, S.M. and Koch, C. "Thalamus." In: *The Synaptic Organization of the Brain*. 4th ed., Shepherd, G. ed., pp. 289–328. New York: Oxford University Press (1998).

Sheth, B.R., Nijhawan, R., and Shimojo, S. "Changing objects lead briefly flashed ones," *Nature Neurosci.* **3**:489–495 (2000).

Shimojo, S., Tanaka, Y., and Watanabe, K. "Stimulus-driven facilitation and inhibition of visual information processing in environmental and retinotopic representations of space," *Brain Res. Cogn. Brain Res.* **5**:11–21 (1996).

Siegel, J.M. "Nacrolepsy," *Scientific American* **282**:76–81 (2000).

Siewert, C.P. *The Significance of Consciousness*. Princeton, NJ: Princeton University Press (1998).

Simons, D.J. and Chabris, C.F. "Gorillas in our midst: Sustained inattentional blindness for dynamic events," *Perception* **28**:1059–1074 (1999).

Simons, D.J. and Levin, D.T. "Change blindness," *Trends Cogn. Sci.* **1**:261–267 (1997).

Simons, D.J. and Levin, D.T. "Failure to detect changes to people during a real-world interaction," *Psychonomic Bull. & Rev.* **5**:644–649 (1998).

Simpson, J. *Touching the Void*. New York: HarperPerennial (1988).

Singer, W. "Neuronal synchrony: A versatile code for the definition of relations?" *Neuron* **24**:49–65 (1999).

Skoyles, J.R. "Another variety of vision," *Trends Neurosci.* **20**:22–23 (1997).

Slimko, E.M., McKinney, S., Anderson, D.J., Davidson, N., and Lester, H.A. "Selective electrical silencing of mammalian neurons in vitro by the use of invertebrate ligand-gated chloride channels," *J. Neurosci.* **22**:7373–7379 (2002).

Smith, S. "Utrocular, or 'which eye' discrimination," *J. Exp. Psychology* **35**:1–14 (1945).

Snyder, L.H., Batista, A.P., and Andersen, R.A. "Intention-related activity in the posterior parietal cortex: A review," *Vis. Res.* **40**:1433–1441 (2000).

Sobel, E.S. and Tank, D.W. "In vivo Ca^{2+} dynamics in a cricket auditory neuron: An example of chemical computation," *Science* **263**:823–826 (1994).

Sobel, N., Prabhakaran, V., Hartely, C.A., Desmond, J.E., Glover, G.H., Sullivan, E.V., and Gabrieli, D.E. "Blindsmell: Brain activation induced by an undetected air-borne chemical," *Brain* **122**:209–217 (1999).

Softky, W.R. "Simple codes versus efficient codes," *Curr. Opinion Neurobiol.* **5**:239–247 (1995).

Solms, M. *The Neuropsychology of Dreams*. Mahwah, NJ: Lawrence Erlbaum (1997).

Somers, D.C., Dale, A.M., Seiffert, A.E., and Tootell, R.B. "Functional MRI reveals spatially specific attentional modulation in human primary visual cortex," *Proc. Natl. Acad. Sci. USA* **96**:1663–1668 (1999).

Sperling, G. "The information available in brief presentation," *Psychological Monographs* **74**. Whole No. 498 (1960).

Sperling, G. and Dosher, B. "Strategy and optimization in human information processing." In: *Handbook of Perception and Performance* Vol. 1. Boff, K., Kaufman, L., and Thomas, J., eds., pp. 1–65. New York: Wiley (1986).

Sperling, G. and Weichselgartner, E. "Episodic theory of the dynamics of spatial attention," *Psych. Rev.* **102**:503–532 (1995).

Sperry, R.W. "Cerebral organization and behavior," *Science* **133**:1749–1757 (1961).

Sperry, R.W. "Lateral specialization in the surgically separated hemispheres." In: *Neuroscience 3rd Study Program*. Schmitt, F.O. and Worden, F.G., eds. Cambridge, MA: MIT Press (1974).

Spinelli, D.W., Pribram, K.H., and Weingarten, M. "Centrifugal optic nerve responses evoked by auditory and somatic stimulation," *Exp. Neurol.* **12**:303–318 (1965).

Sprague, J.M. "Interaction of cortex and superior colliculus in mediation of visually guided behavior in the cat," *Science* **153**:1544–1547 (1966).

Squire, L.R. and Kandel, E.R. *Memory: From Mind to Molecules.* New York: Scientific American Library, Freeman (1999).

Standing, L. "Learning 10,000 pictures," *Quart. J. Exp. Psychol.* **25**:207–222 (1973).

Stapledon, O. *Star Maker.* New York: Dover Publications (1937).

Steinmetz, P.N., Roy, A., Fitzgerald, P.J., Hsiao, S.S., Johnson, K.O., and Niebur, E. "Attention modulates synchronized neuronal firing in primary somatosensory cortex," *Nature* **404**:187–190 (2000).

Steriade, M. and McCarley, R.W. *Brainstem Control of Wakefullness and Sleep.* New York: Plenum Press (1990).

Stern, K. and McClintock, M.K. "Regulation of ovulation by human pheromones," *Nature* **392**:177–179 (1998).

Sternberg, E.M. "Piercing together a puzzling world: Memento," *Science* **292**:1661–1662 (2001).

Sternberg, S. "High-speed scanning in human memory," *Science* **153**:652–654 (1966).

Stevens, C.F. "Neuronal diversity: Too many cell types for comfort?" *Curr. Biol.* **8**:R708–R710 (1998).

Stevens, R. "Western phenomenological approaches to the study of conscious experience and their implications." In: *Methodologies for the Study of Consciousness: A New Synthesis.* Richardson, J. and Velmans, M., eds., pp. 100–123. Kalamazoo, MI: Fetzer Institute (1997).

Stoerig, P. and Barth, E. "Low-level phenomenal vision despite unilateral destruction of primary visual cortex," *Consc. & Cognition* **10**:574–587 (2001).

Stoerig, P., Zontanou, A., and Cowey, A. "Aware or unaware: Assessment of cortical blindness in four men and a monkey," *Cerebral Cortex* **12**:565–574 (2002).

Stopfer, M., Bhagavan, S., Smith, B.H., and Laurent, G. "Impaired odour discrimination on desynchronization of odour-encoding neural assemblies," *Nature* **390**:70–74 (1997).

Stowers, L., Holy, T.E., Meister, M., Dulac, C., and Koentges, G. "Loss of sex discrimination and male-male aggression in mice deficient for TRP2," *Science* **295**:1493–1500 (2002).

Strayer, D.L. and Johnston, W.A. "Driven to distraction: Dual-task studies of simulated driving and conversing on a cellular phone," *Psychol. Sci.* **12**:462–466 (2001).

Stroud, J.M. "The fine structure of psychological time." In: *Information Theory in Psychology.* Quastler, H., ed., pp. 174–205. Glencoe, IL: Free Press (1956).

Strawson, G. *Mental Reality.* Cambridge, MA: MIT Press (1996).

Supèr, H., Spekreijse, H., and Lamme, V.A.F. "Two distinct modes of sensory processing observed in monkey primary visual cortex," *Nature Neurosci.* **4**:304–310 (2001).

Swick, D. and Knight, R.T. "Cortical lesions and attention." In: *The Attentive Brain.* Parasurama R., ed., pp. 143–161. Cambridge, MA: MIT Press (1998).

Swindale, N.V. "How many maps are there in visual cortex," *Cerebral Cortex* **10**:633–643 (2000).

Tallal, P., Merzenich, M., Miller, S., and Jenkins, W. "Language learning impairment: Integrating basic science, technology and remediation," *Exp. Brain Res.* **123**:210–219 (1998).

Tallon-Baudry, C. and Bertrand, O. "Oscillatory gamma activity in humans and its role in object representation," *Trends Cogn. Sci.* **3**:151–161 (1999).

Tamura, H. and Tanaka, K. "Visual response properties of cells in the ventral and dorsal parts of the macque inferotemporal cortex," *Cerebral Cortex* **11**:384–399 (2001).

Tanaka, K. "Inferotemporal cortex and object vision," *Ann. Rev. Neurosci.* **19**:109–139 (1996).

Tanaka, K. "Columnar organization in the inferotemporal cortex." In: *Cerebral Cortex. Vol. 12.* Rockland, K.S., Kaas, J.H., and Peters, A., eds., pp. 469–498. New York: Plenum Press (1997).

Tanaka, K. "Columns for complex visual object features in the inferotemporal cortex: Clustering of cells with similar but slightly different stimulus selectivities," *Cerebral Cortex* **13**:90–99 (2003).

Tang, S. and Guo, A. "Choice behavior of Drosophila facing contradictory visual cues," *Science* **294**:1543–1547 (2001).

Tang, Y.-P., Shimizu, E., Dube, G.R., Rampon, C., Kerchner, G.A., Zhuo, M., Liu, G., and Tsien, J.Z. "Genetic enhancement of learning and memory in mice," *Nature* **401**:63–69 (1999).

Taylor, J.G. *The Race for Consciousness.* Cambridge, UK: MIT Press (1998).

Taylor, J.L. and McCloskey, D.I. "Triggering of preprogrammed movements as reactions to masked stimuli," *J. Neurophysiol.* **63**:439–444 (1990).

Teller, D.Y. "Linking propositions," *Vision Res.* **24**:1233–1246 (1984).

Teller, D.Y. and Pugh, E.N. Jr. "Linking propositions in color vision." In: *Color Vision: Physiology and Psychophysics.* Mollon, J.D. and Sharpe, L.T., eds., London: Academic Press (1983).

Thiele, A., Henning, P., Kubschik, M., and Hoffmann, K.-P. "Neural mechanisms of saccadic suppression," *Science* **295**:2460–2462 (2002).

Thiele, A. and Stoner, G. "Neuronal synchrony does not correlate with motion coherence in cortical area MT," *Nature* **23**:366–370 (2003).

Thier P., Haarmeier, T., Treue, S., and Barash, S. "Absence of a common functional denominator of visual disturbance in cerebellar disease," *Brain* **122**:2133–2146 (1999).

Thomas, O.M., Cumming, B.G., and Parker, A.J. "A specialization for relative disparity in V2," *Nature Neurosci.* **5**:472–478 (2002).

Thompson, K.G. and Schall, J.D. "The detection of visual signals by macaque frontal eye field during masking," *Nature Neurosci.* **2**:283–288 (1999).

Thompson, K.G., and Schall, J.D. "Antecedents and correlates of visual detection and awareness in macaque prefrontal cortex," *Vision Res.* **40**:1523–1538 (2000).

Thorpe, S., Fize, D., and Marlot, C. "Speed of processing in the human visual system," *Nature* **381**:520–522 (1996).

Tolias, A.S., Smirnakis, S.M., Augath, M.A., Trinath, T., and Logothetis, N.K. "Motion processing in the macaque: Revisited with functional magnetic resonance imaging," *J. Neurosci.* **21**:8594–8601 (2001).

Tomita, H., Ohbayashi, M., Nakahara, K., Hasegawa, I., and Miyashita, Y. "Top-down signal from prefrontal cortex in executive control of memory retrieval," *Nature* **401**:699–703 (1999).

Tong, F. and Engel, S.A. "Interocular rivalry revealed in the human cortical blind-spot representation," *Nature* **411**:195–199 (2001).

Tong, F., Nakayama, K., Vaughan, J.T., and Kanwisher, N. "Binocular rivalry and visual awareness in human extrastriate cortex," *Neuron* **21**:753–759 (1998).

Tong, F., Nakayama, K., Moscovitch, M., Weinrib, O., and Kanwisher, N. "Response properties of the human fusiform face area," *Cogn. Neuropsychol.* **17**:257–279 (2000).

Tononi, G. and Edelman, G.M. "Consciousness and complexity," *Science* **282**:1846–1851 (1998).

Tootell, R.B. and Hadjikhani, N. "Where is 'dorsal V4' in human visual cortex? Retinotopic, topographic, and functional evidence," *Cerebral Cortex* **11**:298–311 (2001).

Tootell, R.B., Hadjikhani, N., Mendola, J.D., Marrett, S., and Dale, A.M. "From retinotopy to recognition: Functional MRI in human visual cortex," *Trends Cogn. Sci.* **2**:174–183 (1998).

Tootell, R.B., Mendola, J.D., Hadjikhani, N., Ledden, P.J., Liu, A.K., Reppas, J.B., Sereno, M.I., and Dale, A.M. "Functional analysis of V3A and related areas in human visual cortex," *J. Neurosci.* **17**:7060–7078 (1997).

Tootell, R.B., Reppas, J.B., Dale, A.M., Look, R.B., Sereno, M.I., Malach, R., Brady, T.J., and Rosen, B.R. "Visual motion aftereffect in human cortical area MT revealed by functional magnetic resonance imaging," *Nature* **375**:139–141 (1995).

Tootell, R.B. and Taylor, J.B. "Anatomical evidence for MT and additional cortical visual areas in humans," *Cerebral Cortex* **5**:39–55 (1995).

Tranel, D. and Damasio, A.R. "Knowledge without awareness: An autonomic index of facial recognition by prosopagnosics," *Science* **228**:1453–1454 (1985).

Treisman, A. "Features and Objects: The Fourteenth Bartlett Memorial Lecture," *Quart. J. Exp. Psychology* **40A**:201–237 (1988).

Treisman, A. "The binding problem," *Curr. Opinion Neurobiol.* **6**:171–178 (1996).

Treisman, A. "Feature binding, attention and object perception," *Proc. R. Soc. Lond. B* **353**:1295–1306 (1998).

Treisman, A. and Gelade, G. "A feature-integration theory of attention," *Cogn. Psychol.* **12**:97–136 (1980).

Treisman, A. and Schmidt, H. "Illusory conjunctions in the perception of objects," *Cogn. Psychol.* **14**:107–141 (1982).

Treue, S. and Martinez-Trujillo, J.C. "Feature-based attention influences motion processing gain in macaque visual cortex," *Nature* **399**:575–578 (1999).

Treue, S. and Maunsell, J.H.R. "Attentional modulation of visual motion processing in cortical areas MT and MST," *Nature* **382**:539–541 (1996).

Tsal, Y. "Do illusory conjunctions support feature integration theory? A critical review of theory and findings," *J. Exp. Psychol. Hum. Percept. Perform.* **15**:394–400 (1989).

Tsotsos, J.K. "Analyzing vision at the complexity level," *Behav.Brain Sci.* **13**:423–469 (1990).

Tsunoda, K., Yamane, Y., Nishizaki, M., and Tanifuji, M. "Complex objects represented in macaque inferotemporal cortex by the combination of feature columns," *Nature Neurosci.* **4**:832–838 (2001).

Tully, T. "Toward a molecular biology of memory: The light's coming on!," *Nature Neurosci.* **1**:543–545 (1998).

Tully, T. and Quinn, W.G. "Classical conditioning and retention in normal and mutant Drosophila melanogaster," *J. Comp. Physiol. A* **157**:263–277 (1985).

Tulunay-Keesey, Ü. "Fading of stabilized retina images," *J. Opt. Soc. Am.* **72**:440–447 (1982).

Tulving, E. "Memory and consciousness," *Canadian Psychology* **26**:1–26 (1985).

Tulving, E. "Varieties of consciousness and levels of awareness in memory." In: *Attention: Selection, Awareness and Control. A Tribute to Donald Broadbent.* Baddeley, A. and Weiskrantz, L., eds., pp. 283–299. Oxford, UK: Oxford University Press (1993).

Turing, A. "Computing machinery and intelligence," *Mind* **59**:433–460 (1950).

Ullman, S. "Visual routines," *Cognition* **18**:97–159 (1984).

Ungerleider, L.G. and Mishkin, M. "Two cortical visual systems." In: *Analysis of Visual Behavior.* Ingle, D.J., Goodale, M.A., and Mansfield, R.J.W., eds., pp. 549–586. Cambridge, MA: MIT Press (1982).

Vallar, G. and Shallice, T., eds. *Neuropsychological Impairments of Short-Term Memory.* Cambridge, UK: Cambridge University Press (1990).

Vanduffel, W., Fize, D., Peuskens, H., Denys, K., Sunaert, S., Todd, J.T., and Orban, G.A. "Extracting 3D from motion: Differences in human and monkey intraparietal cortex," *Science* **298**:413–415 (2002).

Van Essen, D.C. and Gallant, J.L. "Neural mechanisms of form and motion processing in the primate visual system," *Neuron* **13**:1–10 (1994).

Van Essen, D.C., Lewis, J.W., Drury, H.A., Hadjikhani, N., Tootell, R.B., Bakircioglu, M., and Miller, M.I. "Mapping visual cortex in monkeys and humans using surface-based atlases," *Vision Res.* **41**:1359–1378 (2001).

VanRullen, R. and Koch, C. "Competition and selection during visual processing of natural scenes and objects," *J. Vision* **3**:75–85 (2003a).

VanRullen, R. and Koch, C. "Visual selective behavior can be triggered by a feed-forward process," *J. Cogn. Neurosci.* **15**:209–217 (2003b).

VanRullen, R. and Koch, C. "Is perception discrete or continuous?" *Trends Cogn. Sci.* **7**:207–213 (2003c).

VanRullen, R., Reddy L., and Koch, C. "Parallel and preattentive processing are not equivalent," *J. Cogn. Neurosci.*, in press (2004).

VanRullen, R. and Thorpe, S. "The time course of visual processing: From early perception to decision making," *J. Cogn. Neurosci.* **13**:454–461 (2001).

van Swinderen, B. and Greenspan, R.J. "Salience modulates 20–30 Hz brain activity in *Drosophila*," *Nature Neurosci.* **6**:579–586 (2003).

Varela, F. "Neurophenomenology: A methodological remedy to the hard problem," *J. Consc. Studies* **3**:330–350 (1996).

Varela, F., Lachaux, J.-P., Rodriguez, E., and Martinerie, J. "The brainweb: Phase synchronization and large-scale integration," *Nature Rev. Neurosci.* **2**:229–239 (2001).

Velmans, M. "Is human information processing conscious?" *Behav. Brain Sci.* **14**:651–726 (1991).

Venables, P.H. "Periodicity in reaction time," *Br. J. Psychol.* **51**:37–43 (1960).

Vgontzas, A.N. and Kales, A. "Sleep and its disorders," *Ann. Rev. Med.* **50**:387–400 (1999).

Vogeley, K. "Hallucinations emerge from an imbalance of self-monitoring and reality modeling," *Monist* **82**:626–644 (1999).

Volkmann, F.C., Riggs, L.A., and Moore, R.K. "Eyeblinks and visual suppression," *Science* **207**:900–902 (1980).

von der Heydt, R., Peterhans, E., and Baumgartner, G. "Illusory contours and cortical neuron responses," *Science* **224**:1260–1262 (1984).

von der Heydt, R., Zhou, H., and Friedman, H.S. "Representation of stereoscopic edges in monkey visual cortex," *Vision Res.* **40**:1955–1967 (2000).

von der Malsburg, C. "The correlation theory of brain function." MPI Biophysical Chemistry, Internal Report 81–2 (1981). Reprinted in *Models of Neural Networks II*, Domany, E., van Hemmen, J.L., and Schulten, K., eds. Berlin: Springer (1994).

von der Malsburg, C. "Binding in models of perception and brain function," *Curr. Opin. Neurobiol.* **5**:520–526 (1995).

von der Malsburg, C. "The what and why of binding: The modeler's perspective," *Neuron* **24**:95–104 (1999).

von Economo, C. and Koskinas, G.N. *Die Cytoarchitektonik der Hirnrinde des erwachsenen Menschen.* Wien, Austria: Julius Springer (1925).

von Helmholtz, H. *Handbook of Physiological Optics.* New York: Dover. (1962). Translation of *Handbuch der physiologischen Optik.* 3 volumes, ed. and trans. by Southall, J.P.C., Hamburg, Voss, 1856, 1860, and 1988.

Von Senden, M. *Space and Sight: The Perception of Space and Shape in the Congenitally Blind Before and After Operation.* Glencoe, IL: Free Press (1960).

Vuilleumier, P., Armony, J.L., Clarke, K., Husain, M., Driver, J., and Dolan, R.J. "Neural response to emotional faces with and without awareness: Event-related fMRI in a parietal patient with visual extinction and spatial neglect," *Neuropsychologia* **40**:156–166 (2002).

Vuilleumier, P., Armony, J.L., Driver, J., and Dolan, R.J. "Effects of attention and emotion on face processing in the human brain: An event-related fMRI study," *Neuron* **30**:829–841 (2001).

Vuilleumier, P., Hester, D., Assal, G., and Regli, F. "Unilateral spatial neglect recovery after sequential strokes," *Neurol.* **46**:184–189 (1996).

Wachtler, T., Sejnowski, T.J., and Albright, T.D. "Representation of color stimuli in awake macaque primary visual cortex," *Neuron* **37**:681–691 (2003).

Wada, Y. and Yamamoto, T. "Selective impairment of facial recognition due to a haematoma restricted to the right fusiform and lateral occipital region," *J. Neurol. Neurosurg. Psychiatry* **71**:254–257 (2001).

Wade, A.R., Brewer, A.A., Rieger, J.W., and Wandell, B.A. "Functional measurements of human ventral occipital cortex: Retinotopy and colour," *Phil. Trans. R. Soc. Lond. B* **357**:963–973 (2002).

Walther, D., Itti, L., Riesenhuber, M., Poggio, T., and Koch, C. "Attentional selection for object recognition—A gentle way." In: *Biologically Motivated Computer Vision*. Bülthoff, H.H., Lee, S.-W., Poggio, T., and Wallraven, C., eds., pp. 472–479. Berlin: Springer (2002).

Wandell, B.A. *Foundations of Vision*. Sunderland, MA: Sinauer (1995).

Wang, G., Tanaka, K., and Tanifuji, M. "Optical imaging of functional organization in the monkey inferotemporal cortex," *Science* **272**:1665–1668 (1996).

Warland, D.K., Reinagel, P., and Meister, M. "Decoding visual information from a population of retinal ganglion cells," *J. Neurophysiol.* **78**:2336–2350 (1997).

Watanabe, T., Harner, A.M., Miyauchi, S., Sasaki, Y., Nielsen, M., Palomo, D., and Mukai, I. "Task-dependent influences of attention on the activation of human primary visual cortex," *Proc. Natl. Acad. Sci. USA* **95**:11489–11492 (1998).

Watanabe, M. and Rodieck, R.W. "Parasol and midget ganglion cells of the primate retina," *J. Comp. Neurol.* **289**:434–454 (1989).

Watkins, J.C. and Collingridge, G.L., eds. *The NMDA Receptor*. Oxford, UK: IRL Press (1989).

Watson, L. *Jacobson's Organ and the Remarkable Nature of Smell*. New York: Plume Books (2001).

Webster, M.J., Bachevalier, J., and Ungerleider, L.G. "Connections of inferior temporal areas TEO and TE with parietal and frontal cortex in macaque monkeys," *Cerebral Cortex* **4**:470–483 (1994).

Wegner, D.M. *The Illusion of Conscious Will*. Cambridge, MA: MIT Press (2002).

Weiskrantz, L. "Blindsight revisited," *Curr. Opinion Neurobiol.* **6**:215–220 (1996).

Weiskrantz, L. *Consciousness Lost and Found*. Oxford, UK: Oxford University Press (1997).

Weller, L., Weller, A., Koresh-Kamin, H., and Ben-Shoshan, R. "Menstrual synchrony in a sample of working women," *Psychoneuroendocrinology* **24**:449–459 (1999).

Wen, J., Koch, C., and Braun, J. "Spatial vision thresholds in the near absence of attention," *Vision Res.* **37**:2409–2418 (1997).

Wertheimer, M. "Experimentelle Studien über das Sehen von Bewegung," *Z. Psychologie* **61**:161–265 (1912).

Wessinger, C.M., Fendrich, R., and Gazzaniga, M.S. "Islands of residual vision in hemi-anopic patients," *J. Cogn. Neurosci.* **9**:203–211 (1997).

Westheimer, G. and McKee, S.P. "Perception of temporal order in adjacent visual stimuli," *Vision Res.* **17**:887–892 (1977).

Whinnery, J.E. and Whinnery, A.M. "Acceleration-induced loss of consciousness," *Archive Neurol.* **47**:764–776 (1990).

White, C. "Temporal numerosity and the psychological unit of duration," *Psychol. Monographs: General & Appl.* **77**:1–37 (1963).

White, C. and Harter, M.R. "Intermittency in reaction time and perception, and evoked response correlates of image quality," *Acta Psychol.* **30**:368–377 (1969).

White, E.L. *Cortical Circuits*. Boston: Birkhäuser (1989).

Wigan, A.L. "Duality of the mind, proved by the structure, functions, and diseases of the brain," *Lancet 1*:39–41 (1844).

Wilken, P.C. "Capacity limits for the detection and identification of change: Implications for models of visual short-term memory." Ph.D. Thesis. University of Melbourne, Australia (2001).

Wilkins, A.J., Shallice, T., and McCarthy, R. "Frontal lesions and sustained attention," *Neuropsychologia* **25**:359–65 (1987).

Williams, D.R., MacLeod, D.E.A., and Hayhoe, M.M. "Foveal tritanopia," *Vision Res.* **21**:1341–1356 (1981).

Williams, D.R., Sekiguchi, N., Haake, W., Brainard, D., and Packer, O. "The cost of trichromacy for spatial vision." In: *Pigments to Perception*. Lee, B. and Valberg, A., eds., pp. 11–22. New York: Plenum Press (1991).

Williams, S.R. and Stuart, G.J. "Dependence of EPSP efficacy on synapse location in neocortical pyramidal neurons," *Science* **295**:1907–1910 (2002).

Williams, S.R. and Stuart, G.J. "Role of dendritic synapse location in the control of action potential output," *Trends Neurosci.* **26**:147–154 (2003).

Williams, T. *The Milk Train Doesn't Stop Here Anymore*. Norfolk, CT: A New Directions Book (1964).

Williams, Z.M., Elfar, J.C., Eskandar, E.N., Toth, L.J., and Assad, J.A. "Parietal activity and the perceived direction of ambiguous apparent motion," *Nature Neurosci.* **6**:616–623 (2003).

Wilson, B.A. and Wearing, D. "Prisoner of consciousness: A state of just awakening following Herpes Simplex Encephalitis." In: *Broken Memories: Neuropsychological Case Studies*. Campbell, R. and Conway, M., eds., pp. 15–30. Oxford, UK: Blackwell (1995).

Wilson, H.R., Levi, D., Maffei, L., Rovamo, J., and DeValois, R. "The Perception of Form: Retina to Striate Cortex." In: *Visual Perception: The Neurophysiological Foundations*. Spillman, L. and Werner, J.S., eds., pp. 231–272. San Diego, CA: Academic Press (1990).

Wilson, M.A. and McNaughton, B.L. "Dynamics of the hippocampal ensemble code for space," *Science* **261**:1055–1058 (1993).

Wittenberg, G.M. and Tsien, J.Z. "An emerging molecular and cellular framework for memory processing by the hippocampus," *Trends Neurosci.* **25**:501–505 (2002).

Wojciulik, E. and Kanwisher, N. "Implicit but not explicit feature binding in a Balint's patient," *Visual Cognition* **5**:157–181 (1998).

Wolfe, J.M. "Reversing ocular dominance and suppression in a single flash," *Vision Res.* **24**:471–478 (1984).

Wolfe, J.M. "'Effortless' texture segmentation and 'parallel' visual search are not the same thing," *Vision Res.* **32**:757–763 (1992).

Wolfe, J.M. "Guided search 2.0: A revised model of visual search," *Psychon. Bull. Rev.* **1**:202–238 (1994).

Wolfe, J.M. "Visual Search." In: *The Psychology of Attention.* Pashler, H., ed., pp. 13–73. Cambridge, MA: MIT Press (1998a).

Wolfe, J.M. "Visual Memory: What do you know about what you saw?" *Curr. Biol.* **8**:R303–R304 (1998b).

Wolfe, J.M. "Inattentional amnesia." In: *Fleeting Memories.* Coltheart, V., ed., pp. 71–94. Cambridge, MA: MIT Press (1999).

Wolfe, J.M. and Bennett, S.C. "Preattentive object files: Shapeless bundles of basic features," *Vision Res.* **37**:25–44 (1997).

Wolfe, J.M. and Cave, K.R. "The psychophysical evidence for a binding problem in human vision," *Neuron* **24**:11–17 (1999).

Wong, E. and Mack, A. "Saccadic programming and perceived location," *Acta Psychologica* **48**:123–131 (1981).

Wong-Riley, M.T.T. "Primate visual cortex: Dynamic metabolic organization and plasticity revealed by cytochrome oxidase." In: *Cerebral Cortex. Vol. 10.* Peters, A. and Rockland, K.S., eds., pp. 141–200. New York: Plenum Press (1994).

Woolf, N.J. "Cholinergic transmission: Novel signal transduction." In: *Neurochemistry of Consciousness.* Perry, E., Ashton, H., and Young, A., eds., pp. 25–41. Amsterdam: John Benjamins (2002).

Wu, M.-F., Gulyani, S.A., Yau, E., Mignot, E., Phan, B., and Siegel, J.M. "Locus coeruleus neurons: Cessation of activity during cataplexy," *Neurosci.* **91**:1389–1399 (1999).

Wurtz, R.H., Goldberg, M.E., and Robinson, D.L. "Brain mechanisms of visual attention," *Sci. Am.* **246**:124–135 (1982).

Yabuta, N.H., Sawatari, A., and Callaway, E.M. "Two functional channels from primary visual cortex to dorsal visual cortical areas," *Science* **292**:297–300 (2001).

Yamagishi, N., Anderson, S.J., and Ashida H. "Evidence for dissociation between the perceptual and visuomotor systems in humans," *Proc. R. Soc. Lond. B* **268**:973–977 (2001).

Yamamoto, M., Wada, N., Kitabatake, Y., Watanabe, D., Anzai, M., Yokoyama, M., Teranishi, Y., and Nakanishi, S. "Reversible suppression of glutamatergic neurotransmission of cerebellar granule cells *in vivo* by genetically manipulated expression of tetanus neurotoxin light chain," *J. Neurosci.* **23**:6759–6767 (2003).

Yang, Y., Rose, D., and Blake, R. "On the variety of percepts associated with dichoptic viewing of dissimilar monocular stimuli," *Perception* **21**:47–62 (1992).

Young, M.P. "Connectional organisation and function in the macaque cerebral cortex. In: *Cortical Areas: Unity and Diversity*, Schüz, A. and Miller, R., eds., pp. 351–375. London: Taylor and Francis (2002).

Young, M.P. and Yamane, S. "Sparse population coding of faces in the inferotemporal cortex," *Science* **256**:1327–1331 (1992).

Yund, E.W., Morgan, H., and Efron, R. "The micropattern effect and visible persistence," *Perception & Psychophysics* **34**:209–213 (1983).

Zafonte, R.D. and Zasler, N.D. "The minimally conscious state: Definition and diagnostic criteria," *Neurology* **58**:349–353 (2002).

Zeki, S. "Color coding in rhesus monkey prestriate cortex," *Brain Res.* **27**:422–427 (1973).

Zeki, S. "Functional organization of a visual area in the posterior bank of the superior temporal sulcus of the rhesus monkey," *J. Physiol.* **236**:549–573 (1974).

Zeki, S. "Colour coding in the cerebral cortex: The responses of wavelength-selective and color-coded cells in monkey visual cortex to changes in wavelength composition," *Neurosci.* **9**:767–781 (1983).

Zeki, S. "A century of cerebral achromatopsia," *Brain* **113**:1721–1777 (1990).

Zeki, S. "Cerebral akinetopsia (Visual motion blindness)," *Brain* **114**:811–824 (1991).

Zeki, S. *A Vision of the Brain*. Oxford, UK: Oxford University Press (1993).

Zeki, S. "The motion vision of the blind," *Neuroimage* **2**:231–235 (1995).

Zeki, S. "Parallel processing, asynchronous perception, and a distributed system of consciousness in vision," *Neuroscientist* **4**:365–372 (1998).

Zeki, S. "Localization and globalization in conscious vision," *Ann. Rev. Neurosci.* **24**:57–86 (2001).

Zeki, S. "Improbable areas in the visual brain," *Trends Neurosci.* **26**:23–26 (2003).

Zeki, S. and Bartels, A. "Toward a theory of visual consciousness," *Consc. & Cognition* **8**:225–259 (1999).

Zeki, S., McKeefry, D.J., Bartels, A., and Frackowiak, R.S.J. "Has a new color area been discovered?" *Nature Neurosci.* **1**:335–336 (1998).

Zeki, S. and Moutoussis, K. "Temporal hierarchy of the visual perceptive systems in the Mondrian world," *Proc. R. Soc. Lond. B* **264**:1415–1419 (1997).

Zeki, S. and Shipp, S. "The functional logic of cortical connections," *Nature* **335**:311–317 (1988).

Zeki, S., Watson, J.D., Lueck, C.J., Friston, K.J., Kennard, C., and Frackowiak, R.S.J. "A direct demonstration of functional specialization in human visual cortex," *J. Neurosci.* **11**:641–649 (1991).

Zeki, S., Watson, J.D., and Frackowiak, R.S.J. "Going beyond the information given: The relation of illusory motion to brain activity," *Proc. Roy. Soc. Lond. B* **252**:215–222 (1993).

Zeman, A. "Consciousness," *Brain* **124**:1263–1289 (2001).

Zhang, K., Ginzburg, I., McNaughton, B.L., and Sejnowski, T.J. "Interpreting neuronal population activity by reconstruction: Unified framework with application to hippocampal place cells," *J. Neurophysiol.* **79**:1017–1044 (1998).

Zihl J., von Cramon, D., and Mai, N. "Selective disturbance of movement vision after bilateral brain-damage," *Brain* **106**:313–340 (1983).

Zipser, D. and Andersen, R.A. "A back-propagation programmed network that simulates response properties of a subset of posterior parietal neurons," *Nature* **331**:679–684 (1988).

Zrenner, E. *Neurophysiological Aspects of Color Vision in Primates: Comparative Studies on Simian Retinal Ganglion Cells and the Human Visual System.* Berlin: Springer (1983).

Index

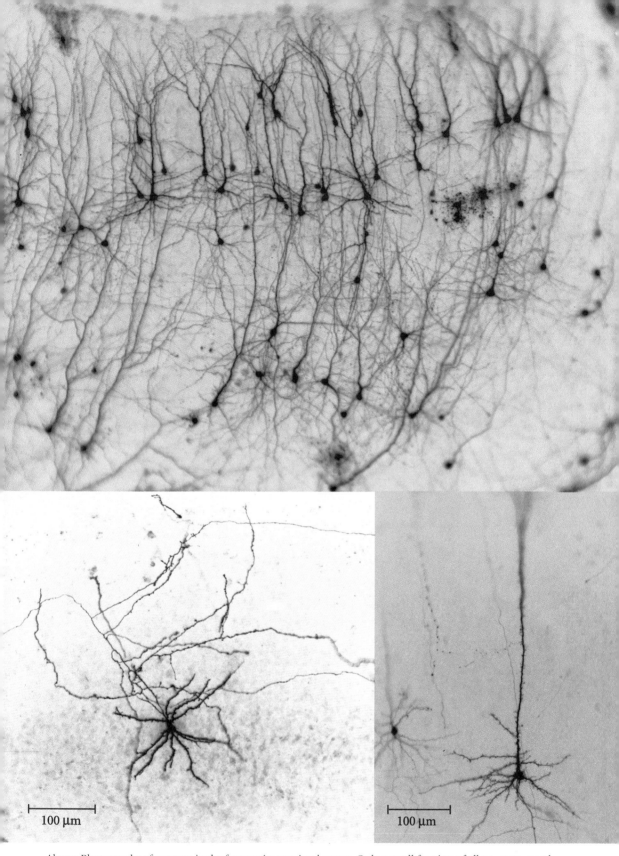

Above: Photographs of neurons in the ferret primary visual cortex. Only a small fraction of all neurons, mostly pyramidal cells, are stained. An inhibitory stellate cell (on the left) and pyramidal neuron (on the right) are shown at higher magnification. Modified from Borrell and Callaway (2002). Opposite page: Photographs of Nissl-stained section of the monkey primary visual cortex. All cell bodies are labeled. The rectangular section is magnified at the top, and five reconstructed neurons (dendrites in red) and one axonal input (on the left) superimposed. From E. Callaway, personal communication. For details, see Blasdel and Lund (1983); Callaway and Wiser (1996); and Yabuta, Sawatari, and Callaway (2001).